Biological Effects of Nonionizing Radiation

Karl H. Illinger, EDITOR

Tufts University

Based on a symposium
sponsored by the Division of
Physical Chemistry
at the 179th Meeting of the
American Chemical Society,
Houston, Texas,
March 25–26, 1980.

ACS SYMPOSIUM SERIES 157

AMERICAN CHEMICAL SOCIETY
WASHINGTON, D. C.   1981

Library of Congress CIP Data
Biological effects of nonionizing radiation.
  (ACS symposium series, ISSN 0097-6156; 157)

  "Based on a symposium sponsored by the Division
of Physical Chemistry at the 179th meeting of the
American Chemical Society, Houston, Texas, March
25-26, 1980."

  Includes bibliographies and index.

  1. Radiation—Physiological effect—Congresses. 2.
Electromagnetism—Physiological effect—Congresses.
  I. Illinger, Karl H., 1934-   . II. American
Chemical Society. Division of Physical Chemistry.
III. Series: ACS symposium series; 157. [DNLM: 1.
Radiation effects—Congresses. 2. Radiation, Nonioniz-
ing—Congresses. QT 162.U4 B615 1980]

QP82.2.R3B527   574.19'15   81-2652
ISBN 0-8412-0634-1 ASCMC8 157 1–342 AACR2
                                           1981

ACS Symposium Series

M. Joan Comstock, *Series Editor*

The organizers of the symposium on which this book is based acknowledge with thanks the partial support in the form of travel funds
provided for 13 of the speakers under the Department of the Navy
Grant N00014-80-G-0031 issued by the Office of Naval Research.

FOREWORD

The ACS Symposium Series was founded in 1974 to provide a medium for publishing symposia quickly in book form. The format of the Series parallels that of the continuing Advances in Chemistry Series except that in order to save time the papers are not typeset but are reproduced as they are submitted by the authors in camera-ready form. Papers are reviewed under the supervision of the Editors with the assistance of the Series Advisory Board and are selected to maintain the integrity of the symposia; however, verbatim reproductions of previously published papers are not accepted. Both reviews and reports of research are acceptable since symposia may embrace both types of presentation.

CONTENTS

Preface vii

1. **Electromagnetic-Field Interaction with Biological Systems in the Microwave and Far-Infrared Region: Physical Basis** 1
   K. H. Illinger

   MOLECULAR DYNAMICS IN AQUEOUS SOLUTION

2. **Dielectric Properties of Water in the Microwave and Far-Infrared Regions** 47
   E. H. Grant, S. Szwarnowski, and R. J. Sheppard

3. **Dielectric Properties of Water in Myoglobin Solution** 57
   E. H. Grant, N. R. V. Nightingale, R. J. Sheppard, and S. R. Gough

4. **Electrical Response of Polymers in Solution** 63
   R. H. Cole

5. **Spectroscopic Determination of the Low-Frequency Dynamics of Biological Polymers and Cells** 83
   L. Genzel, F. Kremer, L. Santo, and S. C. Shen

6. **Long-Range Forces in DNA** 95
   W. N. Mei, M. Kohli, L. L. Van Zandt, and E. W. Prohofsky

7. **Calculated Microwave Absorption by Double-Helical DNA** 101
   M. Kohli, W. N. Mei, L. L. Van Zandt, and E. W. Prohofsky

   DIELECTRIC AND SPECTROSCOPIC PROPERTIES OF
   MEMBRANE SYSTEMS AND BIOLOGICAL TISSUE

8. **Dielectric Properties of Biological Tissue and Biophysical Mechanisms of Electromagnetic-Field Interaction** 109
   H. P. Schwan

9. **Frequency Response of Membrane Components in Nerve Axon** 133
   S. Takashima

10. **A Perturbation Model for Electromagnetic-Field Interaction with Excitable Cellular Membranes** 147
    C. A. Cain

    DIELECTRIC AND SPECTROSCOPIC PROPERTIES
    OF NONEQUILIBRIUM SYSTEMS

11. **Developmental Bioelectricity** 163
    P. Ortoleva

12. **Coherent Processes in Biological Systems** 213
    H. Fröhlich

13. **Coherent Modes in Biological Systems: Perturbation by External Fields** **219**
   F. Kaiser

14. **The Response of Biochemical Reaction Systems to Oscillating Stimuli** **243**
   L. K. Kaczmarek

15. **Nonlinear Impedance and Low-Frequency Dispersion Effects of a Polyelectrolyte Under High Sinusoidal Fields** **255**
   C. J. Hu and F. S. Barnes

16. **Ionic Nonequilibrium Phenomena in Tissue Interactions with Electromagnetic Fields** **271**
   W. R. Adey

17. **Calcium Ion Efflux Induction in Brain Tissue by Radiofrequency Radiation** **299**
   C. F. Blackman, W. T. Joines, and J. A. Elder

A PROTOTYPE SENSORY-SYSTEM EFFECT

18. **The Microwave Hearing Effect** **317**
   J. C. Lin

Index **331**

PREFACE

Considerable advances have been made in recent years in the development of experimental techniques and in the refinement of theoretical models for the interaction of electromagnetic fields with biological systems. The primary objective of this volume is to focus on the current state of these methodologies, and to examine their consequences in elucidating the chemical physics and biophysics of such systems. Four sections trace the development of these topics along a hierarchy of systems of increasing complexity: the ubiquitous milieu of biological structures, water, and macromolecular systems of biological interest; the bulk dielectric and spectroscopic properties of membrane and cellular systems; nonequilibrium properties of biological systems; and the best documented sensory-system effect of nonionizing radiation, the microwave acoustic effect. A brief synopsis of each section is provided below.

In the microwave and far-infrared regions, the dielectric properties of free water dominate the bulk response of biological tissue to electromagnetic fields. Recent accurate determinations of the millimeter-wave complex permittivity of water permit a definitive analysis of the dielectric absorption arising from its rotational diffusion, and provide a connection to its far-infrared absorption stemming from the translational and librational motion of molecular clusters of water. The structure of water in the vicinity of macromolecules is modified by its interaction with such molecular surfaces. Conversely, the structure of macromolecules in aqueous solution is altered by the same interaction. The dielectric properties of water in solution with biopolymers, such as myoglobin, are beginning to be examined in detail, with a frequency resolution heretofore unattainable. The electrical response of biopolymers in aqueous solution, from the regime of low frequencies to the microwave region, is determined by a complex set of interactions. They involve not only the overall rotational diffusion of the macromolecule and the internal rotational diffusion of its segments, but also the dynamically coupled response of its counter-ion atmosphere. New developments in experimental methods and more accurate theoretical models provide an avenue toward the analysis of these interactions. In the far-infrared region, and penetrating into the microwave region, the low-frequency vibrational dynamics of biological polymers arise. The aqueous environment constitutes a refractory experimental system for dielectric spectroscopy and photon (Raman) and phonon (Brillouin) scattering. Nonetheless, recent refinements are beginning to address salient questions concerning the spectroscopic properties of bio-polymers in aqueous solution in the far-infrared and millimeter-wave regions.

Molecular dynamics in aqueous solution embody one sector of the dielectric and spectroscopic properties of biological tissue, and serve as a partial guide toward the analysis of the more complex molecular aggregates and biophysical systems comprised by such structures. A considerable body of information has been amassed on the bulk dielectric properties, into the millimeter-wave region in some cases, and the refinement of mechanisms of electromagnetic-field interaction has been substantial. In parallel, the phenomenology of the (dielectric) frequency response of both artificial and biological membranes has been well documented, particularly in the frequency regime below the microwave region. The dielectric properties of molecular systems in aqueous solution, below the far-infrared region, are characterized by relaxation processes depending only on the nature of the solute molecule and its interaction with the solvent, with a resultant set of (molecular) relaxation times for the dynamical processes involved. In the biological membrane, apart from the modification of the relaxation processes of macromolecules which are embedded in the membrane, additional (biophysical) processes, with characteristic response times, arise from the interactions and biochemical events occurring at this higher level of molecular organization. One set of such characteristic response times has a lower bound dictated by the velocity of ion transport across the membrane. Nonlinear dielectric properties have been invoked for biological membranes in the low-frequency regime. In particular, the voltage–current properties of excitable cellular membranes have been examined in an electromagnetic-field perturbation model, employing the phenomenological Hodgkin–Huxley model as the unperturbed system.

Section 1 *in toto* and aspects of Section 2 treat the equilibrium characteristics of biological tissue and its molecular subsystems. Although the bulk properties of even in vivo biological tissue are dictated by (high-concentration) molecular systems near equilibrium, in order for the in vivo state to be maintained (low-concentration) molecular subsystems obeying steady-state nonequilibrium thermodynamics must exist. While such nonequilibrium systems are not confined to biological structures, they are requisite for biological processes. Section 3 focuses on the dielectric and spectroscopic behavior of nonequilibrium systems. Such biophysical constructs play a crucial role in developmental bioelectricity (the role of intrinsic electric fields in signal propagation and developmental patterns in living systems) over a wide span of morphological complexity, from cellular systems on upward. At the level of what appears to be the irreducible biophysical system exhibiting nonequilibrium dissipative properties, the in vivo biological membrane, coherent processes, and their perturbation by millimeter-wave and far-infrared electromagnetic fields have been studied in theoretical models in some detail. The boson (phonon and photon) distribution associated with chemically pumped, dissipative molecular subsystems is expected to show deviations from the Planckian (equilibrium) distribution, with attendant consequences for the phonon and photon spectroscopy of such systems in the far-infrared region. The same intransigence displayed by the aqueous environment toward the millimeter-wave and far-infrared spectroscopy of biopolymers (Section 1), and the dominance of the bulk properties in the observables, have placed severe limitations on experimental work in this area. In addition to the alterations in the high-frequency spectroscopic properties predicted upon onset of (time-variant) nonequilibrium structures, the response of associated coupled biochemical reaction systems to low-frequency oscillatory stimuli has been examined. Finally, in a category that may be related to nonequilibrium properties in systems consisting of macromolecular polyelectrolytes and ions, the effect of amplitude-modulated electromagnetic fields in the radiofrequency region on Ca^{+2} efflux in biological tissue has been studied extensively. While the mosaic of properties assembled in Section 3 under the rubric of nonequilibrium systems forms, as yet, a far less rigorous structure than that of the more mature fields treated in Sections 1 and 2, even their tentative connection may prove to be suggestive for future development of this field.

At the interface between the areas treated in Sections 1–3 and the virtually unlimited field of nonionizing radiation research involving levels of higher biological complexity, a well-documented effect exists that can be cast into well-defined biophysical models, discussed in Section 4. The microwave acoustic effect involves the auditory-system response to pulsed microwave radiation. The initial step, dielectric interaction with tissue components, can be modeled within the constructs of the previous treatment. However, a higher level of biological organization becomes engaged in subsequent steps of the interaction. The dielectric response is transformed into an (acoustic) compressional wave, and if the (temporal) pulse characteristics of the electromagnetic field are within certain boundaries, the pulses are perceived by the auditory sensory system.

In the attempt to focus the volume on the fundamental chemical physics and biophysics of electromagnetic-field interactions, and to connect hitherto disparate areas of research, an artificial boundary had to be drawn to encompass well-defined aspects of such a focus and hence exclude a multitude of others. In order that the volume may not only depict the state of the art, within its stated objectives, but also stimulate its development, one may only hope that such exclusions will not have been procrustean.

I would like to thank W. H. Flygare for the invitation to organize this symposium, the individual authors for their contributions to this volume, and the Office of Naval Research for its generous support.

K. H. ILLINGER
Tufts University
Medford, Massachusetts 02155

March 11, 1981

Electromagnetic-Field Interaction with Biological Systems in the Microwave and Far-Infrared Region

Physical Basis

K. H. ILLINGER

Department of Chemistry, Tufts University, Medford, MA 02155

The physical basis for the interaction between biological systems and electromagnetic (EM) fields must rest, in part, on the separate dielectric and spectroscopic properties of the molecular constituents and aggregates that comprise the biological system. A fundamental question, to which the simplest answer has frequently been tacitly assumed, is whether this physical basis, even at the cellular level, is completely given by those properties, or whether non-trivial extensions of such a model are necessary to predict all of the salient EM interactions. In spite of certain shortcomings, which continue to evade exact treatment (1), the interaction between EM radiation and ordinary molecular fluids is adequately represented by existing molecular models, and it would appear unlikely that wholly unexpected features will emerge for such systems. While similar considerations apply to the dominant contributions to the attenuation function for biological systems, evidence is gradually accumulating to suggest that the treatment of biological systems (even at the cellular level) exclusively in such terms may be inadequate. In particular, conclusions drawn from such a restrictive model concerning the behavior of biological response functions, as a function of the frequency and intensity of an external field, may, in certain respects, be not only quantitatively inaccurate but qualitatively misleading. Salient physical features, absent in ordinary molecular fluids, may be present in _in vivo_ biological systems, and thus require modeling of additional, non-trivial biophysical processes. These considerations suggest a treatment along the lines presented in Sections 2 and 3 below.

Absorption and Emission of Radiation in Ordinary Molecular Fluids (Equilibrium Systems)

General Theory of Collision Broadening. A molecular component in an ordinary fluid, in the presence of an electromagnetic field $E(\omega,t)$ and the collisional perturbation $V^0(\omega,t)$, due to interactions with other molecules, will experience a total Hamiltonian:

$$H(\omega,t) = H^0 + \mu \cdot E(\omega,t) + V^0(\omega,t) \tag{1}$$

where H^0 is the Hamiltonian for the molecule in the absence of the
EM-field interaction and the intermolecular perturbations described by $V^0(\omega,t)$ and μ is the electric dipole moment. The EM field
can be described by an angular frequency ω, a field strength E_0,
and a distribution over frequencies, $\rho(\omega)$, as follows:

$$E(\omega,t) = E_0(e^{i\omega t} + e^{-i\omega t})\, \rho(\omega) \tag{2}$$

General methods exist (1-7) for determining the complex permittivity $\kappa^*(\omega)$ of a molecule in the presence of collisional pertuba-
tions. Crucial to the form of $\kappa^*(\omega)$, and the attenuation function
$\alpha(\omega)$, descriptive of interaction with an EM field of frequency ω,
is whether the collisional perturbation $V^0(\omega,t)$ occurs on a time
scale which is short, intermediate, or long compared to the period
of the field, $(2\pi/\omega)$. In the limit of collisional perturbations
which are sudden (of very short duration) within the time-frame of
one period of the external field, every collision is effective in
interrupting the absorption-emission process (8), and, in the
limit of a large number of collisions per unit time, as in a fluid,
a totally collision-broadened, relaxation-type spectrum results
(1,9-12). Conversely, in the limit of collisional perturbations
which are of very long duration compared to a period of the EM
field, even in the presence of the large number of collisions, per
unit time, operative in a fluid, a resonant-type spectrum results.
Since the duration of a typical collision in a molecular fluid is
fixed, at a given temperature and pressure, the field frequency ω
becomes the crucial variable in determining the diabatic regime
(relaxation spectrum) and the adiabatic regime (resonance spectrum).
Whether interaction with a field at frequency ω_{ij} leads to a resonant or a relaxation spectrum, in the presence of the intermolecular perturbations described by Eq. (1), can be decided by ex-
aming the status of the inequality (13):

$$f(\omega_{ij}) = \left| \int_0^t (h\omega_{ij})^{-1}\, (dH/dt)\, \{\exp(i\int_0^t \omega_{ij}\, dt'')\}dt' \right| \tag{3}$$

For $f(\omega_{ij}) \gtrsim 1$, a limit attained as ω_{ij} tends toward zero, a relaxation spectrum is obtained; for $f(\omega_{ij}) \ll 1$, a limit attained as ω_{ij}
tends toward ∞, a resonance spectrum is obtained. Although ignor-
ance concerning the detailed form of the time development of the
collisional perturbation in a molecular fluid prevents a sharp
definition of this criterion, Eq. (3) indicates that the regime
of strongly adiabatic interactions (resonant absorption) lies
considerably above ~ 1 cm^{-1} (~ 30 GHz) (14,15). No compelling
experimental evidence (16) exists for resonance absorption in
ordinary molecular fluids below ~ 100 cm^{-1} (~ 3000 GHz)(17-23),
and experimental claims of resonant features in the attenuation
function, at millimeter wavelengths, of biological preparations
(24-25) are made tenuous in view of the difficulty of eliminating

experimental artifacts in the millimeter-wave spectroscopy of fluids.

As a result of these very general considerations, one expects the dielectric response function, as expressed by the complex permittivity, $\kappa^*(\omega)$, or the attenuation function, $\alpha(\omega)$, of ordinary molecular fluids to be characterized, from zero frequency to the extreme far-infrared region, by a relaxation spectrum. To first order, $\kappa^*(\omega)$ may be represented by a sum of terms for individual relaxation processes k, each given by a term of the form:

$$(\kappa^*_k(\omega) - \kappa_{\infty k}) = (\kappa_0 - \kappa_\infty)_k \, (1 + j\omega <\tau_k>)^{-1} \qquad (4)$$

$$\kappa_0 = \lim_{\omega \to 0} \kappa^*(\omega); \quad \kappa_\infty = \lim_{\omega \to \infty} \kappa^*(\omega) \qquad (5)$$

Eq. (4) gives $\kappa^*(\omega)$ for a relaxation process, with a relaxation time $<\tau_k>$ and with zero-frequency and high-frequency limits for $\kappa'(\omega)$ of κ_0 and κ_∞, respectively. Two complicating features render the Debye equation, Eq. (4), approximate, and require emendation: (a) a given relaxation process may be associated with a distribution of relaxation times (9-12), and (b), even for a non-distributed relaxation time, Eq. (4) leads to a physically incorrect high-frequency limit for $\kappa^*(\omega)$ or $\alpha(\omega)$. Empirical functions for a distribution of relaxation times have been applied to a wide variety of molecular (27) and biological (28) fluids, with considerable success. With respect to (b), the Debye equation is consistent with an exponential decay function for the electric dipole moment, thus predicting an instantaneous response to the external field being turned off, a physically untenable assumption (29). Several modifications (1,29-32) have been discussed; the effect of this feature on the interpretation of the millimeter-wave and far-infrared spectrum of $H_2O(\ell)$ will be sketched in Section 2.3. However, even for H_2O, the system with the smallest relaxation time expected in a biological context, deviations from Debye behavior, in the sense of (b) above, are not apparent at frequencies below $\sim$ 100 GHz (15,30). As a result, proper modification having been made in those cases where a distribution of relaxation times obtains, the relaxation-type contributions to the bulk complex permittivity in the microwave region are well understood and have been analyzed in some detail (28,33,34).

The entire analysis presented here has assumed, inter alia, thermal equilibrium among the components of the molecular fluid, and a Planck-type equilibrium for the photons absorbed or emitted in the interactions among the molecules and the external EM field.

The Attenuation Function. The complex permittivity $\kappa^*(\omega)$ and the attenuation function $\alpha(\omega)$ are related by basic electromagnetic theory, and independently of any molecular model, as follows:

$$\alpha(\omega) = (\omega/2)(1/2c) \, [\, \{ \kappa'(\omega)]^2 + [\kappa''(\omega)]^2\}^{1/2} - \kappa'(\omega)]^{1/2} \qquad (6)$$

where c is the velocity of light in vacuo. A closely related quantity is the dielectric conductivity, $\sigma(\omega)$:

$$\sigma(\omega) = \varepsilon_0 \omega \kappa''(\omega) \tag{7}$$

Here, ε_0 is the permittivity of free space. For a simple Debye-type relaxation process, Eq. (4), and owing to the incorrect representation of the high-frequency limit inherent in any expression for $\kappa^*(\omega)$ consistent with an exponential decay function for the electric moment, one obtains for the high-frequency limit of $\alpha(\omega)$ from Eqs. (4) and (6) (30):

$$\lim_{\omega \to \infty} \alpha_{Debye,k}(\omega) = (1/2c)\ [\kappa_0 - \kappa_\infty]_k < \tau_k >^{-1} [\kappa_{\infty k}]^{-1/2} \tag{8}$$

For fundamental physical reasons, the attenuation function for any process must vanish as $\omega \to \infty$. This expectation is borne out by far-infrared measurements of $\alpha(\omega)$ for a variety of molecular systems exhibiting a relaxation-type absorption in the microwave and millimeter-wave region (17-23). While H_2O as a solute in nonhydrogen-bonding solvents also shows this behavior (35), the millimeter-wave and far-infrared spectrum of $H_2O(\ell)$ is complicated by contributions to $\alpha(\omega)$ due to intermolecular vibrations involving a cluster of H_2O molecules (libration and translation), in addition to the high-frequency tail of the relaxation absorption. A heuristic treatment of the general problem (30) makes the relaxation time, Eq. (4), frequency-dependent, such that the limit for $\alpha(\omega)$ in Eq. (8) becomes physically acceptable. Under conditions appropriate to the correct limit, the normalized real and imaginary parts of the complex permittivity and the normalized dielectric conductivity take on the form depicted in Fig. (1). Here, $<\tau_k(0)>$ is the relaxation time in the limit of zero frequency (diabatic limit). Irrespective of the details of the model employed, both $\alpha(\omega)$ and $\sigma(\omega)$ must tend toward zero as $\omega \to \infty$, in contrast to Eq. (8), for any relaxation process. In the case of a resonant process, not expected below the extreme far-infrared region, $\alpha(\omega)$ is given by an expression consistent with a resonant dispersion for $\kappa^*(\omega)$ in Eq. (6), not the relaxation dispersion for $\kappa^*(\omega)$ implicit in Eq. (4). Models for collision-broadened lineshapes have been treated in detail (1-7), in the adiabatic as well as the diabatic limit. As expected, the intermediate case, i.e. strongly damped resonant transitions, is most difficult to treat accurately.

In summary, it is expected that the bulk attenuation function for ordinary molecular fluids is reasonably well represented by relaxation-type processes in the microwave region. At high frequencies, in the region of the extreme far-infrared, deviations from Eq. (4) will occur, even for a process with a single relaxation time. Phenomenologically, as $\omega \to \infty$, the efficiency with which a representative collision interrupts the absorption or emission of radiation in a molecular fluid must decrease toward zero, and the relaxation time in Eq. (4) must become frequency-dependent.

$\underline{H_2O}$: $\underline{The \ Pure \ Liquid}$. Because of the large magnitude of the attenuation of $H_2O(\ell)$ and the ubiquitous presence of water in biological systems, the bulk attenuation function of most biological fluids is dominated by the attenuation due to $H_2O(\ell)$. Until recently, wide gaps existed in the experimental characterization of $\alpha(\omega)$ for $H_2O(\ell)$ in the millimeter-wave and far-infrared region (36-41). These lacunae are now in the process of being filled. Measurements in the extreme far-infrared (6 - 450 cm^{-1}) (42) and a measurement of high precision at 70 GHz (43) on $H_2O(\ell)$ have recently been reported, to complement existing measurements at lower and higher frequencies. Fig. (2) summarizes the measurements of Grant, and Asfar and Hasted, carried out by a high-loss, travelling-wave technique at 70 GHz and reflection-dispersive-Fourier-transform spectroscopy in the far-infrared, respectively. Also represented is the contribution to $\alpha(\omega)$ from the Debye-type relaxation process calculated from the model (30). It would appear that deviations from the Debye-type behavior are not yet operative at 70 GHz. At frequencies above $\sim$150 GHz, the intermolecular vibrations begin to make their contribution, before the asymptotic limit predicted by the Debye model, Eq. (8), is reached. Owing to the complexity of the intermolecular interactions in a strongly hydrogen-bonded liquid, like $H_2O(\ell)$, detailed and unambiguous analysis of the attenuation function above $\sim$100 GHz is difficult to achieve (41,42).

Schematically, the total attenuation function for $H_2O(\ell)$ is given in Fig. 3. The relaxation contribution goes as ω^2 in the low-frequency limit and dominates the attenuation characteristics up to $\sim$100 GHz. The quasi-lattice vibrations involving clusters of strongly interacting molecules begin to contribute, in a preponderant fashion, above $\sim$100 GHz. While the relaxation contribution $\alpha_{REL}(\omega)$, must begin to decrease at frequencies in excess of $\sim$10^3 GHz, the quasi-lattice vibrations persist in a set of very broad bands into the far-infrared, (42), attaining extremely high values for $\alpha(\omega)$. As a result, $H_2O(\ell)$, always present, to some degree, in biological systems, provides very efficient attenuation to EM fields in the millimeter-wave and far-infrared regions. Although millimeter-wave measurements on liquids in the category of highest accuracy are typically single-frequency measurements, and while the far-infrared Fourier-spectroscopic measurements have a finite resolution, neither these nor recent swept-frequency measurements (44) provide any experimental evidence which would compel invoking physical mechanisms other than those sketched in Section 2.1 and 2.2. The broad attenuation due to $H_2O(\ell)$ becomes the more effective as the far-infrared region is reached from lower frequencies. As a result, other possible molecular absorption processes occurring in the interior of a biological system are more strongly shielded by the $H_2O(\ell)$ absorption at higher frequencies in the millimeter-wave and far-infrared range, as indicated

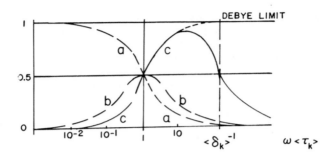

Figure 1.   *Normalized complex permittivity* $\kappa^*(\omega) - j\kappa''(\omega)$ *and conductivity* $\sigma(\omega)$
for a relaxation process of type k.

Curve a: $[\kappa'(\omega) - \kappa_\infty][\kappa_0 - \kappa_\infty]^{-1}$; *Curve b:* $\kappa''(\omega)[\kappa_0 - \kappa_\infty]^{-1}$; *Curve c:* $\sigma(\omega) < \tau_k(0) >$
$[\varepsilon_0(\kappa_0 - \kappa_\infty)]^{-1}$; ω: *the angular frequency;* $< \tau_k(0) >$: *the relaxation time at zero fre-*
quency; κ_0: *the low-frequency limit of* $\kappa'(\omega)$; κ_∞: *the high-frequency limit of* $\kappa'(\omega)$;
$< \delta_k >$: *the average duration of a collision.*

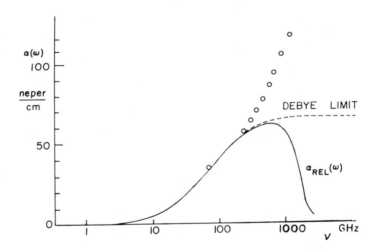

Figure 2.   *Attenuation function for* $H_2O(l)$. $\alpha_{REL}(\omega)$ *is the contribution to the total
attenuation function due to the rotational relaxation, as calculated from the model
in Ref. 30. The circles are the experimental points from Refs. 42 and 43.*

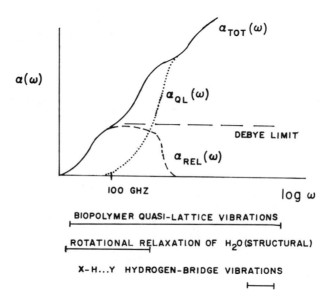

Figure 3. Schematic of the total attenuation function $\alpha_{TOT}(\omega)$, and its contributions, for $H_2O(l)$ at millimeter and far-infrared wavelengths.

$\alpha_{REL}(\omega)$ is the contribution due to the rotational relaxation, and $\alpha_{QL}(\omega)$ is the contribution due to the quasi-lattice vibrations of $H_2O(l)$ clusters. ω is the angular frequency.

schematically in Fig. (3). In particular, quasi-lattice vibrations of biopolymeric systems (Section 2.6) and the vibrations of
the bridge-heads (X,Y) of hydrogen-bonded systems X-H...Y (14)
fall into this category. Thus, the unusually strong molecular
interactions present in $H_2O(\ell)$ produce broad attenuation in a
frequency range ($\gtrsim 100$ cm^{-1}) where the onset of (damped) resonant-
type absorption occurs for non-hydrogen-bonded liquids (17) and
for the quasi-lattice vibrations of polymeric systems. In contrast, in the low-frequency ($\gtrsim$ 1GHz) regime, contributed to virtually exclusively by the $H_2O(\ell)$ relaxation spectrum, $\alpha(\omega)$ falls
off as ω^2. Whereas resonant processes in $\alpha(\omega)$ are not expected
as $\omega \to 0$, Eq. (3), in any system, there exists a (relaxation) absorption process of potential interest in biological systems, in
a region where the $H_2O(\ell)$ absorption, per unit concentration, is
not wholly dominant, i.e. the rotational relaxation of structural H_2O, in the region near $\sim$1GHz. Approaches to the dynamics
of that process will be traced in Section 2.4.

In spite of the complexity of the analysis of the millimeter-
wave and far-infrared spectrum of $H_2O(\ell)$, the principal contribu-
tor to the bulk attenuation function of typical biological systems in this frequency range, no compelling experimental evidence
or theoretical constructs exist to disqualify the assumption that
this system is a complex, but typical, collision-broadened system whose fundamental features (1) are well understood.

Free and Structural Water in Biological Systems. The same
salient physical property that renders the millimeter-wave and
far-infrared spectrum of $H_2O(\ell)$ complex, the hydrogen-bonded
interactions among H_2O molecules in the pure liquid, generates an
additional complexity when H_2O interacts with other molecular
systems also capable of hydrogen-bonded interaction. Although
considerable controversy exists concerning the detailed properties of structural H_2O, it is well recognized that hydrogen-
bonded interactions among H_2O molecules, biologically-important
molecules, and the biological membrane play a crucial role in
biological systems (45,46). The hydrogen-bond interaction exhibits energetics intermediate between those characteristic of
ordinary molecular interactions and weak chemical interactions
and, importantly, possesses directional properties not so fully
articulated in the first. In a mixture of biopolymers, ions and
H_2O, in vitro, as well as in an actual biological context, the
total number of H_2O molecules will be distributed in a complicated fashion over sites which range from loci within essentially
pure clusters of H_2O molecules (the "free" water) and sites directly interacting with other molecular entities (the "structural"
water). Clearly, the instantaneous distribution and the dynamics
of the set of H_2O molecules among such sites, of which these are
the extreme cases, are exceedingly complex. With respect to the
contribution to the total attenuation function, $\alpha(\omega)$, due to
structural H_2O, one requires knowledge of the concentration of

structural H_2O for a given system, the average value of the
relaxation time, and a measure of the distribution of relaxation
times. The fact that many energetically different binding sites
for an H_2O molecule exist in a system with a set of hydrogen-
bonded interactions in different molecular environments (at the
surface of biopolymers or the membrane) would suggest a distribution of relaxation times.

The ab initio calculation of the rotational relaxation time,
even for a pure liquid, is a taxing problem, since it requires
reasonably accurate representation of the interactions experienc-
ed by the molecule from its neighbors, while it responds to the
external EM field. Such a calculation exists for $H_2O(\ell)$ (47),
showing reasonable agreement with the observed complex permittivity $\kappa^*(\omega)$. Structural water, because of the variety of interactions present in this system, has not been examined in this
fashion. Rather, the reverse procedure, extraction of the contribution to $\kappa^*(\omega)$ due to structural H_2O, has been followed (48-50).
Since different tissue types show different free water – structural water ratios, results from one type of tissue to another
may not be transferable. Both the interpretation of the dielectric response function (51) and the dynamics of the rotational
relaxation of bound water (52-58) are as yet subjects of lively
controversy. The results of Grant et al., interpreted in terms
of a static model of a protein molecule, surrounded by bound water
on its surface and free water at larger distance, (49,50) suggest
the frequency region of the order of a few GHz to constitute the
crossover point below which the structural water is more absorptive, per unit volume, than the free water.

As for all the systems relegated to Section 2, the attenuation function for structural H_2O in the microwave and far-infrared
region, as well as that for free H_2O, can be understood in terms
of collision-broadened, equilibrium systems. While the average
values of the relaxation times, distribution parameters, and the
features of the far-infrared spectra for these systems clearly
differ, the physical mechanisms descriptive of these interactions
are consonant. The distribution of free and structural H_2O molecules over molecular environments is different, and differs for
the latter case with specific systems, as are the rotational dynamics which govern the relaxation responses and the quasi-lattice
vibrational dynamics which determine the far-infrared spectrum.
Evidence for resonant features in the attenuation function for
structural H_2O, which have sometimes been invoked (24-26,59) to
play a role in the microwave and millimeter-wave region, is
tenuous and unconvincing.

Nevertheless, in view of the fact that the stability of biopolymers, in respect of their secondary and tertiary (conformational) structure, is strongly influenced by interactions with
structural H_2O (45), it is of considerable interest to explore
further the features discussed in the penultimate paragraph. Even
for a totally collision-broadened (relaxation-type) initial step

in the uptake of energy from an external EM field by the structural H_2O, one must inquire into the possible subsequent steps
and their effect, if any, on the biological system. Energy input into the structural H_2O molecules, e.g. in the grooves of the
DNA molecule, can be dissipated in at least two ways: (a) interaction with nearest-neighbor H_2O molecules, ions, or any other
molecular species not associated with the biopolymer, and (b)
interaction, in a more direct fashion, with the energetics of the
biopolymer. Apart from electronic excitation, which occurs at
much higher frequencies than those of interest here, vibrational
and rotational excitation of the structural H_2O molecules may
occur. Vibrational frequencies of the bridge-heads (X,Y) of a
typical hydrogen-bonded system X-H...Y are of the order of ∿100
cm^{-1} (∿3000 GHz). At these frequencies, the attenuation function
for $H_2O(\ell)$ has already attained a value of ∿500 neper cm^{-1}, and,
while no measurements exist on the structural-H_2O attenuation
function in the far-infrared, it is expected to be no larger, per
unit volume. In consequence, free H_2O is expected to attenuate
vibrational excitation of the hydrogen-bonded bridge-heads very
effectively. In contrast, in the region of rotational relaxation
of structural H_2O, attenuation of external fields in the interior
of a biological system is not nearly so complete (49,50).

Irrespective of the magnitude of the effective EM field
strength at the locus of a structural-H_2O molecule, it is now requisite to consider the dynamics of the events which may follow
the initial absorptive step by the structural-H_2O molecule. If
the system considered were a simple mixture of absorbing and
mutually interacting molecules, no unusual features were to be
expected. However, the role of structural H_2O is closely tied
to the dynamics of the phase transitions of biopolymers, which
are known to be cooperative (60,61), and may also be implicated
in the phase transitions of biological membranes. As the degree
of cooperativity increases, the effect of a unit field perturbation on the structural H_2O is expected to increase, and the total
randomization of initial energy input is expected to decrease.
Schwarz (62,63) has shown that the static field strength required
to cause a phase transition in a helical polymer, with segmental
dipole moment μ, is $E(0) = 4kT \mu^{-1} \sigma_c$, where σ_c is the cooperativity parameter, k is the Boltzmann constant and T is the temperature. For a totally non-cooperative transition, $\sigma_c = 1$; for
PBLG, $\sigma_c \sim 3 \cdot 10^{-5}$. While this (static-field) model does not apply in any direct sense to the present problem, one may expect
any preferential input into the energetics of the secondary or
tertiary structure of a biopolymer, after initial absorption by
the structural H_2O, to be strongly dependent on the inequality
$\sigma_c \ll 1$. Clearly, a dynamical model, Fig. (4), is required to
examine the effect of an external field $E(\omega,t)$ on a system containing free H_2O, structural H_2O, and a cooperative system, such
as a biopolymer or a membrane. Absorption of energy from the
external EM field by the free H_2O essentially increases the random

collisions with the surface of the cooperative system, while similar absorption by the structural H_2O in principle may cause more
direct perturbation of the cooperative system. While it is clear
that, as $\sigma_c \to 1$, any selective effects will disappear, the magnitude of any such effects for highly cooperative systems is not
known. If they exist, they would lead to a (presumably broad)
frequency-selective alteration in the secondary and tertiary
structure of the cooperative system, in the region suggested by
Grant (49,50), with an attendant possibility of alteration of
biological endpoints, Fig. (4). In addition to the possible
intervention into the secondary and tertiary structure of biopolymers by processes involving the initial uptake of EM energy
by structural H_2O, an analogous possibility exists for the intervention into the structure of membranes. Apart from the effect
of the degree of cooperativity in these phase transitions (biopolymer or biological membrane), it is expected that any external
EM-field effects will be maximal under thermodynamic and chemical
conditions close to the phase-transition point. Alterations in
the ordering of the lipid chains in bovine sphingomylen, monitored by Raman-spectroscopic transitions of the scissoring vibration of the hydrocarbon backbone of the lipid chain, have been
reported (64), in the region of $\sim$2 GHz.

In competition with any selective interactions stemming from
the initial absorption by structural H_2O, there exist, of course,
the interactions arising from absorption by free H_2O, polar side-
chain rotation and amino acids, all having a finite $\alpha(\omega)$ in the
frequency range implicated here. As a result, conformational
changes in biopolymers and/or membranes induced by the structural
H_2O absorption will have to be examined as a function of frequency
in the $\sim$1-10 GHz range, in order to rule out trivial, overall
thermalized effects. In the present context, structural H_2O,
although acting as a component of the collision-broadened, equilibrium fluid, because of its specific role in the cooperative
conformational changes of a biopolymer and/or a membrane, may
constitute an interaction mechanism absent in simple systems,
containing no molecules or molecular aggregates which undergo
cooperative phase transitions. It is of interest to note that
such a possible interaction mechanism is expected to occur in
aqueous dielectrics containing the biopolymer(s) and/or mem-
brane(s) in vitro, although details may be modified by alterations in the conformational structures of the cooperative systems
in in vivo biological systems. Certainly, biochemically actuated
conformational changes in in vivo systems will affect the status
of the (cooperative) phase transitions, and hence the susceptibility of the associated conformations to energy uptake by
structural H_2O. However, appropriately chosen in vitro systems,
containing biopolymers and/or membranes, may display similar
interactions.

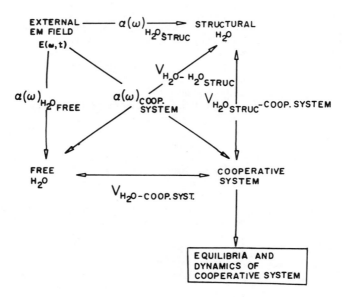

*Figure 4.   Interactions among the free H_2O, the structural H_2O, the cooperative
system, and an external EM field. $\alpha(\omega)$ denotes the various attenuation functions,
and V the intermolecular potentials.*

Aqueous Dielectrics in the Biological Context. To this
point, the interactions, due to molecular systems, that the components of aqueous dielectrics experience have been formally represented by the term $V^0(\omega,t)$ in Eq. (1), where $V^0(\omega,t)$ is the
intermolecular potential in a simple fluid. While the general
considerations we have developed still apply in the biological
context, molecular interactions in situ of a biological environment will differ from V^0. Apart from the more subtle effects on
V due to conformational changes within biological systems, it
is requisite to add another electric field term to Eq. (1). The
biological membrane is the source of a large ($\sim 10^5$ V cm^{-1}) intrinsic electric field, $E_{intr}(\omega,t) = E_1(0) + E_2(\omega,t)$, with its
principal component, $E_1(0)$, at zero frequency. Molecules and
ions inside biological membranes will experience this interaction,
and, in a formal sense, Eq.(1) must be altered to:

$$H(\omega,t) = H^0 + \mu\cdot[E(\omega,t) + E_{intr}(\omega,t)] + V(\omega,t) \qquad (9)$$

Even if we model, for the moment, only the equilibrium aspects of
the aqueous dielectrics in a membrane environment, the large magnitude of $E_{intr}(0)$ indicates that for molecules in that locality
(structural H_2O, biopolymers, ions, in or near the membrane) conditions of dielectric saturation exist. The membrane intrinsic
field plays a pivotal role in the conformation of biopolymers imbedded in the membrane and in membrane transport properties (65-
69), and imparts unusual dielectric properties to molecular systems in the membrane field (70-71). Although the latter are more
farreaching, they indicate, for the purposes of the present discussion, that the complex permittivity, Eq. (4), will differ for
molecules in the presence of the intrinsic membrane field. Presumably, only a small fraction of the components of aqueous dielectrics in a biological context are in the presence of a large
intrinsic field, and the bulk complex permittivity is not strongly affected by it. However, properties of systems in situ of the
membrane intrinsic field can not be analyzed accurately without
taking it into account.

In particular, the analysis of the contribution to $\kappa^*(\omega)$ or
$\alpha(\omega)$ due to the structural H_2O may require explicit modeling of
the membrane intrinsic field, for systems which contain biological
membranes, and an altered $\kappa^*(\omega)$ may obtain for such a case. Although the theory for the static complex permittivity, κ_0 in Eq.
(4), is well-developed (72-74) for the case of dielectric saturation, a general treatment of rotational relaxation, and hence
$\kappa^*(\omega)$, does not appear to exist. The real state of structural
H_2O is, of course, further complicated, with respect to its rotational relaxation, in that, owing to its hydrogen-bonded inter-
action(s) to a substrate, it is a hindered rotor, and Eq. (4)
may have only an approximately correct form. The fact that structural H_2O partakes of a complex environment in the biological
context makes exact modeling of its contribution to $\alpha(\omega)$ difficult.

At least two other species may require the articulation of
the membrane intrinsic field for the description of their contribution to $\kappa^*(\omega)$: ions and biopolymers. The ionic contribution
to the complex permittivity is roughly constant in the microwave
and millimeter-wave region, being associated with large relaxation times (28, 33-34), and is therefore more readily dealt with,
at least in a phenomenological description, than the structural-
H_2O contribution. Rotational motion of biopolymers imbedded in
membranes is highly restricted (75-78), in contrast to their
lateral (translational) diffusion, and hence is not expected to
contribute to $\kappa^*(\omega)$. The quasi-lattice vibrations of biopolymers
may be presumed to interact with the membrane intrinsic field,
and a splitting of degeneracies of the vibrational modes (Stark
effect) may occur. However, these modes are already strongly
overlapping in the frequency regions of interest here (see
Section 2.6) and the main effect of the membrane field will be a
redistribution of intensities over frequency, without large-scale
changes in their contribution to $\kappa^*(\omega)$.

Biopolymers: Rotational Diffusion and Quasi-Lattice Vibrations. The overall rotational diffusion of biopolymer molecules
in aqueous solution contributes to $\alpha(\omega)$ in a constant fashion in
the microwave and millimeter-wave region (28, 33-34), and the rotational diffusion of biopolymers imbedded in biological membranes
is highly restricted, with an associated vanishing contribution
to $\alpha(\omega)$. Polar side chains of biopolymers, as well as the very
complex structures containing polar groups on the surface of membranes (78), however, are expected to show rotational relaxation
in the $\sim$1-10 GHz region. Nonetheless, such rotational-diffusion
events, strongly coupled to the free H_2O, and not directly associated with cooperative phase transitions, should merely contribute
a broad, featureless shoulder to $\alpha(\omega)$ in the microwave and millimeter-wave region.

Of greater potential interest are the quasi-lattice vibrations associated with the biopolymer molecules. Since a molecular system with N atoms exhibits (3N-6) normal modes of vibration, and N $\gtrsim 10^4$ for many biopolymers, a very large number of low-
lying vibrational modes ($\sim$1-100 cm^{-1}) exists. The problem of the
total vibrational analysis of polymers in the unpertubed state
has been attacked (79-83,84-88), and the role of structural H_2O
has been examined in a semi-empirical quantum-mechanical calculation (89). A pervasive problem in the calculation of the low-
frequency tail (terminating near $\sim$1 cm^{-1}) of these vibrations is
the lack of accuracy with which the frequency distribution is
calculable in this limit, compared to reasonably good fit to
experiment in the region $\gtrsim$100 cm^{-1}. As a result, the center frequencies and the width of such vibrations, the more strongly
damped the lower their frequency, is least accurately predictable
in the low-frequency (millimeter-wave) region, where the attenuation function of free H_2O begins to decrease. Raman-spectroscopic

measurements, at frequencies below ∿100 cm^{-1}, have been carried out on α-chymotripsin (90–91) and lysozyme (92). An ingenious method (93) using phase fluctuation optical heterodyne spectroscopy, which evades the problem of direct spectroscopic measurement of a vanishingly small change in attenuation in a high-loss system, has resulted in measurements, between 8–12 GHz, of the absorption of synthetic DNA in aqueous solution; a broad, featureless absorption in this region is found. Crucial to the analysis of the low-frequency tail of these vibrations is the molecular environment of the polymer. As expected from our general considerations of collision broadening, the line-width of a transition, in a given intermolecular environment, will increase as the line frequency decreases, and will depend on V . The vibrational transitions m-n, with frequencies ω_{mn} and transition probabilities $|\mu_{mn}|^2$, will show a damped, resonant-type behavior, for which $\kappa^*(\omega)$ has the form (1,2):

$$[\kappa^*(\omega)-1]=$$

$$\frac{1}{\hbar}\sum_{mn} \rho_m^{(0)}(1-e^{-\hbar\omega_{mn}/kT})\sum_s |\mu_{mn,s}|^2 [A_{mn,s}(\omega)-jB_{mn,s}(\omega)]\frac{E_{int,s}(\omega)}{E_s(\omega)}$$

$$A_{mn,s}(\omega)=8\pi N\frac{\omega_{mn}}{(\omega_{mn}^2-\omega^2)}\left[\frac{-\omega}{2\omega_{mn}^2}\left\{\frac{(\omega_{mn}+\omega_{mn}+\omega}{[1+(\omega_{mn}-\omega)^2\tau_{mn,s}^2]}+\frac{\omega-\omega_{mn})}{[1+(\omega_{mn}+\omega)^2\tau_{mn,s}^2]}\right\}+1\right]$$

$$B_{mn,s}(\omega)=\frac{1}{2}\frac{\omega\tau_{mn,s}}{\omega_{mn}}\left\{[1+(\omega_{mn}-\omega)^2\tau_{mn,s}^2]^{-1}+[1+(\omega_{mn}+\omega)^2\tau_{mn,s}^2]^{-1}\right\}$$

$$s=x,y,z;\quad j=(-1)^{\frac{1}{2}}\tag{10}$$

In Eq. (10), $E_{int,s}(\omega)$ and $E_s(\omega)$ are the s=x,y,z components of the internal electric field and the field in the dielectric, respectively, and $\rho_m^{(0)}$ is the Boltzmann density matrix for the set of initial states m. The parameter τ_{mn} is a measure of the line-width. While small molecules, N<<10^2, in the pure solid show well-defined lattice-vibrational spectra, arising from intermolecular vibrations in the crystal, overlap among the vastly larger number of normal modes for large, polymeric systems, produces broad bands, even in the crystalline state. When the polymeric molecule experiences the molecular interactions operative in aqueous solution, a second feature further broadens the vibrational bands, since the line-width parameters, τ_{mn}, Eq. (10), reflect the increased molecular collisional effects in solution, as compared to those in the solid. These general considerations are borne out by experiment. The low-frequency Raman spectrum of the amino acid cystine (94) shows a line at 8.7 cm^{-1}, in the crystalline solid, with a half-width of several cm^{-1}. In contrast, a careful study of the low frequency Raman spectra of lysozyme (92) shows a broad band (half-width ∿10 cm^{-1}) at 25 cm^{-1},

even in the crystalline state; lysozyme in acetate buffer solution and in aqueous solution shows no spectral features in the
Raman spectrum below a band at 75 cm^{-1} (with half-width $\gtrsim$10 cm^{-1})
attributed to the torsional vibration of the peptide chain. Thus,
existing experimental evidence for biopolymers is consistent with
strongly damped vibrations, even in the pure solid. A measurement
of the complex permittivity of PBLG in the range 1-20 GHz implies
a totally damped (Debye-type) vibration for the lowest vibrational mode (95), involving the longitudinal stretch of the α-helix
that comprises the backbone of this molecule.

In the biological context, biopolymers experience molecular
environments which range from that in dilute solution, in the
free-aqueous phase in intercellular space, to the fluid-mosaic
environment when imbedded in the biological membrane. Needless
to say, specification of the intermolecular potential in the
biological context, with any degree of accuracy, is not feasible.
However, it is expected that the status of collisional broadening
of the biopolymer vibrational transitions encompasses the range
mimicked by the experimental data cited above. Except for the
caveat that the status of the structural H$_2$O and the details of
even the equilibrium features of the membrane environment are not
those of the crystalline solid, one may thus extrapolate the contributions to $\alpha(\omega)$ from such experimental findings. They suggest
that, at millimeter-wave and the extreme far-infrared ranges, biopolymers in the biological context will exhibit broad, highly
overlapping and strongly damped vibrations; in the region above
$\sim$100 cm^{-1}, gradual approach to less severely damped vibrations
is expected, in the same frequency direction in which the attenuation by free H$_2$O rapidly increases the shielding, to external
fields, in the interior of biological structures.

Biological Tissues in vitro. As has been discussed in pre-
ceeding sections, although the general features of the contributions to the bulk attenuation function of aqueous dielectrics
below $\sim$1 GHz are well understood, at higher frequencies, in the
millimeter and far-infrared region, complications are expected to
arise, in principle, which limit the accuracy of extrapolations
from lower-frequency data. In particular, the modeling of the
structural-H$_2$O contribution may be complex (Section 2.4). While
$\alpha(\omega)$ for various types of tissue is well characterized to $\sim$1 GHz
(96), there is a paucity of measurements at higher frequencies
(97-100), some of which tend to indicate that straightforward
extrapolation in terms of simple contributions of the Debye-relaxation type, Eq.(4), may not be accurate. The attempt to analyze
the contribution to $\kappa*(\omega)$ of tissue in vitro due to structural H$_2$O,
even with extended-frequency data in the region above 1 GHz, is, of
course, open to the criticism that in vivo tissue, even in its
equilibrium aspects, may differ from the former. Changes in the
nature of the structural H$_2$O are certainly plausible, but their
magnitude is difficult to assess. Techniques which permit measure-

ment of $\kappa^*(\omega)$ in the region $\gtrsim$1GHz in vivo are one avenue to the
solution of this open question (101–102). Another way in which
in vitro and in vivo tissue will, in principle, differ is the
distribution of biopolymers among various possible conformational
states, and hence one expects alterations in the contribution to
$\kappa^*(\omega)$ due to the biopolymeric system, structural H_2O and ions,
even in the equilibrium sense.

Chemically-Pumped Steady-State (Non-equilibrium) Systems.

A fundamental assumption made in most of dielectric and
spectroscopic theory is that the system interacting with the
external EM field is in thermal equilibrium and, in the presence
of the external EM field, attains a Planck-type distribution for
the photons being exchanged, by absorption and emission, with the
field. Under these conditions, the theory of collision broadening leads to expressions for damped-resonant transitions, Eq. (10),
and, in the limit of diabatic interactions, articulated in Eq. (3),
to that for relaxation transitions, Eq.(4). A Planck-type distribution of the photons implies a Boltzmann distribution of the
molecular species over their energy levels. This generates the
factor $[1-\exp(-\hbar\omega_{mn}/kT]$ in the Van Vleck-Weisskopf Karplus-
Schwinger line-shape function, Eq.(10), of which Eq.(4) is a
special case. A more accurate analysis of the effects of the
Boltzmann distribution on $\kappa^*(\omega)$ has been made (103), accounting
for the fact that in collision-broadened lines the line-frequency
is not a delta function but has a distribution. No major modifications of the form of the analysis implicit in Eqs. (3),(4), and
(10) arises. However, if physicochemical processes occur in a
system which significantly alter the Boltzmann distribution of
systems connected with that species, the ordinary equations of
collision-broadening can no longer be expected to apply to that
species.

As implied in Section 2 above, ordinary molecular fluids,
obeying the equilibrium thermodynamics of closed systems, and
experiencing, apart from the EM field, the effect of non-reactive
collisions, V, are not expected to contain such processes. As a
result, the entire hierarchy of systems discussed in Section 2,
from $H_2O(\ell)$ to biological tissues in vitro, should be susceptible
of at least phenomenological analysis in terms of ordinary aqueous
dielectrics. In fact, the experimental evidence for that assumption is overwhelming and well-documented, and the hypothesis of a
closed, equilibrium system for these cases is reasonable not only
for the dielectric response functions $\kappa^*(\omega)$ or $\alpha(\omega)$, but also
other physicochemical parameters, such as heat transfer, specific
absorption rate, etc. A fundamental question that nevertheless
arises is whether any subsystems occur in an in vivo biological
system which violate these assumptions. Even for the simplest
level of biological organization, the living cell, to which these
considerations shall be limited, the answer is in the affirmative.

Biophysical constructs which have been adduced are sketched in
Sections 3.1 and 3.2, and an analysis of the coupling between
external EM fields and those subsystems not tractable by the
methods of Section 2, is presented in Sections 3.3 and 3.4.

   Dissipative Structures in Biological Systems. Although not
confined to biological entities (104,105), open, dissipative systems occur in living cells, and the irreducible biophysical system, in the in vivo biological context, showing such features, appears to be the biological membrane (106). While the classical
models for the electrical properties of the biological membrane
veil the intrinsic dissipative characteristic, a recent alternative formulation (107) brings it more sharply into focus. Descriptions of membrane properties in terms of irreversible, nonequilibrium thermodynamics have been given (106,108). For our
purposes here, it suffices to consider the in vivo biological membrane (its components and attendant biophysical processes) as a
chemically pumped, open, steady-state system. Furthermore, the
biochemical reactions which provide energy for the membrane system may, in general, be associated with a sequence of feedback
loops linking the steady-state concentrations of oscillatory biochemical reactions(109-111). Under such conditions, the simple
(equilibrium-type) perturbations due to non-reactive collisions
[V in Eq. (9)] are replaced, for the membrane subsystem (including
biopolymers, structural H_2O and ions), by much more complicated
interactions, which may exhibit novel features. In contrast to
the fully elaborated fabric of the theory of (non-reactive) collision broadening of ordinary molecular fluids, models for EM-
field interactions with dissipative systems are still in the
developmental stage. Ross and coworkers (112-115) have discussed
the effect of frequency-dependent perturbations on oscillatory
chemical reactions in a general fashion. A direct study of perturbation by an electric field of the chemical-wave system of the
(oscillatory) Belousov-Zhabotinskii reaction has recently been
carried out (116). In a more general sense, an application has
been made to the analysis of the ELF-field perturbation of limit-
cycle systems (117-118). Similarly to the status of current
theoretical models, confirmatory experimental data are as yet
sparse for the EM-field interactions with biological systems, and
will require fuller corroboration and extension. In contrast to
the EM-field interaction models, structural models for the biological membrane are now in a full state of development (78,77,
119-124), the fluid-mosaic model of Singer and Nicolson (78), with
some modification (77), being generally accepted. These detailed
structural models, describing the spatial and dynamical organization of the membrane components, will no doubt play a role in more
physical extensions of the formal theory (Section 3.2) when those
are developed.
   The foregoing considerations indicate that in vivo biological
entities, even at the cellular level, must be considered as a mix-

ture of an equilibrium system and dissipative subsystem (s), Fig. (5). Thus, the total attenuation function has the components:

$$\alpha_{TOT}(\omega) = \alpha(\omega) + \alpha_{DIS}(\omega) \qquad (11)$$

where $\alpha(\omega)$ is the contribution by the equilibrium system, analysable in terms of the concepts in Section 2, and $\alpha_{DIS}(\omega)$ is the contribution by the dissipative subsystem (s), approaches to whose behavior will be discussed in Section 3.4 below. In an analogous fashion, we may define a set of biological-response functions, of type i:

$$\beta_{i,TOT}(\omega) = \beta_i(\omega) + \beta_{i,DIS}(\omega) \qquad (12)$$

Since the energy uptake by the equilibrium system is related to $\alpha(\omega)$, the contribution, $\beta_i(\omega)$, to the biological response function by EM-field interactions with the equilibrium system is expected to parallel $\alpha(\omega)$, at least in a qualitative sense. That is to say, contributions to biological response functions arising from the interaction with the equilibrium system are expected to show the broad features exhibited by $\alpha(\omega)$, with the possible exception of a somewhat narrower response due to interaction with structural H_2O, as discussed in Section 2.4 . The relationship between the contribution to the attenuation function, $\alpha_{DIS}(\omega)$, and the biological response function, $\beta_{i,DIS}(\omega)$, due to EM-field interactions with the dissipative subsystems, is not directly predictable. In consequence, it is possible that in frequency regimes where interactions between the EM-field and the dissipative system(s) are operative, the bulk attenuation function, $\alpha_{TOT}(\omega)$, or the attenuation function in the absence of the dissipative structures, $\alpha(\omega)$, may not always be an infallible guide to the presence or absence of biological effects, expressed by $\beta_{i,DIS}(\omega)$.

A special case of such a circumstance is that $\alpha_{DIS}(\omega)$ takes on a vanishing value, such that $\alpha_{TOT}(\omega) \cong \alpha(\omega)$, while $\beta_{i,DIS} \neq 0$. Even if $\alpha_{DIS}(\omega)$ does not vanish, it may be a taxing experimental problem to detect, for a given signal-to-noise ratio in attenuation measurements, a contribution $\alpha_{DIS}(\omega) << \alpha(\omega)$ due to the dissipative structure, when the equilibrium-structure contribution is that of a high-loss fluid. Irrespective of the attenuation coefficient per unit volume, the concentration of the dissipative subsystem(s) will typically be small, compared to that of the high-loss equilibrium system. As a result, several factors conspire (see also, Section 3.4) to undo the parallelism between the attenuation function and the biological response functions, a connection which is roughly valid for the equilibrium system. Detailed physical models, which are requisite to predict the magnitudes of $\alpha_{DIS}(\omega)$ and $\beta_{i,DIS}(\omega)$, and hence establish their relationship, do not exist as yet. Finally, it must be recognized that the status of the dissipative system, with respect to chemical events (steady-state concentrations and kinetics of various

biochemical reactions) and the energy states of the membrane system (biopolymers, structural H_2O and ions), will, in general,
change as temporal structures in cell growth and development occur.
As a result, while the attenuation function and the biological
response functions for the equilibrium system are time-independent,
$\alpha_{DIS}(\omega)$ and $\beta_{i,DIS}(\omega)$ will be a function of biochemical kinetic
processes in the dissipative subsystem(s).

   The Fröhlich Vibrational Model. As an elaboration of an
earlier hypothesis (125) concerning the existence of a branch of
polar vibrational modes in biopolymers and/or regions of the biological membrane, Fröhlich has constructed a formal theory (70-71,
126-137) for the distribution of photons for such a system in the
presence of energy input from the thermal bath. If the absorption
and emission of photons from a system containing a set of vibrational modes k, is associated with non-linear, coupled photon
transitions, an excitation of the lowest mode analogous to a
Bose-condensation (138) results. Such excitations would have important consequences for the establishment of selective interactions among the chemical species partaking of biochemical processes. For the purpose of this discussion, the treatment has
consequences for the spectroscopic functions and provides one
avenue toward discussing the biological response functions. It
was thought originally that the low-frequency vibrations of biopolymers (Section 2.6) (90-91) played a direct role in such excitations (139). Subsequently (92), such vibrations were shown to
be associated with intermolecular vibrations of the biopolymers
and not to persist in aqueous solution. It would appear from this
that (random) thermal energy (as available from non-reactive, and
hence, chemically non-specific collisions) supplied to biopolymeric systems is not sufficient to cause the Bose-condensation
type of excitation. In fact, in a formal sense, the Fröhlich
model contains similar conditions to those required for oscillatory chemical reactions, i.e. (chemical) pumping and non-linear
interaction terms (110-111). These, and the additional requirement for oscillatory chemical reactions, reaction(s) subject to
feedback, do not obtain for biopolymers or membranes in a purely
chemically-nonreactive collisional environment, but are appropriate to the in vivo biological membrane. Although this feature is
not explicitly incorporated into the Fröhlich vibrational model,
oscillatory, limit-cycle behavior has been invoked (136-137) to
account for the extremely narrow frequency selectivity of experimental biological response function reported for cell growth rate,
Section 3.3 below.
   The Fröhlich vibrational model does not address itself directly to the problem of the interaction between an external EM-field
and the dissipative subsystem, but rather to the internal redistribution of photons and phonons upon excitation of the Bose-
condensation state. In particular, the frequencies, ω_k, of the
(coherent) vibrations are availalbe only within the framework of a

heuristic estimate. Selection rules for photon-induced transitions due to an external EM field are not attainable from the
model in any facile manner, since the description of the vibrational states and the non-linear interactions is purely formal.
Furthermore, if the experimental data on cell growth rates (Section 3.3) are an accurate guide, the extremely narrow frequency-
dependence of the biological-response functions $\beta_{i,DIS}(\omega)$ is to be
understood in terms of oscillatory, limit-cycle mechanisms. Nonetheless, the model provides an incisive formal insight into what
may, in detail, be subsystems of great complexity and subtlety.

Fröhlich considers a set of polarization waves, of frequen-
cies $\omega_1 < \omega_2 \ldots < \omega_j \ldots < \omega_k \ldots < \omega_z$, in interaction with a thermal bath,
and in the presence of energy being supplied from the latter at a
rate $S_k = dE_k/dt$ to the k modes, Fig. (6). The number of photons,
n_k, in each one of the vibrational modes of the system, is associated with vibrational states $v_k = 0,1,2..$, for the molecular
subsystem in the k'th mode. The distribution of the total number
of photons, $N = \sum_k n_k$, will depend on the nature of the photon
exchange among the k vibrational modes of the subsystem and the
thermal bath. If the exchange of photons, associated with vibrational transitions $v_k \to v_k \pm 1$, of the subsystem with the equilibrium
system (the thermal bath) involves only independent, first-order
processes, the rate equations for the time derivatives of the number of quanta in each mode, n_k, are given by:

$$\dot{n}_{k,1} = S_k - \phi_k \left[n_k e^{(\hbar\omega_k/kT)} - (n_k + 1) \right]$$

$$k = 1,2,3,\ldots z, \tag{13}$$

where the ϕ_k are the transition probabilities for exchanges of
single quanta, $\hbar\omega_k$, between the subsystem and the equilibrium system. If, in addition to first-order processes, described by Eq.
(13), there exist second-order processes $[v_k \to v_k \pm 1; v_j \to v_j \pm 1]$ which
are non-linearly connected, the rate equations for the number of
photons in each mode k become:

$$\begin{cases} \dot{n}_k = S_k - \phi_k [n_k e^{(\hbar\omega_k/kT)} - (n_k + 1)] \\[6pt] \quad -\sum_{j \neq k} \chi_{jk} [n_k(n_j+1) e^{(\hbar\omega_k/kT)} - (n_k+1) n_j e^{(\hbar\omega_j/kT)}] \\[6pt] \quad -\sum_{j \neq k} \lambda_{jk} [n_k n_j e^{[\hbar(\omega_k + \omega_j)/kT]} - (n_k+1)(n_j+1)] \\[6pt] k = 1,2,3,\ldots z \end{cases} \tag{14}$$

Here, χ_{jk} and λ_{jk} are transition probabilities for the non-linear
exchange of two quanta, $\hbar\omega_k$ and $\hbar\omega_j$, between the subsystem and the
equilibrium system, which is the source of the energy inputs, per
unit time, S_k. After a steady state has been reached in the exchange of photons between the subsystem and the equilibrium system,

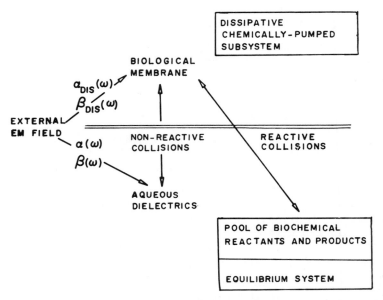

Figure 5. Schematic of an external EM field interaction with the equilibrium system and the dissipative subsystem. $\alpha(\omega)$ and $\beta(\omega)$ are the attenuation function and the biological-response function for the equilibrium system, respectively; $\alpha_{DIS}(\omega)$ and $\beta_{DIS}(\omega)$ are the same functions, respectively, for the dissipative subsystem; ω is the frequency of the EM field.

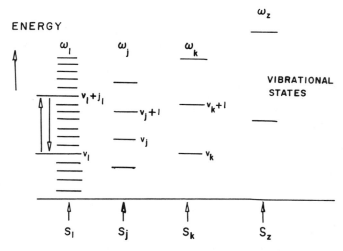

Figure 6. Vibrational states and representative photon-induced transitions for the set of vibrations $\omega_1, \omega_2 \ldots \omega_k, \ldots \omega_z$ in the Fröhlich vibrational model.

v_k *is the vibrational quantum number of the k'th mode, ω_k its frequency, and S_k the rate of the (chemically pumped) energy transfer into the modes k of the dissipative subsystem by the surroundings.*

$\dot{n}_k=0$, for each vibrational mode k. Neglecting the dependence of the transition probabilities on the modes (j,k) and summing over all k in Eq. (14), one obtains:

$$\sum_k S_k = \sum_k [n_k e^{(\hbar\omega_k/kT)} - (n_k+1)][\phi + \lambda \sum_j (n_j e^{(\hbar\omega_j/kT)} + (n_j+1)] \quad (15)$$

The total number of photons in the k modes of the subsystem is given by:

$$\sum_k n_k = N \quad (16)$$

Eqs. (14)-(16) permit a formal solution (70,71,136-137) of the coupled differential equations, Eq. (14), for the number of photons, n_k, at steady state conditions, in the modes k:

$$n_k = 1 + \frac{S_k}{[\phi + \chi \sum_j (n_j e^{(\hbar\omega_j/kT)}) + \lambda \sum_j (n_j+1)]} [e^{(\hbar\omega_k+\mu)/kT} -1]^{-1} \quad (17)$$

Here, μ is a quantity dependent on the magnitude of the non-linear coefficients χ and λ, Eq. (14), on the details of the distributions n_j, and independent of the terms S_k, as follows:

$$[1-e^{-(\mu/kT)}] = (\chi-\lambda)\frac{\sum_j [n_j e^{(\hbar\omega_j/kT)} - (n_j + 1)]}{[\phi + \chi \sum_j n_j e^{(\hbar\omega_j/kT)} + \lambda \sum_j (n_j+1)]} \quad (18)$$

For $(\chi - \lambda)=0$, as in the absence of non-linear terms $(\chi=\lambda=0)$, the pumped modes k acquire a Planck-type distribution, $\mu=0$, modified only by the term S_k, and consistent with the set of rate equations, Eq. (13),

$$n_{k,1} = \{1 + \frac{S_k}{\phi}\} [e^{(\hbar\omega_k/kT} -1]^{-1} \quad (19)$$

Thus, even in the presence of pumping, of energy S_k, from the thermal bath into the modes k, a Planck-type distribution of photons over the modes k, and hence a Boltzmann-type distribution of molecular systems over vibrational states $(v_1,v_2...v_j,..v_k,..v_z)$ results from linear systems.

In contrast, for a non-linear system, $(\chi-\lambda)>0$, $\mu>0$, the distribution, Eq. (17) differs in a salient fashion from the modified Planck distribution, Eq. (19). For a somewhat more specialized model, $\lambda<<\chi$, Eqs. (17) and (15) reduce to:

$$n_k = \{1+S_k \frac{(\phi)}{\sum_j S_j} \frac{1}{\chi} (1-e^{-(\mu/kT)})\}[e^{(\hbar\omega_k-\mu)/kT} -1]^{-1} \quad (20)$$

and

$$\sum_k S_k = \phi \sum_k [n_k e^{(\hbar\omega_k/kT)} - (n_k + 1)] \quad (21)$$

Since $n_k > 0$, Eq. (20) and the definition of μ in Eq. (18) require:

$$\hbar\omega_1 > \mu \geq 0 \tag{22}$$

where ω_1 is the frequency of the lowest vibrational mode, v_1. As a result of Eqs. (20), (21), and (22), the total number of photons in all the k vibrational states of the subsystem is given by the upper limit:

$$N = \sum_{k=1}^{z} n_k \leq \{1 + S_m \frac{(\phi)}{\overline{\Sigma S_j}} [1 - e^{-(\hbar\omega_1/kT)}]\} \sum_{k=1}^{z} [e^{[(\hbar\omega_k - \mu)/kT]} - 1]^{-1} \tag{23}$$

where S_m is the largest of the terms S_k. Eq. (23) must be consistent with the implication of Eq. (21) that the total number of photons in the subsystem increases proportionally to ΣS_k. This obtainsonly if μ in the sum on the rhs of Eq. (23) closely approaches $\hbar\omega_1$, such that the number of photons in state 1, of lowest frequency ω_1, becomes much larger than any other number n_k, as energy pumping, $S = \Sigma S_k$, increases. This condensation of the photons into the lowest-frequency state is formally equivalent to the Bose condensation (138), and μ, Eq. (18), plays a role analogous to the chemical potential in the Einstein condensation of a Bose-Einstein gas.

A fundamental prediction of the Fröhlich model then is that in subsystems which exchange photons with a thermal bath, in the nonlinear manner given by the set of Eqs. (14) and quantified by the magnitude of μ in Eq. (18), a condensation of photons into the lowest-frequency vibration occurs as the rate of energy pumping from the thermal bath increases above a threshold value, S_0:

$$n_1 >> n_{k \neq 1}, \quad S > S_0 \tag{24}$$

Condensation of the photons into the lowest vibrational state of the subsystem has implications concerning the distribution of molecular systems over the vibrational states, and hence will affect the contribution to the spectroscopic functions due to these vibrations. This aspect will be discussed in Section 3.4. Fröhlich has given a heuristic estimate of the frequency domain in which polarization waves in a system of dimension x will be supported as an elastic deformation of velocity v, $v \sim (c/x)$, $\omega = 2\pi v$ (70, 71, 136-137). Although different types of biological membranes show marked differences in dimensions (77, 78, 119-124), and a single parameter is clearly insufficient for an accurate description, $x \sim 10^{-6}$ cm. If v is taken to be 10^5 cm sec^{-1}, 100 GHz is the order of magnitude of v expected for such processes. The threshhold value, S_0, for onset of the Bose condensation has been estimated theoretically (140-141) to be of the order of $\sim 10^{-2}$ mWcm^{-2}; however, it is important to recall that S refers to the energy coupling between the thermal bath and the subsystem, and extrapolation to the effect of other perturbations, e.g. external EM fields, may not be rigorous.

If we now suggest a correspondence between the formal model of Fröhlich and the dissipative subsytem(s) and the equilibrium system discussed in Section 3.1, one may consider the processes which are operative, including interactions with an external EM field, as depicted schematically in Fig. (7). No compelling experimental evidence exists that the equilibrium system made up of the ordinary aqueous dielectrics, Sections 2.3 to 2.7, shows the Bose-condensation which arises in the Fröhlich theory. In fact, even systems of sufficient complexity to exhibit low-lying vibrational modes and structural subtlety to play a direct role in biochemical reactions at the interface between biochemical and biological processes [α-chymotrypsin (90-91), lysozyme (92) and DNA (93)], fail to show features not predicted by the methods of Section 2. Since collisional perturbations, even when non-reactive, will provide a source of the energy inputs, S_k, this implies the absence of non-linear terms ($\chi=0, \lambda=0$), Eq. (14), for such systems.

In contrast, it is not unexpected that dissipative structures in the sense of (106) which are linked by a set of biochemical reactions, and characterized by chemically-pumped steady states, rather than being connected only by non-reactive collisions, may exhibit the non-linear behavior of coupled photon-exchange processes requisite for the Bose-condensation. Interconnected photon exchange, with the non-linear effects in Eq. (14), has a physical basis in the behavior of dissipative structures although, as Fröhlich suggest (136), specific molecular subsystems with large non-linear terms in Eq. (14) may be the result of highly specialized biochemical-biological selection. Dissipative structures may be connected with subsystems showing non-linear photon exchange with the equilibrium system in a general fashion, but the magnitude of the non-linear terms may depend crucially on the nature of the molecular systems involved.

Occurence of the Bose-condensation, Eq. (24), into the vibrational mode v_1, implies vibrational excitation of the system into states $v_1 = 1, 2, \ldots$ While the intensity of absorption-emission lines gives information only about the difference in the number of molecules per cm^3 in the upper and lower states connected by the photon, the intensities of Raman lines, in elastic light scattering at frequencies $(\omega_0 \pm \omega_{mn})$, permit determination of the ratio of the number of molecules per cm^3 in the excited state n and the lower state m. This ratio is given by (142):

$$(N_n/N_m) = [I(\omega_0 + \omega_{mn})/I(\omega_0 - \omega_{mn})] \, (\omega_0 - \omega_{mn})^{-4} \, (\omega_0 + \omega_{mn})^{-4} \quad (25)$$

where $I(\omega_0 + \omega_{mn})$ and $I(\omega_0 - \omega_{mn})$ are the integrated intensities of the anti-Stokes and Stokes lines, respectively. Since the Bose condensation, Eq. (24), implies a ratio N_n/N_m larger than

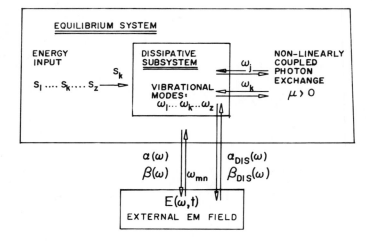

Figure 7. Formal representation of the interaction of an external EM field with the dissipative subsystem in the Fröhlich vibrational model (μ is the nonlinear coupling parameter (Equation 17); the other quantities have the same meaning as in Figures 5 and 6)

in the case of a Boltzmann-type distribution of molecular systems over states,

$$(N_n/N_m)_B = [\exp -(\hbar\omega_{mn}/\underline{k}T], \tag{26}$$

experimental evidence for a ratio N_n/N_m in excess of the
Boltzmann ratio, Eq. (26), would provide confirmatory evidence
of an excitation of the type predicted by Eq. (24). Measurements
of the intensities in the region ~ 100 cm^{-1} for active cells of
E. coli B (143,144) have reported excitation in excess of the
Boltzmann ratio, and that the relevant frequencies ω_{mn} are a
function of temporal changes (of the order of tens of minutes)
in the cells. Corroborative experiments on this and similar
systems would be of considerable interest. Since the Boltzmann
ratio, Eq. (26), tends toward unity as $(\hbar\omega_{mn}/\underline{k}T) \ll 1$, determinations of the experimental ratio, via Eq. (25), are the more con-
vincing, given a finite error in the measurement of relative
Raman intensities in aqueous systems (92), the higher the
frequency, ω_{mn}.

Biological Response Functions. As argued in Section 3.1,
energy absorption from an external EM field coupling to an equilibrium system, and hence closely related to the bulk attenuation
function, $\alpha(\omega)$, is not expected to show frequency-selective effects of a pronounced sort, since the bulk attenuation function
of ordinary aqueous dielectrics is not expected per se to show
such features. Furthermore, although the biological response
to the temperature rise caused by absorption of EM radiation in
the bulk system will not be linear over an extended range of ΔT,
a rough correspondence between $\alpha(\omega)$ and biological response functions, $\beta_i(\omega)$, should obtain.
The excitation of a Bose-type condensation as predicted by
Fröhlich (Section 3.2), and the existence of dissipative structures in the more general sense of Section 3.1, provide for the
possibility of effects for which the considerations of Section 2
no longer hold. While strongly frequency-selective features are
not expected for either $\alpha(\omega)$ or $\beta_i(\omega)$, quasi-resonant interactions with external harmonic perturbations of the dynamical
variable(s) of non-linear, dissipative subsystems are possible
(112-115). Such interactions might then manifest themselves in
a quasi-resonant, frequency-selective (frequency-response width
<<response frequency) interaction with a global biological end-
point, e.g. cell growth rate, if the dynamical variables of
linked biochemical reactions couple with the external EM field.
Although such effects are possible even with systems involving
very simple molecular species (110-116), one may speculate that,
in the case of certain types of biochemical systems, which involve, among other interactions, conformational changes in biopolymers during the chemical reaction, the frequency regime for
such effects may lie in the millimeter-wave and far-infrared

region. Similar conclusions inhere, of course, in the Fröhlich model (70-71,136-137).

As with the accurate measurement of the attenuation function, severe experimental difficulties are associated with reliable measurements of biological response functions, even for simple cellular systems, in the millimeter-wave region. The most completely documented study to date (145-147) provides a foundation for an experimental field as yet in its infancy, and places earlier work (148-156) into clearer perspective. A highly frequency-selective bimodal distribution (rate decreases and rate increases) is reported for the growth rate of yeast cells of type Saccharomyces cerevisiae for EM-fields in the 41-42 GHz range, at power levels ∿1 mWcm^{-2}. Since cell growth rate is measured simultaneously, in a crossed-beam experiment utilizing light scattering in the thermostated, stirred solution, standing-wave artifacts should be efficiently suppressed. Owing to the extreme narrowness of the response width (∿10 MHz), spectroscopic resolution (∿5 MHz) of the cavity-controlled BWO and frequency measurement are perhaps the experimental parameters most susceptible to further improvement. In particular, the accuracy of the overall biological statistics would be increased if resolution in the frequency domain were improved by an order of magnitude or more. Frequency-stabilization techniques for broad-band sources in the millimeter-wave region have been described (157-159), and the attainable spectroscopic resolution (γ 10^2 kHz) will make such experimental refinements possible. Simultaneous improvement in the biological statistics of the growth rate, at fixed frequency, and the more fine-grained data for the overall biological statistics afforded by improvements in spectroscopic resolution [FM-ing of source (short-term and long-term)<<frequency response width] are a primary research objective.

The extreme narrowness of the biological-response function suggested by these experimental studies has, at present, no quantitative theoretical explanation, although limit-cycle behavior has been invoked (135-137). In fact, earlier, low-resolution studies (150-153) had appeared to be consistent with transitions (presumably involving biopolymeric systems) collision-broadened by the structural H$_2$O, with linewidths thus expected to be of the order of the inverse of the relaxation time for structural H$_2$O, ∿0.3 GHz. The much narrower response width found in (145-147) implies experimentally that collision-broadening concepts (Section 2) are invalid, even in a qualitative sense, as a model for this type of EM-field interaction. It is of interest to note that the artifactual effects of short-term and long-term FM-ing on a frequency-selective bimodal distribution are more complex than the simpler artifactual broadening of a line in ordinary spectroscopy. For a source signal, with a given amount of short-term FM-ing, which drifts in a random manner over the frequency range in which the bimodal distribution occurs, average distribution patterns for the growth-rate function (which requires monitoring for time of the order of hours) will depend on the temporal details of the drift pattern. Frequency stabilization appears not to have been employed in the earlier studies (148-155). Assuming that experimental refinements of the type suggested above will not erase the validity of the current findings (i.e. compromise, rather than improve the credibility of the overall biological statistics), even the purely phenomenological cataloguing of the frequencies of the extrema of the biological response functions for a given system would provide a set of biophysical parameters of considerable interest. While no detailed theoretical models exist at present to analyze (let alone, predict) these frequencies, they may carry fine-grained information on biophysical and biochemical processes in in vivo cellular systems. In fact, Fröhlich has suggested (136-137) that, owing to the possibility that evolutionary processes have played a dominant role in selecting the molecular systems which show the Bose-condensation, vibrations connected with that mechanism may be pervasive in many types of biological tissue, not only simple cellular entities.

The connection between the vibrational frequencies reported in the Raman spectra of in vivo cellular systems (143,144) and the frequencies associated with the extrema in the biological response functions (145-156) is not understood in any detail. From the experimental point of view, it should be noted that the resolution of millimeter-wave spectroscopy (with phase-locked frequency stabilization) is far superior to that of ordinary Raman spectroscopy. It remains to be established whether the large linewidths found in the Raman spectra of in vivo cellular systems (143,144) ($\sim$10 cm^{-1} for the lines near $\overline{120 \text{ cm}^{-1}}$, and $\sim$20 cm^{-1} for the lower-frequency lines) are due, in part, to the limited resolution of Raman spectroscopy and inaccuracies introduced by procedures which subtract the background of the strong (rotational-anisotropy) scattering of H_2O near the Rayleigh line (92), or whether they accurately represent the actual linewidth. The detailed nature and extent of collision broadening for the system showing the Bose-condensation is not known. In addition, it is possible that more than a single frequency contributes to the spectra of such systems, and a complex overlapping line-spectrum may result, even in the absence of collisional broadening. More generally, a serious impediment to the firm establishment of a correspondence between the low-frequency Raman transitions and the characteristic frequencies of biological response functions at millimeter wavelengths is the accelerating decrease in the accuracy of the Raman spectra of aqueous systems as $(\omega_0 \pm \omega_{mn})$ approaches the Rayleigh line, ω_0, for $\omega_{mn} \underset{\sim}{<} 10$ cm^{-1} ($\underset{\sim}{>} 300$ GHz).

The Attenuation Function. In contrast to the existing experimental evidence which would suggest that the biological response fucntions $\beta_{i,DIS}(\omega)$ may have sharply frequency-selective features at millimeter wavelengths (145-147), $\sim$1 cm^{-1}, and that the Raman lines of in vivo cellular systems are consistent with a Bose-condensation predicted by the Fröhlich model, at far-infrared wavelengths, $\sim$100 cm^{-1}, (143,144), firm experimental data on the attenuation function $\alpha_{DIS}(\omega)$ do not yet exist, in any frequency region of interest. In consequence, there are no substantive experimental guides toward relating $\alpha_{DIS}(\omega)$ and $\beta_{i,DIS}(\omega)$. It has already been cautioned in Section 3.1 that the parallelism between these functions, operative for the equilibrium-system being perturbed by an external EM-field, may not persist for the dissipative subsystem. We shall attempt here to examine the more detailed implications of the Bose-condensation predicted by Fröhlich on those contributions to $\alpha_{DIS}(\omega)$ which are associated with photon-induced transitions, among the vibrational states $(v_1, v_2, \ldots v_k \ldots v_z)$, excited by an external EM-field.

The integrated intensity of a spectroscopic transition, associated with the absorption and emission of a photon ω_{mn}, is given by:

$$\alpha_{mn} = (8\pi^3/3hc)(N_m - N_n)\omega_{mn}|\mu_{mn}|^2 \qquad (2\,7)$$

Here, N_m and N_n are the number of molecular species per cm^3 in the lower and the higher energy state, respectively, and $|\mu_{mn}|$ is the dipole-moment matrix element for the transition. While the distribution of molecules over the states m and n affects the Raman intensities in the manner given by Eq. (25), the intensities of absorption-emission lines go as Eq. (2 7). A general vibrational transition between two states of the system described in Section 3 2 is characterized by the initial and final states, $(v_1, v_2, \ldots v_j, \ldots v_k \ldots v_z)$=m, and $(v_1+j_1, v_2+j_2, \ldots v_j+j_j, \ldots v_k +j_k, \ldots v_z+j_z)$=n, with: $j_k = \pm 1, \pm 2, \ldots$ Which of the transitions m↔n have a non-vanishing dipole-moment matrix element depends on the variation of the potential energy, $V(Q_1, Q_2, \ldots Q_j, \ldots Q_k, \ldots Q_z)$, and vibrational normal coordinates (Q_k) which describe the vibrational distortion of the system. In a formal fashion, one may expand V and μ in a Taylor series about the equilibrium position $(Q_1 = Q_2 = \ldots Q_j = \ldots Q_k = \ldots Q_z) = 0$: (160):

$$V(Q) = V(0) + \sum_k (\partial V/\partial Q_k)_0 + \tfrac{1}{2} \sum_j \sum_k (\partial^2 V \partial Q_j \partial Q_k)_0 + \cdots \qquad (2\,8)$$

and

$$\mu_s(Q) = \mu_s(0) + \sum_k (\partial \mu_s/\partial Q_k)_0 + \tfrac{1}{2} \sum_j \sum_k \partial^2 \mu_s (\partial Q_j \partial Q_k)_0 + \cdots \qquad (29)$$

s = x,y,z

If only the first derivatives in the dipole-moment function and the second derivatives (k=j) in the potential function are retained, the strict harmonic-oscillator-linear-dipole-moment approximation, the selection rules are strict:

$\Delta v_k = (v_k + j_k) = \pm 1$, $\Delta v_j = (v_j + j_j) = 0$, $j \neq k$. A photon-induced transition via an external field occurs only for a given fundamental frequency, for $\omega = \omega_k$, between adjacent vibrational states, v_k and $(v_k \pm 1)$. Non-vanishing terms, to higher order in Eq. (28), mechanical anharmonicity, and non-linear terms in the dipole-moment function, Eq. (29), lead to breakdown in these strict selection rules, and frequencies other than the set, $\omega_{mn} = \omega_1, \omega_2$, $\omega_j \cdots \omega_k \cdots \omega_z$, become observable in the dipole-allowed spectrum. For systems of the complexity envisaged in the Fröhlich model, biopolymers and/or portions of the membrane, the magnitude of the terms in Eqs. (28) and (29) is difficult to ascertain, and non-vanishing higher-order terms are not unexpected. Even if the set of vibrations is mechanically uncoupled (161), i.e. terms of the form $[\partial^2 V(Q)/\partial Q_k \partial Q_j] = 0$, $k \neq j$, non-linear terms in μ make the related photon-induced transitions non-vanishing. The Raman intensities, Eq. (25), can be expressed in a similar fashion in terms of the derivatives of the components of the polarizability tensor, α_{tt}, t=x,y,z with respect to the vibrational coordinates:

$$I(\omega_0 \pm \omega_{mn}) = (64\pi^4/3hc^3) (\omega_0 \pm \omega_{mn})^4 |P_{mn}|^2 \tag{30}$$

$$\alpha_{tt}(Q) = \alpha_{tt}(0) + \sum_k (\partial \alpha_{tt}/\partial Q_k)_0 + \tfrac{1}{2} \sum_j \sum_k (\partial^2 \alpha_{tt}/\partial Q_j \partial Q_k)_0 + \ldots \tag{31}$$

Analogous arguments apply in this case, the strict harmonic-oscillator-linear-polarizability approximation limiting the non-vanishing intensities to: $\omega_{mn} = \omega_k$, i.e. inelastic scattering of a fundamental quantum $\hbar\omega_k$. As in the photon-induced absorption-emission spectrum, even for vanishing mechanical coupling among the k vibrations, non-linear terms in Eq. (31) will permit non-zero intensities for transitions, ω_{mn} other than the fundamental frequencies ω_k. In the limit of nearly harmonic vibrations for each of the k normal modes, i.e. all terms in Eq. (28) beyond the second-derivatives (k=j) zero, the frequencies ω_{mn} in Eqs. (27) and (30), are the harmonics: $\omega_{mn} = j_k \omega_k$, $j_k = 1,2,3,\ldots$

A detailed analysis (165) of the spectroscopic properties, under certain restrictive conditions (linear dipole-moment, harmonic-oscillator approximation for a non-interacting set of z normal modes), of the Fröhlich model provides the following results. The terms $\alpha(\Delta v_k = j_k)$, the intensities integrated over all possible transitions $v_k \leftrightarrow v_k \pm j_k$, are invariant with the number of photons in the mode ω_k, $n(\omega_k)$, Eq. (20), hence provide no information concerning the onset of the Bose condensation, and preclude facile assignment of the frequencies ω_k. This prediction is borne out by the negative results (44,166) obtained in a careful search for quasi-resonant features in the attenuation function of biological fluids in the millimeter-wave region. The terms, $[I(\omega_0 + \omega_k j_k)/I(\omega_0 - \omega_k j_k)]$, Eq. (25), while dependent on the form of $n(\omega_k)$, are insensitive to the value of j_k, in the low-frequency limit, $n(\omega_k) \ll 1$. In contrast, a single emissivity term, $\varepsilon(\omega_1)$, is predicted to exhibit behavior saliently different from all the others, $\varepsilon(\omega_1 j_1)$, $j \neq 1$ and $\varepsilon(\omega_j j_k)$, $k \neq 1$, each of the latter being essentially blackbody terms, $\varepsilon(\omega) \cong 1$. Thus, in spite of the experimental problems concerning the determination of the photon and phonon emissivity, this experimental variable would appear to provide the most direct route to the quantification of the Fröhlich model. In general, direct photon or phonon spectroscopic determinations of millimeter-wave and far-infrared properties of in vivo biological systems possess the not inconsiderable advantage of providing biophysical information at the molecular-systems level, while global biological endpoints (e.g. cell growth rate) are, by their very nature, integrative effects, not currently susceptible of complete analysis.

While the effects on infrared and Raman intensities of general systems due to non-Planckian redistributions (non-Boltzmann distribution for molecular systems) of photons with vibrational excitation have been assessed (165), the exact details of the present problem are considerably more complex, depending on the parameters of the Fröhlich model (S_k, ϕ_k, and μ). However, in a rough manner, the foregoing analysis points to the possibility that the pragmatically desirable protocol, i.e. establishment of frequencies $\alpha_{DIS}(\omega)$ from measurements of the total attenuation function $\alpha_{TOT}(\omega)$, Eq. (11), and subsequent determination of biological-response functions $\alpha_{i,DIS}(\omega)$ at such frequencies, may not be feasible in a general way. This is to say that a one-to-one correspondence between measurable contributions to the attenuation function and the frequencies for extrema in the $\beta_{i,DIS}(\omega)$ may not always obtain, a complication not found in interactions between the equilibrium system and the EM field. Even for vibrational modes with finite absorption coefficients the low concentration of the dissipative systems and the limitations in accuracy of swept-frequency measurements in determining relative attenuation (perhaps no better than 0.2 dB in a typical average value of tens of dB for aqueous systems and appropriate pathlengths) conspire to make difficult direct measurements of $\alpha_{DIS}(\omega)$. As a result, the parallel between features (attainable by standard dielectric measurements) in the total attenuation function and the biological-response functions is no longer as strong a corollary of general energy-coupling mechanisms as it is for interactions with the equilibrium system, Section 2.

The preceeding discussion has dealt with the qualitative effects of the Bose-condensation on the attenuation function, $\alpha_{DIS}(\omega)$. In general, we require the frequencies ω_{mn} and matrix elements $|\mu_{mn}|$ and $|p_{mn}|$, for all the possible transitions, $m \leftrightarrow n$, among the vibrational states postulated by Fröhlich, in order to characterize the resulting absorption spectra, Eq. (27), Raman spectra, Eq. (30), and the phonon spectra. As indicated in the above, the formal theory does not provide a complete guide to either of these quantities. In fact, it is not known whether the vibrational modes ω_k in the model involve portions of the biological membrane or (portions of) biopolymeric systems. Qualitatively, a relationship between the unperturbed low-frequency vibrational modes of biopolymers, ω_k^0, (Section 2.6) and the vibrational modes involving the Bose-condensation may exist. In this sense, the frequency range predicted for the quasi-lattice vibrations of biopolymers (79-89), $\sim$1-100 cm^{-1} ($\sim$30-3000 GHz), may be thought of as the frequency regime in which EM-field interactions with the dissipative system are most likely to occur. In a formal way, one may think of the frequencies of the unperturbed system as generating the phonon vibrational modes in situ of the membrane environment. Characterization of the non-linear coefficients (χ, λ) and quantification of the frequencies and spectroscopic assignments will require articulation of detailed features of the dissipative subsystem.

Conclusions.

We have attempted to trace fundamental characteristics of the interaction between biological systems and EM fields, with an overview with respect to well-established phenomena and a sharper focus on more recent experimental and theoretical studies, which appear to require the application of new concenpts and promise the expansion of biophysical information attainable by experiment. On this basis, an assessment is offered of research objectives which may prove to be promising as advances beyond the present state of the art.

(i) Because of the dominant role played by the attenuation due to free H_2O in the millimeter-wave and far-infrared spectra of biological systems, measurements of the attenuation function $\alpha(\omega)$ for $H_2O(\ell)$ in the region above 50 GHz are of considerable interest, to complement recent measurements (42-44). Although techniques of highest accuracy, in the millimeter-wave region, will presumably involve impedance-matched, single-frequency measurements and require demanding mechanical precision, the accuracy of existing broad-band techniques at millimeter wavelengths and in the far-infrared may be capable of improvement. Nevertheless, it is expected that precision measurements of $\alpha(\omega)$ for $H_2O(\ell)$ will be required to determine, in connection with (ii) below, the contribution of structural H_2O to $\alpha(\omega)$ or $\kappa^*(\omega)$.

(ii) In order to quantify the contribution to $\alpha(\omega)$ or $\kappa^*(\omega)$ of structural H_2O in biological systems, and further test the hypothesis of Grant (48-50) concerning the attenuation functions of structural H_2O and free H_2O, accurate measurements for well-defined tissues of known structural H_2O content, of $\kappa^*(\omega)$ in the region $\sim$1-10 GHz would be of interest. One of the problems in the analysis of structural H_2O in biological systems in general (45,46 51-58) is that different physical methods give different assessments of the equilibrium concentration, and, in particular, of the rotational mobility of structural H_2O in the same system. Accurate determination, via (i) and (ii) of the dielectric increment due to structural H_2O might help to elucidate this question. A fundamental advantage of the dielectric-relaxation method is, of course, that it probes directly in the time domain of the rotational relaxation process, in contrast to nuclear magnetic resonance measurements.

(iii)   While the dielectric increment due to structural H_2O is, in itself, of basic interest, more germane to the question of EM-field interactions with biological systems are the consequences of initial energy coupling to structural H_2O. As an intermediate case, which may mimic aspects of biological systems, the effect EM-field interaction in the frequency region implicated by Grant (49,50) on the equilibrium structure and structural dynamics of biopolymers should be examined. While the status of a biopolymer in vitro is expected (Section 3) to differ from the actual biological environment, such experiments may serve as a guide.

(iv)   In order to analyze experiments of type (iii), other than in a purely phenomenological fashion, the model sketched in Section 2.4 requires quantification.

(v)   The effects of EM fields in the region ∿1-5 GHz on systems containing membranes interacting with structural H_2O have begun to be examined (64,168). In these experiments, as well as those suggested in (iii), it is necessary to differentiate between effects due to increase in the thermal energy of the entire membrane environment (including the free H_2O) and any effects more directly associated with the structural H_2O. Deviations from a parallelism between the extent of structural alterations of the membrane and the bulk attenuation function would imply the intervention of the structural H_2O, especially if such deviations concur with the dielectric increment due to structural H_2O. As a result, measurements over a range of frequencies, at constant E_0, would provide the most convincing protocol. Measurements of this type, particularly with model systems which closely mimic the biological membrane, are of continuing interest.

(vi)   A general question in dielectric theory, and one related to the problem of the rotational relaxation of molecular species in situ of the membrane field, is the effect of a large static electric field, $E_{intr}(0)$, on the behavior of $\kappa^*(\omega)$ for relaxation absorption, Eq. (4). Although theoretical treatments exist for saturation effects on the permittivity of fluid dielectrics, a general treament for $\kappa^*(\omega)$ for membrane systems does not appear to be available (169).

(vii)   A phenomenon related to (vi) is the effect of the membrane electrostatic field on the vibrational states of bipolymeric systems. Splitting of degeneracies of vibrational states and perturbation of the normal-mode frequencies ω_k^0 are possible. In addition, distortion of the molecular charge distribution in a large static field, $E_{intr}(0)$, Eq. (9), may alter the coefficients in Eqs. (29) and (31), which determine the infrared and Raman transition probabilities. Estimates of these effects would provide an approach to the analysis of the altera-

tion of the vibrational spectrum of biopolymers (Section 2.6)
in situ of the membrane intrinsic field.
(viii) Application of the general formalism (112–116) of
frequency-dependent perturbations on systems containing oscillatory chemical reactions may provide an avenue toward the analysis of the extremely narrow, quasi-resonant behavior of the biological-response function reported in in vivo cellular systems
(145–147). It is not clear at present what the physical and biochemical prerequisites for non-vanishing terms, Eq. (18), in the
Fröhlich model, are, except that they must reflect non-linear
interactions between the subsystem, capable of the vibrations
$(\omega_1, \omega_2, \ldots \omega_z)$ in the frequency regime $\sim$1–100 cm^{-1}, and the thermal
bath. If the thermal bath interacts with the subsystem in terms
of linked, oscillatory biochemical reactions, containing feedback loops, behavior of biological-response functions in the
manner of (145–147), as well as the Bose-condensation, might be
predictable in terms of a common physical model (111).
(ix) As already indicated in Section 3.3, corroboration of
the measurements (145–147) of the effect of low-level EM fields
at millimeter wavelengths on cellular growth rate, with increased
spectroscopic resolution and long-term frequency stability (157–
159), is of crucial interest. The credibility of the overall biological statistics would be enhanced by an improvement in the
frequency domain with such an experimental protocol. In particular, experimental points in the frequency regions well within
the extrema of the cellular-growth response function would increase the confidence in the biological statistics. If the
extreme narrowness of the frequency dependence of biological-
response functions in the millimeter-wave range reported in (145–
147) is characteristic of such behavior, the methods of high-
resolution millimeter-wave spectroscopy (157–159, 167) will be
required for the analysis of such systems rather than those of
ordinary dielectric-measurement methodology. The latter places
less stringent requirements on short-term and long-term FM-ing
of the source, as well as on frequency measurement, since $\kappa^*(\omega)$
for ordinary molecular fluids is not expected to show resonant
behavior at these frequencies.
(x) Corroboration and extension of the Raman-spectroscopic
measurements on in vivo cellualr systems (143, 144) is clearly
of interest. Such measurements would provide direct evidence for
the existence of the Bose-condensation predicted in the Fröhlich
model, in the case of cellular systems (167). Fröhlich has postulated (136–137) that the Bose-condensation may be a pervasive
phenomenon, existing not only in cellular systems but in biological tissue in general. One possible source of experimental
artifacts in measurements of this type is the Rayleigh scattering
from the inhomogeneous suspensions that make up cellular and/or
tissue preparations. For an accurate assessment of Raman lines
with $\omega_{mn} \lesssim 20$ cm^{-1}, the methods of (92) may, in addition, be required.

(xi) As discussed in Section 3.4, the connection between
the frequencies implicated in those cases where non-Boltzmann
excitation is suggested by experiment (143,144), $\omega_{mn} \sim 100$ cm^{-1},
and those associated with reported quasi-resonant behavior in
cellular growth rate (145-147), $\omega_{mn} \sim 1$ cm^{-1}, is not understood in
any detail at present. In order to examine any such connection,
one might measure the intensities of the Raman-active transitions
(x) as a function of perturbation by millimeter-wave EM fields.
Changes in the intensity of the Raman-active lines with non-
Boltzmann intensities, as a function of the frequency of the
millimeter-wave EM field, would indicate an interference in the
status of the Bose-condensation by the EM field. Techniques
similar to those employed in (64) could be adapted to this purpose. If the Bose-condensation plays the direct role in cellular
regulatory function envisaged by Frohlich (135-137), then EM-
field perturbations, at low level, at the associated frequencies
would be of particular importance in the understanding of cellular
regulatory function. In fact, such measurements might eventually
make possible diagnostic and/or therapeutic applications of
millimeter-wave EM-fields.

(xii) Measurements of the type suggested in (iii) would
give an assessment of changes in the conformational structure
and equilibria of biopolymers induced by EM fields in the range
which is thought to involve an initial absorption step into the
rotational relaxation of structural H_2O. While such effects are
possible even for in vitro systems, it is of interest to inquire
whether initial energy uptake by the structural H_2O leads, owing
to its interaction with in vivo biopolymeric systems, to a perturbation of the vibrational modes ω_k, and , in particular, the
status of the Bose-condensation. The requisite experiment is
the monitoring of the intensity of the Raman-active transition,
ω_1, as a function of low-level EM-field irradiation in the range
~ 1-10 GHz, in a crossed-beam experiment analogous to the monitoring of the membrane Raman modes (64).

(xiii) Initial absorption by structural H_2O may also, in
principle, affect the frequency-dependence of biological-response
functions at millimeter wavelengths, by interfering in the conformation equilibria and dynamics of the biopolymers which are
associated with the dissipative subsystem. It would be of interest to examine the frequency dependence of biological response
functions, along the lines in (ix), coupled by low-level irradiation by an EM-field in the ~ 1-10 GHz range, as a function of frequency. While the experiments proposed in (iii) relate to biopolymers in a chemically non-reactive, equilibrium environment,
those in (xii) and (xiii) address themselves to the biopolymeric
system as a component of the dissipative subsystem in vivo.

(xiv) As discussed in some detail in Section 3.4, several
circumstances conspire to make difficult the extraction of the
contribution to the total attenuation function of $\alpha_{DIS}(\omega)$ by conventional attenuation measurements, even if the transition pro-

babilities are non-vanishing. This is an unfavorable situation since the other parameters which give access to the characteristic frequencies, i.e. the biological-response functions, typically require a large set of point-by-point measurements, as a function of frequency, and thus are extraordinarily cumbersome as a search technique for the relevant frequency regions. In fact, the converse protocol would, of course, be the most desirable: location of the characteristic frequencies by spectroscopic measurements, and subsequent determination of the parameters $\beta_{i,DIS}(\omega)$ in the freuqncy ranges indicated. While extraction of the small contribution $\alpha_{DIS}(\omega)$ for in vivo cellular systems at millimeter wavelengths may be vitiated by the experimental signal-to-noise ratio in swept-frequency measurements of $\alpha_{TOT}(\omega)$, this goal might be achievable by using modulation techniques which preferentially perturbthe dissipative system and do not substantially alter the equilibrium system. If the detection system for the attenuation measurement is frequency-tuned and phase-locked to a harmonic perturbation of the dissipative system, extraction of $\alpha_{DIS}(\omega)$ may become feasible (167).

(xv) The highly detailed fine-structure in the frequency dependence of the growth-rate function for cellular systems (145-147) is not assignable, within the formal framework of existing theory. A guide toward phenomenological assignments of possibly interconnected processes associated with extrema in $\beta_{i,DIS}(\omega)$ would be provided by the use of double-resonance or multiple-resonance measurements, i.e. measurement of $\beta_{i,DIS}(\omega)$ with an EM-field at one of the characteristic frequencies of the fine-structure, and, in the case of double resonance, a second EM-field varied across the entire frequency range of interest. If corroborated, these highly frequency-dependent biological endpoints could provide deep insights into the dynamics of the dissipative biochemical subsystems, and provide an avenue toward the understanding of the biophysics of cell regulatory function.

LITERATURE CITED

1. For an incisive review of the general problem, see: Van Vleck, J.H. and Huber, D.L. Rev. Mod. Phys. 1977, 49, 939.

2. Van Vleck, J.H. and Weisskopf, V.F. Rev. Mod. Phys. 1945, 17, 227.

3. Van Vleck, J.H. and Margenau, H. Phys. Rev. 1949, 76, 1211.

4. Fröhlich, H. Nature 1946, 157, 478.

5. Fröhlich, H. "Theory of Dielectrics"; Oxford University Press: London, 1949; p. 173.

6.   Karplus, R.; Schwinger, J. Phys. Rev. 1948, 73, 1020.
7.   Debye, P. "Polar Molecules": Chemical Catalog Co., New York,
     1929, Chap. 5.
8.   Trindle, C.O.; Illinger, K.H. J. Chem. Phys. 1967, 46, 3429.
9.   Hill, N.E.; Vaughan, W.E.; Price, A.H.; Davies, M. "Dielec-
     tric Properties and Molecular Behavior   Van Nostrand-
     Reinhold, London, 1969.
10. Grant, E.H.; Sheppard, R.J.; South, G.P. "Dielectric Behavior
     of Biological Molecules in Solution": Oxford, England:
     Clarendon, 1978.
11. Cole, R.H. Progr. in Dielectrics 1961, 3, 47.
12. Illinger, K.H. Progr. in Dielectrics 1962, 4, 37.
13. Margenau H.; Lewis, M. Rev. Mod. Phys. 1959, 31, 569.
14. Illinger, K.H. "Interaction between Microwave and Millimeter-
     Wave Electromagnetic Fields and Biological Systems: Molecular
     Mechanisms", in "Biological Effects and Health Hazards of
     Microwave Radiation", Proc. Intern. Symposium, Czerski, P. et.
     al., Eds. (Polish Medical Publishers Warsaw, 1974) p. 160.
15. Illinger, K.H. "Millimeter-Wave and Far-Infrared Absorption
     in Biological Systems", in "The Physical Basis of Electro-
     magnetic Interactions with Biological Systems", Proceedings
     of a Workshop Univ. of Maryland, Taylor, L.S; Cheung, A.Y.
     Eds., June 1977, p. 43.
16. See also, Ref. (12), p. 88.
17. Goulon, J.; Rivail, J.L.; Fleming, J.W.; Chamberlain, J.;
     Chantry, G.W. Chem. Phys. Lett. 1973, 18, 211.
18. Chamberlain, J.; Asfar, M.N.; Davies, G.H.; Hasted, J.B.;
     Zafar, M.S. IEEE Trans. MTT-22, 1974, 1028.
19. Asfar, M.N.; Hasted, J.B.; Zafar, M.S.; Chamberlain, J. Chem.
     Phys. Lett. 1975, 36, 69.
20. Asfar, M.N.; Chamberlain, J.; Chantry, G.W. IEEE Trans. IM-25
     1976, 290.
21. Asfar, M.N.; Hasted, J.B.; Chamberlain, J. Infrared Phys.
     1976, 16, 301.
22. Asfar, M.N.; Honijk, D.D.; Passchier, W.F.; Goulon, G. IEEE
     Trans. MTT-25, 1977, 505.
23. Asfar, M.N.; Hasted, J.B. J. Opt. Soc. Am. 1977, 67, 902.
24. Webb, S.J.; Booth, A.D. Nature 1969, 222, 1199.
25. Webb, S.J.; Booth, A.D. Science 1971, 174, 72.
26. Stamm, M.E.; Winters, W.D.; Morton, D.L.; Warren, S.L.
     Oncology 1974, 29, 294.
27. Havriliak, S.; Negami, S. J. Polym. Sci. Part C 1966, 14, 99.
28. Schwan, H.P. in "Advances in Biological and Medical Physics",
     Vol. V, Lawrence, J.H.; Tobias, C.A. Eds. Academic Press,
     New York, 1957, p. 147.
29. See also, Shore J.E.; Zwanzig, R. J. Chem. Phys. 1975, 63,
     5445.
30. Illinger, K.H., in "Biological Effects of Electromagnetic
     Waves", Compilation of Selected Papers, 1975 Annual Meeting
     USNC/URSI, HEW Publication (FDA) 77-8011, p. 169.

31. Calderwood, J.H.; Coffey, W.T.; Morita, A.; Walker, S. Proc. Roy. Soc. Lond. 1976, A352, 275.

32. Evans, G.J.; Evans, M.W.; Calderwood, J.H.; Coffey, W.T.; Wedgam, G.H. Chem. Phys. Lett. 1977, 50, 142.

33. Schwan, H.P., in "The Physical Basis of Electromagnetic Interactions with Biological Systems", Proceedings of a Workshop, Univ. of Maryland, Taylor, L.S.; Cheung, A.Y. Eds., June, 1977, p. 91.

34. Schwan, H.P.; Foster, K.R. Proc.IEEE 1980, 68, 104.

35. Pardoe, G.W.F.; Gebbie, H.A. in Symposium on Submillimeter Waves, Polytechnic Institute of Brooklyn, 1970, p. 643.

36. Hasted, J.B., in Franks, F., Ed., "Water. A Comprehensive Treatise": Plenum Press, New York, 1972, Vol. I, Chap. 7.

37. Walrafen, G.E. ibid. Vol. I, Chap. 5.

38. Hasted, J.B. ibid., Vol. II, Chap. 7.

39. Pottel, R. ibid., Vol. III, Chap. 6.

40. Hasted, J.B. "Aqueous Dielectrics": Chapman and Hall, London, 1973, Chap. 2.

41. Schwan, H.P.; Sheppard, R.J.; Grant, E.H. J. Chem. Phys. 1976, 64, 2257.

42. Asfar, M.N.; Hasted, J.B. J. Opt. Soc. Am. 1977, 67, 902.

43. Grant, E.H. Abstracts of Scientific Papers, 1977 International Symposium on the Biological Effects of Electromagnetic Waves, USNC/URSI, 1977, p. 27.

44. Ghandi, O.P.; Hill, D.W.; Partlow, L.M.;Johnson, C.C.; Stensaas, L.J. ibid., p. 26.

45. Cooke, R.; Kuntz, I.D. Ann. Rev. Biophys. Bioeng. 1974, 3 95.

46. Berendsen, H.J.C. in Franks, F. Ed., "Water. A Comprehensive Treatise": Plenum Press, New York, 1972, Vol. V., Chap. 6.

47. Rahman, A.; Stillinger, F.H. J. Chem. Phys. 1971, 55, 3336.

48. Grant, E.H.; Mitton, B.G.R.; South, G.P.; Sheppard, R.J. Biochem. J. 1974, 139, 375.

49. Grant, E.H.; Sheppard, R.J.; South, G.P. Proc. 5th European Microwave Conference, Hamburg, 1975, p. 366.

50. Grant, E.H. in "The Physical Basis of Electromagnetic Inter-Actions with Biological Systems", Proceedings of a Workshop, Univ. of Maryland, Taylor, L.S.; Cheung, A.Y. Eds., June 1977, p. 113.

51. Schwan, H.P.; Foster, K.R. Biophysical J. 1977, 17, 193.

52. Beall, P.T.; Hazelwood, C.F.; Rao, P.N. Science 1976, 192, 904.

53. Brownstein, K.R.; Tarr, C.E. Science, 1976, 194, 213.

54. Foster, K.R.; Resing, H.A.; Garroway, A.N. Science, 1976, 194, 324.

55. Chang, D.C.; Woessner, W.E. Science, 1977, 198, 1180.

56. Resing, H.A.; Foster, K.R.; Garroway, A.N. Science 1977, 198, 1182.

57. Wilkinson, D.A.; Morowitz, H.J.; Prestegard, J.H. Biophys. J. 1977, 20, 169.
58. Packer, K.J. Phil. Trans. R. Soc. Lond., 1977, B278, 59.
59. Webb, S.J. Ann. New York Acad. Sci. 1975, 247, 327.
60. Zimm, B.H.; Bragg, J.K. J. Chem. Phys. 1959, 31, 526.
61. Engel, J.; Schwarz, G. Angew. Chem. Int. Ed. 1970, 9, 389.
62. Schwarz, G. in "Functional Linkage in Biomolecular Systems" Schmitt, F.O.; Schneider, D.M.; Crothers, D.M. Eds.; Raven Press, New York, 1975, p. 32.
63. Schwarz, G. Ann. New York Acad. Sci. 1977, 303. 190.
64. Sheridan, J.P.; Priest, R.; Schoen, P.; Schnur, J.M. in "The Physical Basis of Electromagnetic Interactions with Biological Systems", Proceedings of a Workshop, Univ. of Maryland, Taylor, L.S.; Cheung, A.Y. Eds., June 1977, p. 145.
65. Ehrenstein, G.; Lecar, H. Ann. Rev. Biophys. Bioeng. 1972, 1, 347.
66. Taylor, R.E. Ann. Rev. Phys. Chem. 1974, 25, 387.
67. Armstrong, C.M. Quart. Rev. 1974, 7, 179.
68. McLaughlin S.; Eisenberg, M. Ann. Rev. Biophys. Bioeng. 1975, 4, 335.
69. Ehrenstein, G. Phys. Today 1976, 29, 33.
70. Fröhlich, H. Proc. Nat. Acad. Sci. 1975, 72, 4211.
71. Fröhlich, H. Revista del Nuovo Cim. 1977, 7, 399.
72. Fuller-Brown, W. "Dielectrics", Handbuch der Physik 17, 1, Flügge, S. Ed., Springer Verlag, Berlin, 1956.
73. Böttcher, C.J.F. "The Theory of Dielectric Polarisation", 2nd Ed., Vol. 1, Elsevier, Amsterdam, 1973 .
74. Coffey, W.T.; Scaife, B.K.P. Proc. Roy. Irish Acad. 1976, 76A, 195.
75. McConnell, H.M. in "Functional Linkage in Biomolecular Systems:, Schmitt, F.O.; Schneider, D.M.; Crothers, D.M. Eds., Raven Press, New York, 1975, p. 123.
76. Nicolson, G.L. ibid., p. 137.
77. Singer, S.J. ibid., p. 103.
78. Singer, S.J.; Nicolson, G.L. Science 1972, 175, 720.
79. Abe, Y.; Krimm, S. Biopolymers 1972, 11, 1817.
80. Fanconi, B.; Peticolas, W.L. Biopolymers, 1971, 10, 2223.
81. Fanconi, B. J. Chem. Phys. 1972, 57, 2109.
82. Fanconi, B. Ann. Rev. Phys. Chem. 1980, 31, 265.
83. Itoh, K.; Shimanouchi, T. Biopolymers 1970, 9, 383.
84. Prohofsky, E.W. in "The Physical Basis of Electromagnetic Interactions with Biological Systems", Proceedings of a Workshop, Univ. of Maryland, Taylor, L.S.; Cheung. A.Y., Eds., June 1977, p. 133.
85. Prohofsky, E.W. Phys. Lett. 1977, 63A, 179.
86. Eyster, J.M.; Prohofsky, E.W. Phys. Rev. Lett. 1977, 38, 371
87. Eyster, J.M.; Prohofsky, E.W. Biopolymers 1977, 16, 965.
88. Prohofsky, E.W.; Eyster, J.M. Phys. Lett. 1974, 50A, 329.
89. Perahia, D.; Jhon, M.S.; Pullman, B. Biochem. Biophys.Acta 1977, 47, 349.

90. Brown, K.G.; Erfurth, S.C.; Small, E.W.; Peticolas, W.L.
     Proc. Nat. Acad. Sci. 1972, 69, 1467.
91. Peticolas, W.L. Ann. Rev. Phys. Chem. 1972, 23, 93.
92. Genzel, L.; Keilmann, F.; Martin, T.P.; Winterling, G.;
     Yacoby, Y.; Fröhlich, H.; Makinen, M.W. Biopolymers 1976,
     15, 219.
93. Swicord, M.L. Abstracts, Second Annual Meeting, Bioelectro-
     magnetics Society, San Antonio, TX, 14-18 September 1980,
     Abstract 56.
94. Weissberger, A.; Rossiter, B.W. "Physical Methods of Organic
     Chemistry. Part IIIB, Vol. I": Wiley-Interscience, 1972,
     p. 112.
95. Davies, M.; Maurell, D.; Price, A.H. Trans. Faraday Soc.
     1972, 67, 1041.
96. Kritikos, H.N.; Schwan, H.P. IEEE Trans. BME-19, 1972, 53.
97. Masszi, G.; Szijarto, Z.; Grof, P. Acta Biochim. Biophys.
     Acad. Sci. Hung. 1976, 11, 129.
98. Lin, J.C. IEEE Trans. BME-22 1975, 74.
99. England, T.S. Nature 1950, 166, 480.
100. Herrick, J.F.; Jelatis, D.G.; Lee, G.M. Fed. Proc. 1950, 9,
     60.
101. Stuchly, M.A.; Stuchly, S.S.; Gajda, G; Brady, M.M. Abstracts
     Second Annual Meeting, Bioelectromagnetics Society, San
     Antonio, TX, 14-18 September 1980, Abstract 90.
102. Burdette, E.C.; Seals, J.; Toler, J.C.; Cain, R.L.; Magin,
     R.L. IEEE MTT-S International Microwave Symposium Digest,
     1977, 344.
103. Huber, D.L.; Van Vleck, J.H. Rev. Mod. Phys. 1966, 38, 187.
104. Prigogine, I. "Introduction to the Theory of Irreversible
     Processes": New York, Interscience, 1967, 3rd. Ed.
105. Glansdorff, P.; Prigogine, I. "Thermodynamic Theory of
     Structure, Stability and Fluctuations": Interscience-Wiley,
     New York, 1971.
106. "Membranes, Dissipative Structures, and Evolution", Nicolis,
     G.; Lefever, R. Eds., Adv. Chem. Physics 1975, 29, 1-374.
107. Strandberg, M.W.P. J. Theor. Biol. 1976, 58, 33.
108. Blumenthal, R.; Changeux, J.P.; Lefever, R. J. Membrane
     Biol. 1970, 2, 351.
109. Ortoleva, P.; Ross, J. in ref.(106), p. 49.
110. Noyes, R.M.; Field, R.J. Ann. Rev. Phys. Chem. 1974, 25, 95.
111. See also: Kaiser, Fr. Z. Naturforsch. 1979, 34a, 134.
112. Ortoleva, P.; Ross, J. J. Chem. Phys. 1971, 55, 4378.
113. Gilbert, R.; Hahn, H.; Ortoleva, P.; Ross, J. J. Chem. Phys.
     1973, 57, 2672.
114. Ortoleva, P.; Gilbert, R.; Ross, J. J.Chem.Phys. 1973, 58,
     3625.
115. Nitzan, A.; Ross, J. J.Chem. Phys. 1974, 60, 3134.
116. Showalter, K.; Noyes, R.M.; Turner, H. J. Am. Chem. Soc. 1979,
     101, 7463.
117. Kaczmarek, L.K. Biophys. Chem. 1976, 4, 249.

118. Kaiser, Fr. Phys. Lett. 1977, 62A, 63.
119. Jain, M.K. "The Bimolecular Lipid Membrane": Van Nostrand-Reinhold, 1972.
120. Weissmann, G.; Claiborn, R.; Eds., "Cell Membranes": HP Publishing Co.., New York, 1975.
121. Bretscher, M.S. ; Raff, M.C. Nature 1975, 258, 43.
122. Quinn, P.J. "The Molecular Biology of Cell Membranes": University Park Press, Baltimore, 1976.
123. Rothmann, J.E.; Lennard, J. Science 1977, 195, 743.
124. Abrahamsson, S.; Pascher, I. "Structure of Biological Membranes", Nobel Foundation Symposium 1977, 34 (Nobel Foundation Symposium Series).
125. Fröhlich, H. Intern J. Quantum Chem. 1968, 2, 641.
126. Livshits, M.A. Biofizika 1972, 17, 726.
127. Wu, T.M.; Austin, S. Phys. Lett. 1977, 64A, 151.
128. Wu, T.M.; Austin, S. Phys. Lett. 1978, 65A, 74.
129. Kollias, N.; Melander, W.R. Phys. Lett. 1976, 57A, 102.
130. Vermiglio, G.; Tripepi, M.G. Phys. Lett. 1977, 60A, 263.
131. Cooper, M.S. Phys. Lett. 1978, 65A, 71.
132. Fröhlich, H. Phys. Lett. 1968, 26A, 402.
133. Fröhlich, H. Phys. Lett. 1972, 39A, 153.
134. Fröhlich, H. Phys. Lett. 1975, 51A, 21.
135. See also, Genzel, L. Phys. Lett. 1978, 65A, 371.
136. Fröhlich, H. IEEE Trans. MTT-S, Special Issue on Microwaves in Medicine, with Accent on the Application of Electromagnetics to Cancer Control", 1978.
137. Fröhlich, H. "Advances in Electronics and Electron Physics", Vol. 53 85 (Academic Press, New York, 1980).
138. For a general discussion, see: ter Haar, D. "Elements of Statistical Mechanics": Rinehart and Co., New York, 1954, p. 209 ff.
139. Fröhlich, H. Phys. Lett 1973, 44A, 385.
140. Bhaumik, D.; Bhaumik, K.; Dutta-Roy, B. Phys. Lett. 1976, 56A 145; 1976, 59A, 77.
141. Bhaumik, D.; Bhaumik, K,; Dutta-Roy, B.; Engineer, M.H. Phys. Lett. 1977, 62A, 197.
142. Placzek, G. Z. Physik 1931, 70, 84.
143. Webb, S.J.; Stoneham, M.E.; Fröhlich, H. Phys. Lett. 1977, 63A, 407.
144. Webb, S.J.; Stoneham, M.E. Phys. Lett. 1977, 60A, 267.
145. Grundler, W.; Keilmann,F.; Fröhlich, H. Phys. Lett 1977, 62A, 463.
146. Grundler, W.; Keilmann, F. Z. Naturforsch. C (in press).
147. Keilmann, F. Proceedings of NATO Advanced STudy Institute "Coherence Spectroscopy and Modern Physics", Versilia, 1977.
148. Webb, S.J.; Dodds, D.E. Nature 1968, 218, 74.
149. Webb, S.J.; Booth, A.D. Nature 1969, 222, 199.
150. Devyatkov, N.D. Sov. Phys. - Uspekhi (Translation) 1974, 16, 568.
151. Sevast'yanova L.A.; Vilenskaya, R.D. ibid, 1974, 16, 570.

152. Smolyanskaya, A.Z.; Vilenskaya, V.L. ibid., 1974, 16, 571.
153. Kirelev, R.I.; Zalynvoskaya, N.P. ibid., 1973, 15, 464.
154. Blackman, C.F.; Benane, S.G.; Weil, C.M.; Ali, J.S. Ann. New York Acad. Sci. 1974, 247, 352.
155. Bertaud, A.J.; Dardalhon, M.; Rebeyrotte, N.; Averbeck, D. Compt. Rend. Acad. Sci. (D) (Paris)1975, 281, 843.
156. See also: Webb, S.J. Physics Reports 1980, 60, 202.
157. Hines, M.E.; Collinet, R.J.; Ondria, J.G. IEEE Trans MTT-16, 1968, 738.
158. Daprowski, J.; Smith, C.; Bernues, F.J. Microwave J. October 1976, p. 41.
159. Henry, R.S. Rev. Sci. Instrum. 1976, 47, 1020.
160. Herzberg, G. "Molecular Spectra and Molecular Structure. II. Infrared and Raman Spectra of Polyatomic Molecules": Van Nostrand, New York, 1945, p. 259.
161. See also, Ref. (71)(136).
162. Illinger, K.H.; Freeman, D.E. J. Molec. Spectrosc. 1962, 9, 191.
163. Rubin, R.J. ; Shuler, K.E. J. Chem. Phys. 1957, 26, 137.
164. Gordy, W.; Cooke, R.L. "Microwave Molecular Spectra": Interscience, New York, 1970.
165. Illinger, K.H. National Radio Science Meeting (USNC/URSI), June 1979, Seattle, Washington; Abstracts,p. 467.
166. Lee, R.A.; Hagmann, M.J.; Gandhi, O.P.; Tanaka, I.; Hill,D.W.; Partlow, L.M. National Radio Science Meeting (USNC/URSI), June 1979, Seattle, Washington; Abstract, p. 463.
167. For a further discussion of the experimental limitations attendant to both attenuation and Raman-spectroscopic measurements, see: Gandhi, O.P.; Athey, T.W.; Illinger, K.H.; Motzkin, S.; Partlow, L.M.; Sheridan, J.P. Proc. IEEE 68, Vol. 1, January 1980.
168. Allis, J.W.; Jinha, B.L. Abstracts, Second Annual Meeting, Bioelectromagnetics Society, San Antonio, TX, 14-18 September 1980, Abstract 126.
169. See also, Kasprowicz-Kielich B.; Kielich, S. Adv. Molec. Relaxation Processes 1975, 7, 275.

RECEIVED December 29, 1980.

MOLECULAR DYNAMICS IN AQUEOUS SOLUTION

Dielectric Properties of Water in the Microwave and Far-Infrared Regions

E. H. GRANT, S. SZWARNOWSKI, and R. J. SHEPPARD

Physics Department, Queen Elizabeth College, London, W8 7AH, U.K.

The dielectric behaviour of pure water has been the subject of study in numerous laboratories over the past fifty years. As a result there is a good understanding of how the complex permittivity $\hat{\epsilon} = \epsilon' - \jmath\epsilon''$ varies with frequency from DC up to a few tens of GHz and it is generally agreed that the dielectric dispersion in this range can be represented either by the Debye equation or by some function involving a small distribution of relaxation times. At these frequencies the variations of $\hat{\epsilon}$ with frequency are due to relaxation phenomena and may be described by equations appropriate to classical physics. In the far infrared and at higher frequencies resonance-type phenomena which can be accounted for on quantum principles, have been observed and well documented. Interest therefore lies in the frequency region between around 20–200GHz where measurements are sparse and, where they have been reported, relate to isolated frequencies and temperatures only. Prior to the commencement of the present work, the highest microwave frequency at which values of complex permittivity of water were available as a function of temperature was 35GHz ([1]). In the far infrared the principal work in existence was that of Asfar and Hasted ([2]) who measured the dielectric properties of water at 19–20°C in the frequency range 170GHz–13THz, using interferometric techniques. In the present investigation it was therefore decided to measure the complex permittivity of water at 70GHz over a range of temperatures in the hope that combining the 70GHz results with those previously obtained at higher and lower frequencies would enable a better understanding of the dielectric behaviour of water in this relatively unexplored frequency region, thus helping to fill the final gap in the knowledge of how the

0097-6156/81/0157-0047$05.00/0

dielectric properties of water vary with frequency from DC to
the visible region.   Determining the complex permittivity
of water at 70GHz poses problems in that the attenuation is
very high which, coupled with the small dimensions of the
waveguides, necessitates the taking of special precautions in
order to obtain high accuracy.

Experimental Procedure

The waveguide system used to measure the dielectric
parameters of water and other lossy liquids has been
described previously (3).   Basically it involves the
measurement of the power profile of a wave reflected from a
movable short circuit as it traverses the liquid under test.
The variation of the amplitude of the reflected wave with the
distance moved by the short circuit is related directly to the
complex permittivity of the liquid contained in the
experimental cell.   A computer program has been written to
evaluate ϵ' and ϵ'' from the measured amplitude variation.
In order to obtain high precision it is necessary to measure
the distances moved by the plunger very accurately and this
has been achieved by a worm drive and lever mechanism of
high mechanical stability which enables the plunger to be
located to a precision of 0.001mm.   Other important
requirements are good frequency stability, a high signal to
noise ratio and detector crystal characteristics which are
independent of power level.   All these features have been
incorporated into the present system (3).

Results and Discussion

The values measured for water at 70GHz at different
temperatures are shown in Table I.   Both ϵ' and ϵ'' are
seen to increase with increasing temperature, which is
typical behaviour for a pure polar liquid at frequencies well
in excess of the relaxation frequency.

In the first instance the data were combined with those
obtained by other workers at lower frequencies (4-15) and an
analysis was carried out.   The combined values of ϵ' and ϵ''
were fitted to a Cole-Cole dispersion relationship in order to
find the best value for α and ϵ_∞ at each temperature.   The
Cole-Cole dispersion equation is

$$\hat{\epsilon} = \epsilon_\infty + \frac{\epsilon_s - \epsilon_\infty}{1 + (j\omega\tau)^{1-\alpha}} \quad (1)$$

where ϵ_s is the static permittivity and τ is the dielectric

Table I.   The complex permittivity of water at 70GHz.
(The errors correspond to the 95% confidence intervals)

$T/^{\circ}C$	ϵ'	$\Delta\epsilon'$	ϵ''	$\Delta\epsilon''$
0.3	7.49_3	0.08	11.46_0	0.09
1.0	7.59_0	0.09	11.82_3	0.10
5.0	8.12_6	0.11	13.03_1	0.11
10.2	8.60_1	0.08	14.46_7	0.12
15.0	9.20_5	0.10	15.80_6	0.13
20.0	9.92_6	0.10	17.55_9	0.14
25.0	10.82_7	0.14	19.14_1	0.16
30.0	12.05_8	0.15	20.84_1	0.17
35.0	13.00_5	0.13	21.90_9	0.20
40.0	14.54_1	0.16	23.32_2	0.19
45.0	15.86_8	0.22	24.80_6	0.22
50.0	17.41_2	0.17	25.50_3	0.21

relaxation time at the appropriate temperature.   The parameter ϵ_∞ is the value of the permittivity to which ϵ' would be asymtotic at high frequencies in the <u>absence of further dispersion</u>.   As shown later in this paper this assumption does not hold for water and so in practice never appears as a plateau and its value is model-sensitive.   The parameter designated by α is a measure of any distribution of relaxation times which may exist, and for the case of a single relaxation time $\alpha = 0$ and equation (1) becomes the Debye equation.

The results of the fit are shown in Table I where it is seen that at most temperatures the 95% confidence limit for α overlaps zero and hence there is little deviation from single relaxation time behaviour according to this analysis.   Another inference is that the value of ϵ_∞ deduced from this procedure probably decreases with increasing temperature but the most important conclusion is that the relaxation time τ is not particularly sensitive to the model chosen, the values obtained agreeing to within experimental error irrespective of whether the value of α was allowed to be fitted as an unknown parameter, or whether it was clamped at zero (Debye case).

Table II therefore summarises the dielectric behaviour of water as evaluated from curve-fitting the measured permittivity data taken at frequencies up to 70GHz.   Extra information which emerges by consideration of the new 70GHz results alone will now be obtained by examining the variation with temperature of the function $F = (\epsilon_s - \epsilon') (\omega \epsilon'')^{-1}$.   If the dielectric behaviour of water at this frequency can be entirely accounted for by the Debye equation then F is equal to the relaxation time (τ).   If there is any departure from single relaxation time behaviour then $F \neq \tau$; for example if the experimental data at 70GHz could be described by a Cole-Cole relationship then F would equal $\tau + \omega^{-1}\alpha\left[\frac{\pi}{2} - \omega\tau \ln(\omega\tau)\right]$ as shown previously (16).   The values of F as calculated from the results in Table II are shown in Figure 1 together with the values of the relaxation time τ obtained from Table II, which are in agreement with the literature values of relaxation time. A clear departure from Debye behaviour is observed below room temperature i.e. the values of ϵ' and ϵ'' at 70GHz do not conform to a single Debye dispersion.   Therefore some other process must be involved which is operative at the high frequency end of the principal dispersion.   The discrepancy in Figure 1 cannot be accounted for by the proposition that the principal dispersion can be characterised by a distribution of

2. GRANT ET AL. *Dielectric Properties of Water* 51

Table II   Water permittivity data fitted to various models
(The errors correspond to the 95% confidence intervals)

T/°C	Debye τ/ps	$\Delta\tau$/ps	Cole-Cole τ/ps	$\Delta\tau$/ps	Debye ε_∞	$\Delta\varepsilon_\infty$	Cole-Cole ε_∞	$\Delta\varepsilon_\infty$	Cole-Cole α	$\Delta\alpha$
0	17.64	0.28	17.69	0.32	5.02	0.63	5.37	0.95	0.001	0.012
5	14.75	0.14	14.71	0.15	6.09	0.36	5.85	0.49	0.004	0.006
10	12.84	0.17	12.76	0.19	5.20	0.56	4.69	0.83	0.008	0.009
20	9.43	0.08	9.32	0.10	5.35	0.40	4.53	0.60	0.010	0.006
25	8.27	0.06	8.21	0.07	5.57	0.30	5.11	0.44	0.006	0.004
30	7.24	0.08	7.19	0.11	4.89	0.50	4.48	0.85	0.005	0.008
35	6.56	0.06	6.52	0.11	5.41	0.42	5.01	0.89	0.006	0.009
40	5.90	0.07	5.87	0.11	4.94	0.57	4.65	0.93	0.003	0.008
50	4.78	0.05	4.77	0.08	4.58	0.52	4.44	0.85	0.001	0.007

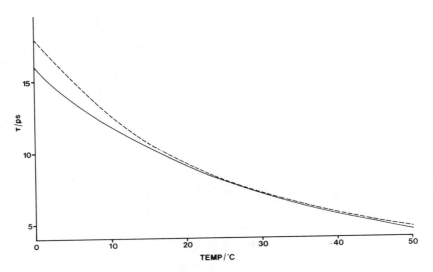

Figure 1.   Departure of τ from the literature values ((– – –) literature values of τ; (———) τ calculated from the present 70-GHz data using the Debye model)

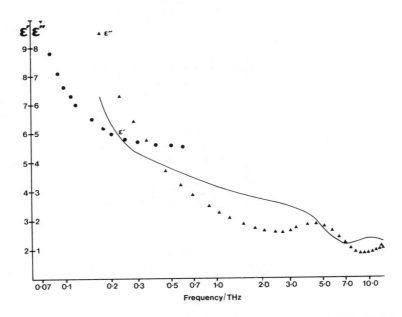

Figure 2.   Complex permittivity of water at frequencies above 70 GHz ((▼) from the present 70-GHz study; (⊙) ε' calculated from the Debye model using τ = 9.3 ps, ε_s = 80.1, and ε_∞ = 5.5; data of Asfar and Hasted (2): (———) ε'; (▲) ε'')

relaxation times.   The value of α required to account for the value of F at 0°C would be 0.06 which is far in excess of the value indicated in Table II.   The explanation must therefore lie elsewhere.

For a dispersion region having a relaxation mechanism underlying it a lowering in the temperature corresponds to a decrease in the relaxation frequency.   For water at 0°C the relaxation frequency is 9GHz, i.e. a factor of eight lower than the frequency of measurement in the present work.   Therefore measurements on water carried out at 70GHz at the lower temperatures correspond to points approaching the high frequency tail of the main dispersion region.   The presence of a small subsidiary dispersion in the far infrared could therefore affect the values of ϵ' and ϵ'' below room temperature without having any effect at higher temperatures.   This proposal will now be examined in further detail.

Dielectric dispersion in pure water in the far infrared

Reliable permittivity data at frequencies in excess of around 100GHz are rather sparse but one study that has been carried out is that due to Asfar and Hasted (2) where occur measurements at approximately 19°C.   Their values of ϵ' together with the present 70GHz point and values of ϵ' calculated by assuming a Debye type relaxation for the main dispersion are shown in Figure 2.   The ϵ'' data of Asfar and Hasted are also indicated in this Figure, and it may be seen that resonance absorption due to effects such as hindered translation begin to occur at around 2THz.   At frequencies below this, variations of ϵ' and ϵ'' are consistent with classical-type phenomena.

To determine the nature of the dispersion curve at frequencies between the main dispersion and resonance regions the data contained in references (4-15) at 20°C were combined with the 70GHz values and the permittivity results of Asfar and Hasted up to frequencies less than 2THz.   The combined data were then fitted to the equation

$$\hat{\epsilon} = n^2 + \frac{\epsilon_s - \epsilon_\infty}{1 + j\omega\tau_1} + \frac{\epsilon_\infty - n^2}{1 + j\omega\tau_2} \qquad (2)$$

which represents a sum of two Debye dispersion regions.   The lower frequency dispersion, which has a relaxation time τ_1 and a static permittivity ϵ_s, corresponds to the main dispersion region.   The higher frequency region has a low frequency permittivity of ϵ_∞ and a small amplitude of $\epsilon_\infty - n^2$.

Table III.   A two component fit to the microwave data and the
infrared data of Asfar and Hasted

Parameter	Value	95% Confidence Interval
ϵ_s	80.10_3	Parameter held constant
ϵ_∞	5.74	0.31
n^2	3.34	0.38
τ_1	9.48 ps	0.07 ps
τ_2	0.25 ps	0.08 ps

The high frequency limit of ϵ' for this second process is therefore n^2. The result of the fit is shown in Table III where the mean values of the various parameters and their associated 95% confidence intervals are given. Considering the small amplitude of the second dispersion both in absolute terms and in relation to the main dispersion the parameters ϵ_∞, n^2 and τ_2 are quite well defined, and therefore it may be concluded that the double Debye representation is an acceptable description of the dielectric behaviour of water up to around 2THz. Other alternative interpretations are clearly possible but no attempt has been made here to follow these up at this stage. What is clear is that a small subsidiary dispersion region in the far infrared is necessary to account for all the presently available permittivity data, and that such a dispersion is centred around 650GHz and has an amplitude of about 2.4 in comparison with that of the principal dispersion which is approximately 75.

Whether or not a relaxation phenomenon could exist at frequencies as high as hundreds of GHz could be a matter for discussion. However the inertia of the water molecule is fairly low and at 20°C a number of zero bonded and singly bonded molecules (which can rotate without surmounting an appreciable potential barrier) would be expected to exist on thermodynamical grounds in sufficient quantities to account for the small observed dispersion.

Literature Cited

1. Grant,E.H.; Shack,R.J. Brit.J.Appl.Phys.1976, 18, 1807
2. Asfar,N.M.; Hasted,J.B. J.Opt.Soc.Am. 1977, 67, 902
3. Szwarnowski,S.; Sheppard,R.J. J.Phys.E 1977. 10. 1163
4. Collie, C.H.; Hasted.J.B.; Ritson,D.M. Proc.Phys. Soc. 1948, 60, 145
5. Lane,J.A.; Saxton,J.A. Proc.Roy.Soc.A. 1952, 213,400
6. Cook,H.F. Brit.J.Appl.Phys. 1952, 3, 249
7. Hasted,J.B.; El Sabeh, S.H.M. Trans.Faraday Soc. 1953, 49, 1003
8. Buchanan,T.J.; Grant,E.H. Brit.J.Appl.Phys.1955,6,64
9. Grant,E.H.; Buchanan,T.J.; Cook,H.F. J.Chem.Phys. 1957, 26, 156
10. Sandus,O; Lubitz,B.B. J.Phys.Chem. 1961, 65, 881
11. Van Loon,R; Finsy,R. J.Phys.D. 1975, 8, 1232

12. Bottreau,A.M.; Marzat,C.; Lacroix ,Y., Dutuit,Y.
        J.Microwave Power 1975, 10, 297
13. Schwan,H.P.; Sheppard,R.J.; Grant,E.H.; J.Chem.Phys.
        1976, 64, 2257
14. Pottel, H. In Hasted,J.B., "Aqueous Dielectrics";
        Chapman & Hall: London 1973
15. Malmberg,C.G.; Maryott, A.A. J.Res.Natl.Bur.Stand.(U.S)
        1956, 56, 1
16. Grant,E.H. J.Phys.Chem. 1969, 73, 4386

RECEIVED December 1, 1980.

3

Dielectric Properties of Water in Myoglobin Solution

E. H. GRANT, N. R. V. NIGHTINGALE, and R. J. SHEPPARD
Physics Department, Queen Elizabeth College, London, W8 7AH, U.K.

S. R. GOUGH

Division of Chemistry, National Research Council of Canada,
Ottawa, Ontario, Canada, K1A OR9

Biological material has a high aqueous content and it is acknowledged that the physical properties of the water are different from those of pure liquid water.   This has given rise to the respective terms "bound" water and "free water" although, of course, the terms are purely relative.   The actual properties of the water in biological solution are however subject to controversy and there is still considerable disagreement about its nature.   One method of investigation is to determine the dielectric properties of an appropriate biological material over a frequency range from around 100 MHz or lower right up to high microwave frequencies, and in the present paper some recent measurements on myoglobin solutions are described. The determinations, which were made at $20°C$ on solutions of concentration 200 mg/ml, over a frequency range 0.6 - 15000 MHz represent the first stage of a comprehensive programme to measure the dielectric properties of water in solution.   Owing to the difficulty of measuring accurately the conductivity at the low frequency end of this range only the ϵ' values were used in the analysis.   Over the frequency range 0.6 to 100 MHz bridge apparatus was used;   the methods having been previously described (1,2).   At frequencies between 250 - 15000 MHz the permittivity determinations were made using coaxial line apparatus.   Between 250 - 4000 MHz methods were used which involve a coaxial line cell having a sliding inner conductor with a protruding probe which detects the electric field strength as a function of distance within the liquid sample.   The cell construction and the appropriate techniques of measurement have been described previously(3-6). In the overlapping range 1500-15000 MHz the results were obtained using a coaxial line cell terminated by a movable short circuiting plunger(7).

0097-6156/81/0157-0057$05.00/0
© 1981 American Chemical Society

The solutions were prepared at a concentration of 200mg/ml by dissolving sperm whale myoglobin (Miles Laboratories (PTY) Limited) in de-ionised water.   The samples were electro-dialysed before measurement to reduce the ionic conductivity. Full details of the solution preparation procedure have appeared previously (8).   The permittivity measurements were obtained at 20°C using sample cells thermostatically controlled to $\pm$ 0.1°C. The determinations were made at 45 frequencies and the mean value of ϵ' at each frequency is shown in Figure 1.

Interpretation of dielectric data on myoglobin solution

In order to analyse the results in Figure 1 it is necessary to make various assumptions about the nature of the processes involved at a molecular level.   Basically there are two types of polar molecule present - myoglobin and water - and there-fore a simple approach would be to represent the information by two dispersion regions.   Since, however, the water molecules adjacent to the macromolecules have dielectric properties different from those in the bulk of the fluid (1,9) a more realistic interpretation is to consider two separate dispersion regions for the water i.e. three dispersions in total. Further refinements would be possible by subdividing the water into more than two categories since it is an oversimplified picture to consider the water molecules as either rigidly bound to the myoglobin on the one hand, or in an identical state to those in pure water on the other.   From work carried out previously on myoglobin (8) at frequencies within the dispersion region of the myoglobin molecule it is known that this dispersion may not be characterised by a Debye dispersion, and therefore the present data were fitted to three relaxation regions consisting of a Cole-Cole dispersion to represent the myoglobin followed by two Debye dispersions to account for the water.   The Cole-Cole spread parameter for the myoglobin was found to be 0.15 $\pm$ 0.03;   the values of the relaxation time and dielectric increment are shown in Table I.

Table I. Dielectric increments and relaxation frequencies for the myoglobin solution

(Temperature 20°C; Concentration 200mg/ml; Errors are the 95% confidence intervals)

Dispersion	Dielectric increment (Δ)	Relaxation frequency/MHz (f_R)
β	34 $\pm$ 5%	2.2 $\pm$ 7%
δ	3.6 $\pm$ 11%	583 $\pm$ 22%
γ	59.0 $\pm$ 0.4%	14274 $\pm$ 1.6%

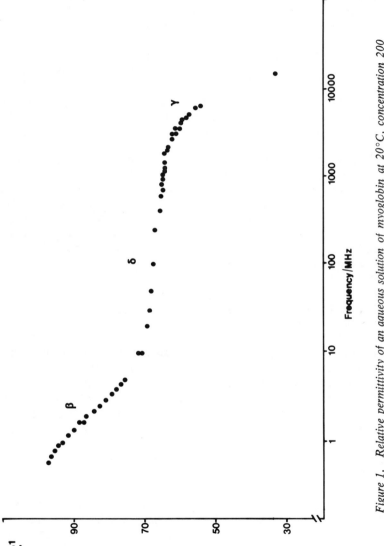

Figure 1. Relative permittivity of an aqueous solution of myoglobin at 20°C, concentration 200 mg/mL

Attempts made to fit two dispersions only failed on account of
the unacceptably high root mean square deviation.   In an
attempt to fit four dispersions it was found that the parameters
were highly correlated which means that although the possibility
of four dispersions is not precluded there is not sufficient
evidence from the present experiments to demonstrate their
existence.

The values of the parameters indicated for the β dispersion
(myoglobin) and δ dispersion (water immediately adjacent to the
myoglobin) are in good agreement with those concluded
previously from work carried out at frequencies between 0.2 -
1300 MHz (8,10). For the γ dispersion, however it is found
(Table I) that the relaxation frequency is significantly less than
the literature value for pure water of 16.7 ± 0.1 GHz which has
been verified in our laboratory (7) using the same apparatus
as that employed for the present myoglobin studies.   Moreover
this conclusion is not affected by the model used to represent
the data.   For example, if the δ and γ dispersions are each
represented by a Cole-Cole distribution the mean values of all
the parameters in Table I are unchanged to within experimental
error and the confidence intervals of the values of the Cole-Cole
spread parameter overlap zero in both cases.   The value of
in this case is now 14.2 ± 0.3 GHz as compared with 14.3 ± 0.2 GHz
in Table I and 16.7 ± 0.1 GHz for pure water.

Molecular interpretation of myoglobin solution data

Our results imply that very little of the bulk water
component of the solution has dielectric properties the same
as those of pure water.   On molecular grounds this appears
to be a reasonable conclusion.   For a 20% solution of
myoglobin the molecules would on average be separated by a
distance of around one molecular radius (~ 1.5 nm).   This
distance could be occupied by about five water molecules and
thus no water molecule would on average be further away from
a macromolecule than the third shell.   This lowering in
relaxation frequency of the bulk water component of a biological
solution from that of pure water is an established phenomenon
and was observed in the early 1950's by Cook (11,12) and by
Haggis, Hasted and Buchanan (13) although the rigour of the
conclusions was hampered by the presence of measurements at a
few frequencies only.   It is well known that organic solutes
in general modify the properties of bulk water.   For instance
an addition of 20% by weight of tetrohydrofuran to water
increases the water dielectric relaxation time by over 50% as a
result of structural modification of the hydrogen-bonded network

(14). It is not surprising that biological macromolecules impose a similar stabilizing effect. A similar proposal concerning the increasing of the water relaxation time was made recently by Masszi, Szuarto and Gaf (15) from conductivity measurements made on muscle tissue but in this case the highest frequency of measurement was 4GHz which is too low to provide unambiguous evidence in respect of the characteristics of the dispersion. Other work on muscle tissue carried out by Foster, Schepps and Schwan (16) at $1^{\circ}C$ came to the opposite conclusion, namely, that the bulk water relaxation frequency was not significantly different from that of pure water at that temperature. This is at variance with the present work although the differences in the temperature and in the material being studied may be at least part of the explanation of the apparent discrepancy.

The amount of tightly bound water (water of hydration) present in the myoglobin solution can be calculated from the amplitude of the δ dispersion using a method previously described (1,10). From the value of 3.6 for this parameter (Table I) a value of hydration of 0.15 ± 0.02 unit mass of water per unit mass of myoglobin is obtained. Considered as a volume fraction of the total water content this would amount to about 4%, which compares well with the figure of 5% recently proposed for muscle fibres by Foster, Schepps and Schwan (16).

Acknowledgements

We would like to thank the United States Office of Naval Research (Physiology Program Grant No. N00014-77-G-0075) for supporting NRVN and the National Research Council of Canada for the provision of sabbatical leave for SRG.

Literature Cited

1. Grant,E.H; Sheppard,R.J; South,G.P: "Dielectric behaviour of biological molecules in solution"; Oxford University Press, 1976.
2. Essex,C.G; South,G.P; Sheppard,R.J; Grant,E.H; J.Phys.E 1975, 8, 385
3. Grant,E.H; Keefe S.E. Rev.Sci.Instrum 1968, 39, 1800
4. Sheppard,R.J; J.Phys.D 1972, 5, 1576
5. Sheppard,R.J: Grant,E.H: J.Phys.E 1972, 5, 1208
6. Szwarnowski,S; Sheppard,R.J. J.Phys.E 1979, 12, 937
7. Nightingale,N.R.V; Szwarnowski,S; Sheppard,R.J; Grant,E.H; Submitted to J.Phys.E
8. South,G.P; Grant,E.H; Proc.R.Soc.Lond.A. 1972, 328,371

9.   Pennock, B.E; Schwan, H.P; J.Phys.Chem 1969, 73, 2600
10. Grant, E.H; Mitton, B.G.R; South, G.P; Sheppard, R.J.
                          Biochem J. 1974, 139, 375
11. Cook, H.F. Brit.J.Appl.Phys. 1951, 2,295
12. Cook, H.F. Brit.J.Appl.Phys. 1952, 3, 249
13. Haggis, G.H; Hasted, J.B; Buchanan, T.J. J.Chem.Phys.
                          1952, 20, 1452
14. Gough, S.R. J.Soln.Chem. 1978, 8, 371
15. Masszi, G; Szverto, A; Graf, P. Biophys.Acad.Sci.Hung.
                          1976, 129
16. Foster, K.R; Schepps, J.L; Schwan, H.P. Biophys.J.1980,
                                        29, 271

RECEIVED February 3, 1981.

4

Electrical Response of Polymers in Solution

ROBERT H. COLE

Chemistry Department, Brown University, Providence, RI 02912

The title of this paper, chosen for brevity, is both too short and too comprehensive. No attempt is made to give anything like a comprehensive survey of existing knowledge about biopolymer solutions, as excellent reviews can be found in the recent book by Grant, Sheppard, and South (1) and the earlier article by G. Schwarz (2). The preceding and following papers for this symposium, by Grant and by Schwan, also serve this purpose as well as presenting some newer developments, leaving the opportunity to discuss here some other recent developments which seem of present interest and future usefulness.

In conventional dielectric measurements, one observes the Maxwell polarization or electric moment density P(t) which is induced by an applied electric field E(t), and from this the complex permittivity ε^* as a function of frequency $f = \omega/2\pi$ of the field. For a system of charges e_i in volume V with displacement z_i in the field direction z, P is given by

$$P(t) = <\sum_i e_i z_i \rho(t)>/V \qquad (1)$$

where the angle brackets denote a macroscopic average with the distribution function $\rho(t)$ of displacements and momenta in the presence of E(t), and V is the volume of the system. In linear response theory, the effect of the applied field on the dynamics and $\rho(t)$ is obtained formally from the interaction energy $H_1(t)$ with the field, which with suitable caveats about internal field effects can be written for the dielectric case as

$$H_1(t) = \sum_i e_i z_i E(t) \qquad (2)$$

The evaluation for effects linear in E(t) leads to an expression for P(t) of the form (3,4,5),

$$P(t) = \frac{1}{kTV} \int_{-\infty}^{t} dt' \frac{dE(t')}{dt'} <(\sum_i e_i z_i(t'))(\sum_i e_i z_i(t-t')\rho_o> \qquad (3)$$

where the correlation function in the angle brackets is of displacements $z_i(t-t')$ evolving from $z_i(t')$ and averaged over the
equilibrium distribution ρ_o in the absence of the field.

For an applied field $E(t) = E\exp(i\omega t)$, the complex susceptibility $\chi^*(i\omega) = P(t)/E(t) = [\epsilon^*(i\omega) - 1)]/4\pi$ is expressed as

$$\chi^*(i\omega) = \frac{1}{kTV} L[-\dot{\Phi}(t)] \tag{4}$$

where L denotes the Laplace transform integral with variable
$s = i\omega$ and the dipole correlation function $\Phi(t)$ is given by

$$\Phi(t) = <(\textstyle\sum_i e_i z_i(o))(\textstyle\sum_i e_i z_i(t)\rho_o> \tag{5}$$

Equations (3) or (4), with refinements as necessary for
"local field" effects, are an appropriate and useful basis for
discussion of various models of non-conducting solutions of biological species considered in I. In many cases, however, solutions of interest have appreciable ionic concentrations in the
natural solvent medium and the polymer or other solute species
may also have net charges. Under these conditions, the electrical response is better considered in terms of the total current
density $J_t(t)$ defined and expressed by linear response theory as

$$\underline{J}_t(t) = <\textstyle\sum_i' e_i \dot{z}_i(t)\rho(t)>/V = \frac{1}{kTV} \int_{-\infty}^t$$

$$dt'E(t')<(\textstyle\sum e_i \dot{z}_i(t')(\textstyle\sum e_i \dot{z}_i(t-t')\rho_o> \tag{6}$$

As the current correlation function in the time integral has sums
over all charge velocities $\dot{z}_i$, effects of cross terms between
ionic and molecular motions appear which cannot be identified or
separated by electromagnetic measurements. In addition to static
solvation and saturation effects on permittivity often considered
in biological contexts, Hubbard and Onsager have pointed out
"kinetic depolarization" effects which need to be considered. In
II, we discuss experimental evidence and implications of the
theoretical predictions of such effects.

The usefulness of electrical response measurements of solutions is not limited to effects linear in applied field. Transient birefringence induced by polarizing electric fields (the
transient or dynamic Kerr effect) has given valuable information
about biopolymers in solution; the effect must by symmetry be an
even function of $E(t)$, beginning with terms in $E^2(t)$. In both
cases, a response theory treatment of transient behavior meets
with difficulties not encountered in linear problems, but recent
progress in deriving correlation function expressions for such
effects is described in III.

The most extensive information about dielectric properties
of solutions has come from measurements at frequencies from 10^2
to 10^6 Hz because of the relative ease and accuracy of measure-

ments in this range. Microwave measurements at 10^9 Hz and above, though not without difficulties, have given information about very fast processes, but there has been a comparative dearth of results in the intermediate range from 10^6 to 10^9 Hz because of technical difficulties. Developments in time domain techniques which overcome many of these and have much promise for obtaining further useful information are described briefly in IV.

I.   Permanent and Fluctuating Dipoles.

Solutions of many proteins, synthetic polypeptides, and nucleic acids show large increases in permittivity $\varepsilon^*(\omega)$ over that of solvent, normally aqueous, at sufficiently low frequencies $f = \omega/2\pi$ of steady state AC measurements, but with dispersion and absorption processes which may lie anywhere from subaudio to megahertz frequencies. Although our interest here is primarily in counterion fluctuation effects as the origin of polarization of aqueous DNA solutions, we first summarize some relevant results of other models for biopolymers.

The observed frequency dependent behavior of biopolymer solutions often resembles that of polar liquids and their solutions in nonpolar solvents, the most conspicuous differences being the very large effects of small concentrations of solute and the much lower frequencies. The classic theory of Debye (6) for polar liquids and solutions assumes N independent permanent dipoles of moment μ reorienting in an applied field $E(t) = E\exp(i\omega t)$ with effects of torques of the surroundings represented by a rotational diffusion constant D. This model leads to an expression of the form

$$\varepsilon^* - \varepsilon_\infty = \frac{(4\pi N\mu^2/3kTV)A}{1 + i\omega\tau_D} \tag{7}$$

where A represents an effective internal field factor and ε_∞ contributions of induced polarization plus any solvent background polarization without dispersion at frequencies of interest. Debye obtained his result by solving a forced diffusion equation (i.e., with torque of the applied field included) for the distribution of dipole coordinate $\mu_z = \mu\cos\theta$, with θ the polar angle between the dipole axis and the field, and the same result for the model follows very simply from equation (3) using the time dependent distribution function in the absence of the field (5). The relaxation time τ_D is given by $\tau_D = 1/2D$, which for a molecular sphere of volume v rotating in fluid of viscosity η becomes

$$\tau_D = 3\eta v/kT$$

For such biopolymers as globular proteins with many dipolar groups contributing to a resultant μ, the theory provides a simple understanding of the observed behavior: the large values of

$\varepsilon^* - \varepsilon_\infty$ are attributable to moments much larger than for small
polar molecules and the lower frequencies of relaxation to large
values of volume ν and hence τ_D of even relatively small proteins. The pioneer experimental work of Oncley and associates
(7) confirmed these predictions with derived values of μ and τ_D
of reasonable and proper magnitude for a variety of proteins.
Deviations from the simple Debye relaxation function
$(1 + i\omega\tau_D)^{-1}$, or "line shape", were found, and in some cases the
observed relaxations could be fitted by assuming a sum of two,
or possibly three, such functions resulting from non-spherical
shapes of the molecules with two rotational diffusion constants
for different axes of rotation as a result (theory of Perrin (8)).

In some cases, observed breadths of the ε' dispersion in
frequency are too great to be fitted by a small number of Debye
functions with reasonable range of τ_D from considerations of
shape and size distribution. A case in point is the relaxation
of β-lactoglobulin in 0.48 to 2.5 molar aqueous glycine solution,
which was studied in considerable detail over a wide range of
protein concentration by Shaw and co-workers (9). They found
that increasing concentrations from 1 to 10 percent produced increasingly large deviations from the Debye eq. 7 which could,
however, be fitted by the empirical Cole-Cole (10) "circular
arc" function

$$\varepsilon^* - \varepsilon_\infty = \frac{(\varepsilon_s - \varepsilon_\infty)}{1 + (i\omega\tau)\beta} \tag{9}$$

with values of β decreasing from 0.92 to 0.81 (and to 0.60 for
liquid crystals with 325 g/ℓ of protein). The effects of molecular interaction are evidently considerable even at the lowest
concentration, making extrapolation to "independent" molecules
difficult.

For solutions of nucleic acids and polyelectrolytes such as
polypeptides, an increasing body of results indicates the importance of displacements of counterions along the linear chains of
the charged polymers as an important source of polarization.
The case of DNA in the double helix form is of especial interest
because dipoles along the oppositely directed helical strands
cancel to leave little or no resultant dipole moment. The observed dielectric increments, i.e., excess of permittivity over
that of solvent water, are very large, however, and reach a static
value only at audio or subaudio frequencies, showing the neces-
sity of some mechanism of considerable charge displacements
which develop slowly.

There have been numerous investigations of DNA solution
polarization using a variety of techniques of low frequency measurements. The problem is made difficult because of the appreciable ionic conductance of the solutions with or without added
salt. The polarization currents $\partial P/\partial t$, equal to $i\omega P$ for an A.C.
field, make increasingly small contributions to the total current

$J_t = J + i\omega P$ at low frequencies, and in many cases of biological
interest, there is the more serious problem of "electrode polarization" resulting from accumulation of ionic space charge.

In experiments of M. S. Tung (11) and R. J. Molinari in the
writer's laboratory, these difficulties were overcome reasonably
well by use of lock-in amplifiers as current detector for the
output of a low-frequency four-terminal bridge originally developed for other purposes (12) and considerably upgraded since.
In this instrument current through the unknown solution is compared with balancing in phase and quadrature currents derived
from the negative of the potential drop between two probe electrodes in the solution, the latter obtained with a minimum of
space charge effect by using circuitry drawing currents of less
than 10^{-11} ampere. The objectives of the experiments were to
test predictions of counterion polarization models, especially
as embodied in the McTague and Gibbs (13) treatment of static
polarization by equilibrium statistical mechanics.

In Tung's experiments, aqueous solutions of calf thymus DNA
from commercial sources with average molecular weights in the
range 10^6 to 10^7 were measured from 10 Hz to several kHz with or
without added salts (NaCl and $BaCl_2$). Some of the results are
shown in Figure 1. In Figure 1(a), dispersions of ε' (real part
of ε^*) at 5, 15, and 25C extrapolated to zero frequency show
that the static permittivities _increase_ with increasing temperature, which is contrary to the $1/T$ dependence expected for permanent dipole polarization, as in eq 7, but can be explained as
a consequence of polyion polarization.

As the fraction of polyion negative charge sites occupied by
counterions is expected to lie between 0.5 and 1.0, one expects,
and the McTague-Gibbs theory predicts, that increasing temperature results in a reduced number of counterions and increased
freedom for polarization from their displacements in the field,
and the experimental results are in agreement with the theory.
Also, under these conditions, adding positive ions to the solution medium should _decrease_ the static permittivity, because when
more than half the available sites are occupied an increase in
this number by adding salt will reduce the number of "vacancies"
available for displacements by the field. Experimentally, it was
found that the extrapolated static permittivity of 3.75×10^{-4} M
DNA solutions with average molecular weight 2×10^6 decreased
from 3500 for no added salt to 2600 for a 4×10^{-5} NaCl solution.
Even larger decreases were found for $BaCl_2$ solutions. Evidence
that the large effects are peculiar to the double helical form
comes from their near disappearance after denaturation, as by
heating to 85-95C (11).

A comparison of either the dispersion ε' or the complex
plane loci of ε^* with the Debye relaxation function in eq 7 shows
that the experimental curves extend over much broader ranges of
frequencies, a behavior typical also of other polyelectrolyte
systems and described within their accuracy by the empirical cir-

cular arc function, eq 9. The results for DNA of Tung and other
investigators (14, 15, 16) correspond to values of β of about
0.7. Choices of β between 0.5 and 1.0 can represent data for a
considerable number and variety of non-biological dielectric
materials, as first shown in (10) and since found in other cases
too numerous to be listed here. The number and variety of attempts at theoretical explanations of such behavior is also too
great to be summarized briefly. The writer's opinion is that the
more promising of these involve cooperative or many-body interactions between the individual dipoles or displaceable charges
and their neighbors, as in the theory of Shore and Zwanziy for
linear polymers (17) and the stochastic treatment of "hopping"
charge transport in amorphous solids by Scher and coworkers (18).

In most of the studies of DNA solutions, including those
just discussed, the molecular weight or helix length distribution was unknown or ill-defined and even the average values were
poorly defined. Experiments by R. J. Molinari in this laboratory
were undertaken as a first step in obtaining dielectric information on better defined samples. These were prepared by using gel
electrophoresis chromatography as the most suitable technique
available at the time for obtaining "sized" fractions in moder-
ately large quantities. Five such fractions were obtained, with
average molecular weights M_r(ave) from 0.20 to 1.9 x 10^6 and
roughly 2 to 1 range or less in molecular weight of each. These
were measured in dilute solutions with concentrations C_p, as referred to 7.9 percent phosphorus, in the range 2 to 9 x10^{-5}
moles (p)/liter and stabilized by using 10^{-4} N KCl as solvent.

Observed dispersions ε' for four sized fractions with average molecular weights $\bar{M}_r$ from 0.44 to 1.85 x 10^6 Dalton at concentrations C_p 8 to 9 x10^{-5} are shown in Figure 1(b). Within
experimental error, the values of $\Delta\varepsilon_s/C_p$, where $\Delta\varepsilon_s$ is the increment of static permittivity for added solute, were independent
of concentration but increased linearly with molecular weight,
as predicted by the McTague-Gibbs theory for molecular weights
below about 10^6 Dalton.

The relaxation frequencies of the fractionated sample solutions increased roughly as the square of molecular weight, as
predicted by several models of counterion fluctuations (2), (19),
(20). Surprisingly, however, the breadths of the relaxation
functions were, if anything, slightly greater than for previous
measurements of unfractionated native DNA (β∿0.65 versus 0.7)
with no distinguishable molecular weight dependence. The anomaly
may be the result of different starting materials or combined
errors, but in any case the breadth for the sized fractions cannot be reasonably explained in terms of their relatively narrow
molecular weight distributions.

Three processes by which counterion polarizations of DNA and
polypeptides can relax have been discussed in the literature (19,
20), with different conclusions as to the parts they play in determining the observed low frequency behavior. The three are:

direct ion hopping between surface sites, transfer by exchange
with the solvent, rotation of the helix axis r with respect to
space axis z. Van der Touw and Mandel ([20]) have pointed out that
if these processes operate independently with decay functions
$\exp(-k_i t)$, the correlation function $\Phi(t)$ of eq 5 will also be an
exponential, $\exp(-kt)$, with overall rate k the sum of the separate rates for the processes involved.

In such a case, no conclusion about the mechanisms can be
reached from the form of $\Phi(t)$ and the observed rate will be determined primarily by the fastest process. By extension of the
argument, one easily sees that marked deviation of any of the
parallel processes from exponential decay will be reflected in
the overall rate with possible change in the functional form.
Thus, if the rotation is described by $\exp(-2D_r t)$ as in Debye-
Perrin theory, and the ion displacements by a non-exponential
$\Psi(t)$, one finds from eq 5 that $\Phi(t) = \exp(-2D_r t)\Psi(t)$ and the frequency response function $\sigma(i\omega) = L\Phi(t) = \psi(i\omega^r + 2D_r)$ where
$\psi(i\omega) = L\Psi(t)$. This kind of argument can be developed further,
but suffices to show the difficulties in unambiguous interpretation of observed relaxation processes. Unfortunately, our present knowledge of counterion mobilities and our ability to assess cooperative aspects of their motion are both too meagre to
permit any very definitive conclusions for DNA and polypeptides.

The low frequency relaxation in DNA shows no signs of any
separable contributions of different processes, but a distinct
faster relaxation at megahertz frequencies and much smaller amplitude has been found. Mandel and Van der Touw ([21]) have proposed that this results from more localized counterion displacements within double helical segments separated by "nicks" which
are traversed or bypassed only with greater difficulty. Tung,
Molinari, Cole, and Gibbs suggested that it could result from
transverse ion displacements around the shorter circumference
([22]) of the double helix, i.e., at right angles to the axis.
Here again there is no unambiguous interpretation and further experiments are needed.

Finally, in this section, the possible role of counterion
displacements in relaxation of globular proteins should be mentioned. These can result in fluctuating dipole moments $\delta\mu_i$ in
addition to permanent moments μ_i along principal molecular axes.
If their relaxations are independent and separately exponential
with rate constants k_{Ci} and k_{Di}, response theory formulation
gives the complex permittivity in the form

$$\varepsilon^*(i\omega) = \frac{4\pi N}{3kTV}\left[\sum_i \frac{\mu_i^2}{1 + i\omega/k_{Di}} + \sum_i \frac{<\delta\mu_i^2 \rho_0>}{1 + i\omega/(k_{Ci} + k_{Di})}\right] \quad (10)$$

Fluctuating moments thus produce a relaxation proportional
to their mean square value at a faster rate than that of permanent dipole rotations because of the added effect of the rotations
in relaxing the $\delta\mu_i$ correlations. Although it seems to be gener-

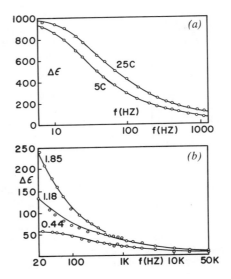

Figure 1. (a) Dispersion curves vs. log frequency of 6.2×10^{-4}M solutions of DNA (molecular weight 9×10^6) at 5C (and 25C) and (b) dispersion curves of fractionated samples at concentrations $C_p \cong 8.5 \times 10^5$. Numbers by curves are average molecular weight $\overline{M}_r \times 10^{-5}$.

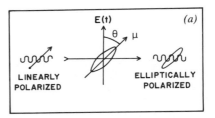

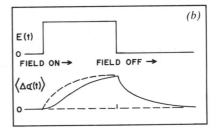

Figure 2. (a) Observation of Kerr effect: linearly polarized light from left is partially depolarized by molecules oriented in the bias field E(t), resulting in time-dependent birefringence $< \Delta\alpha(t) >^{\sim}$ and (b) birefringence $< \Delta\alpha(t) >$ following application and removal of bias field E(t). Asymmetry produced by permanent dipole torques results in the difference from the dashed curve for the field-on response.

erally accepted that for relatively small globular proteins the fluctuation polarization is much smaller than the dipole contributions and not resolvable experimentally (cf. G. Schwarz ($\underline{2}$)), Scheider ($\underline{23}$) has advanced a further argument against its playing a significant role. Starting with a forced rotational diffusion equation including torques of the applied field on the dipoles μ_i and $\delta\mu_i$, Scheider obtained an expression differing from eq 10 by having factors $k_{Ci}/(k_{Ci} + k_{Di})$ multiplying the $\delta\mu_i^2$ terms. He then argues that if the effect of these terms is to be resolvable in frequency, one needs k_{Ci} appreciably smaller than k_{Di} and that then these factors make the $\delta\mu_i^2$ contributions negligible. South and Grant ($\underline{24}$) have criticized Scheider's development on the ground that he failed to take proper account of the effect of the applied field on the counterion displacements in the torque function used. Their correction for this exactly cancels the Scheider factors and results in eq 10, obtained by response theory methods. Proper treatment of the kinetics of polarization involving ionic displacements can be treacherous, as discussed in other contexts in III, but it appears to the writer that eq 10 is the correct one for the model.

II. Kerr Effect Relaxation

This electro-optical effect, commonly observed as transient changes in optical birefringence of a solution following application, removal, or reversal of a biasing electric field E(t), has been used extensively as a probe of dynamics of biopolymer solutions, notably by O'Konski, and is a valuable tool because it gives information different in form, but related to, results from conventional dielectric relaxation measurements. The state of the subject to 1975 has been comprehensively presented in two review volumes edited by O'Konski ($\underline{25}$). The discussion here is confined to an outline of a response theory treatment, to be published in more detail elsewhere, of the quadratic effect. The results are more general than earlier ones obtained from rotational diffusion models and should be a useful basis for further theoretical and experimental developments.

The simplified schematic in Figure 2a shows the essential features of the effect. Optically anisotropic molecules in the solution are preferentially oriented by the applied field E(t), resulting in a difference of refractive indices for components of polarized light parallel and perpendicular to the bias field which is measured as a birefringence. The basic theoretical problem is to evaluate this effect in terms of anisotropies of polarizability $\Delta\alpha_i$ referred to molecular axes which produce a time dependent effect when the molecules are preferentially oriented by the field. For no anisotropy in absence of the field, the effect must be an even function of field strength, and at low fields proportional to E^2. A remarkable feature of the effect is that for molecules with permanent dipole moments the response af-

ter applying a constant field can be and often is different in
form from that following its removal, as shown in Figure 2b.

The classic theory of Benoit ($\underline{26}$) provided the first understanding of the effect, and with various elaborations has been a
principal basis for interpretation of observed transient behavior. Benoit assumed axially symmetric molecules with difference
$\Delta\alpha = \alpha_p - \alpha_s$ of polarizabilities parallel and perpendicular to
this axis and dipole moment μ along it. The forced rotational
diffusion equation with torques $-\Delta\alpha E^2(t)(3\sin\theta\cos\theta)$ and
$-\mu E(t)\sin\theta$ of the bias field was then solved for the time dependent distribution function $\rho(t)$ through terms of order E^2. Apart
from geometrical and optical field factors not dependent on the
dynamics, the relevant quantity is $\Delta\alpha<P_2(\cos\theta)\rho(t)>$, where the
second Legendre polynomial $P_2(\cos\theta) = (1/2)(3\cos^2\theta-1)$ is the result of transformation of the polarizability from molecular to
space fixed axes. Benoit's results when a constant field E is
turned on or off at $t = 0$ can be written

(a) Field off

$$<\Delta\alpha P_2\rho(t)> = \frac{1}{15}\beta\Delta\alpha(\Delta\alpha + \beta\mu^2)E^2[\exp(-6D_r t)] \qquad (11)$$

(b) Field on

$$<\Delta\alpha P_2\rho(t) = \frac{1}{15} \beta\Delta\alpha(\Delta\alpha + \beta\mu^2)E^2[1 - \exp(-6D_r t)] -$$

$$\frac{3}{4} \frac{2}{15} \Delta\alpha\beta^2\mu^2 [\exp(-2D_r t)- \exp(-6D_r t)] \qquad (12)$$

In these equations, D_r is the appropriate rotational diffusion coefficient and $\beta = 1/kT$ results from thermal averaging.
The asymmetry of the two responses, given by the second term of
the field on expression, clearly results from permanent dipole
torques but involves both dipole relaxation with $\tau_D = 1/2 D_r$ and
polarizability with relaxation time $\tau_\alpha = 1/6 D_r = \tau_D/3$, both for
rotational diffusion.

Benoit's model and results give insight into the effects op-
erating and have been widely used, both in the original form and
as extended to lower molecular symmetry in the field off case.
There are, however, serious limitations of the model: there is
no way of accounting for observed deviations from simple exponential response functions, no account is taken of joint correlations, and the relation $\tau_\alpha = \tau_D/3$ from diffusion theory is often
not found from experiments giving estimates of $P_1(\cos\theta)$ and
$P_2(\cos\theta)$ correlations. We now outline here a more general formal
treatment with less restrictive assumptions which both shows the
role of dipole torques quite explicitly and provides a basis for
analysis of different models.

In the response theory approach, we start with the Liouville
equation for $\rho(t)$

$$\frac{\partial \rho(t)}{\partial t} + L(t)\rho(t) = 0$$

and take as the Liouville operator for the problem

$$L(t) = L_0 + L_1(t) + L_2(t)$$

$$L_1(t) = - \mu E(t) \sum_i \sin\theta_i \frac{\partial}{\partial p\theta_i}$$

$$L_2(t) = - \Delta\alpha E^2(t) \sum_i 3\sin\theta_i \cos\theta_i \frac{\partial}{\partial p\theta_i}$$

where L_0 is the Liouville operator in the absence of applied field and the sum over all units i leads to joint correlation terms.

The first order effect of $L_2(t)$ is obtained exactly as in linear response theory and generates the counterpart of terms in $(\Delta\alpha)^2$ in eqs 11 and 12. The new problem comes in obtaining the second order effect of the dipole torque operator $L_1(t)$ for terms in E^2, as one must then evaluate the consequences of operations of the form

$$L_1(t)\rho_0 P_{1i}(-t) = L_1(t)\rho_0 e^{-tL_0}\cos\theta_i =$$

$$e^{-tL_0}\cos\theta_i L_1(t)\rho_0 + \rho_0 L_1(t) e^{-tL_0}\cos\theta_i$$

The operation $L_1(t)\rho_0$ is equal to $-\beta\mu E(t)\rho_0 \dot{P}_1$ (dot denoting time derivative) as in linear response theory. The operation $L_1(t)P_{1i}(-t)$ is evaluated at $t = 0$ in the field off case and hence is zero, but in the field on case one must evaluate $(\partial/\partial p\theta_i)\exp(-tL_0)\cos\theta_i = (\partial/\partial p\theta_i)\cos\theta_i(-t)$ for $t \neq 0$ which does not vanish. The ansatz used which reduces its consequences to a simple and useful form is that the effect of an increment in initial momentum $p\theta_i$ in the ensemble average is produced by the increments in $\theta_i(t)$ at time t which are in the initial direction $\theta_i(0)$. With this and some manipulation of the averages, one finally obtains as the generalization of Benoit's equations

(a) Field off

$$<\Delta\alpha P_{2i}\rho(t) = \frac{1}{3}\beta(\Delta\alpha)^2 E^2 <\rho_0 P_{2i}\sum_i P_{2i}(t)> +$$
$$\frac{1}{2}\beta^2 \Delta\alpha\mu^2 E^2 <\rho_0 P_{2i}[\sum_i P_{1i}(t)]^2 > \qquad (13)$$

(b) Field on

$$\langle \Delta\alpha P_{2i}\rho(t) = \frac{1}{3}\beta(\Delta\alpha)^2 E^2 \langle \rho_0 P_{2i}[\sum_i P_{2i} - \sum_i' P_{2i}(t)]\rangle$$
$$+ \frac{1}{2}\beta^2\Delta\alpha\mu^2 E^2 \langle \rho_0 P_{2i}[(\sum_i P_{1i})^2 - (\sum_i P_{1i}(t))^2]\rangle \qquad (14)$$
$$- \frac{3}{4}\beta^2\Delta\alpha\mu^2 E^2 \langle \rho_0 P_{2i}\sum_i P_{1i}(t) \sum_i[P_{1i} - P_{1i}(t)]\rangle$$

These results are now in terms of correlation functions of $P_2(t)$ and, in the field on cases, of $P_1(t)$, as in linear dielect-ric and other response theories. The asymmetry given by the last term of the field on expression reveals the interesting possibil-ity of obtaining both P_2 correlations (from the field off re-sponse) and P_1 correlations (from the asymmetry). One easily verifies that Benoit's result is obtained for diffusional reor-ientations, as then $\langle \rho_0 P_2 P_2(t)\rangle = (1/5)\exp(-6D_r t), \langle \rho_0 P_2 P_1^2(t)\rangle = (2/15)\exp(-6D_r t)$, and $\langle \rho_0 P_2^2 P_1 P_1(t)\rangle = (2/15)\exp(-2D_r t)$, but this form of dynamics is $\underline{not}$ assumed in the development and effects of joint correlations are included in eqs.13 and 14.

This outline of the response theory has for simplicity been limited to molecules with axial symmetry of μ and $\Delta\alpha$ and to the field on, field off cases, but can be extended in both respects without basic difficulties. Detailed comparisons with experiment have not yet been made, but it already is clear that Kerr effect relaxation data can now provide more valuable and better defined information about orientational dynamics of biopolymers and other molecules than was previously possible. With the increasing ac-curacy and time resolution of digital methods, it should be pos-sible to study not only slow overall rotations of large mole-cules (microseconds or longer) but small conformational effects and small molecule reorientations on nano and picosecond time scales. Moreover, one can anticipate the possibilities, for simple problems at least, of extending response theory to other quadratic and higher order effects of strong electric fields on observable responses.

III. High Frequency Polarization.

The polarizations attributable to biopolymers in solution are of course both coupled to the solvent medium and superposed on polarizations attributable to the solvent. The usual pattern of dispersion, as discussed by Schwan in the paper following this one, is indicated schematically in Fig. 3(a): the β relaxation or relaxations of biopolymers are found at frequencies from a few hertz to a few tens of megahertz, while the γ relaxation is for small solvent molecules at gigahertz frequencies, e.g., for aque-ous solutions not far from the 18 GHz relaxation frequency (8 picosecond relaxation time) of pure water. In the few cases for which the intermediate frequency range has been studied in enough detail by sufficiently precise methods, notably in the laboratories of H. P. Schwan and E. H. Grant, clear evidence has been found for a δ dispersion between the β and γ dispersions and of much smaller amplitude than either. The reasons for attributing the δ dispersion to solvent molecules somehow bound to the biopolymer have been discussed in detail in the book of Grant, Sheppard, and South (1), together with theoretical models of the solvation. Here we consider only some implications of recent developments in understanding of electrolyte solution polarization which can be significant for biopolymer solutions which have appreciable ionic conductivity, and in such cases may in particular modify current inferences about solvation from the observed γ and δ dispersions.

The effects of ion concentrations in aqueous and other electrolytic solvents in reducing the "static" permittivity of the solution and changing its relaxation time has been reviewed by Hasted (27) and by Lestrade, Badiali, and Cachet (28), together with discussion of various explanations of the decrements and relaxation shifts. Until recently, the explanations of the decrements have for the most part been by static models such as dielectric saturation of a solvent continuum in the Coulomb fields near the ions, more specific binding or solvation layers of solvent molecules, and mixture models of ionic spheres of low permittivity in a polar continuum of high permittivity. In 1977, Hubband and Onsager (29,30) first presented a unified treatment of the kinetic effects of ion and solvent dipole interactions by taking into account in a self-consistent way two aspects which had previously been considered by Born (31) and by Zwanzig (32, 33). Their treatment recognizes both the delayed relaxation response of solvent dipole polarization to the changing fields of moving ions and the response of ionic charge displacements to changing dipole relaxation fields. Both effects are found to be proportional to solvent relaxation time τ_D, and for their original hydrodynamic continuum model Hubbard and Onsager obtained the result that the decrement $\Delta\varepsilon_s$, defined as the difference of solution and pure solvent static permittivities, is given (in electrostatic units) by the remarkably simple formula

$$\Delta\varepsilon_s = -2\pi[(\varepsilon_s - \varepsilon_\infty)/\varepsilon_s](p + p')\tau_D\sigma_o \qquad (15)$$

The effect of ion concentrations appears only through the ionic conductivity σ_o, as the parameters p and p' for the ionic and dipole depolarization contributions to $\Delta\varepsilon_s$ are either 2/3 or 1 for "slip" or "stick" boundary conditions at the ion surface, and the factor $(\varepsilon_s - \varepsilon_\infty)/\varepsilon_s$ accounts for the dipole contribution $(\varepsilon_s - \varepsilon_\infty)$ to the sum ε_s of dipole and induced dipole (ε_∞) polarizations of solvent.

Although Hubbard and Onsager derived eq 15 in a different way, the kinetic decrement is from the linear response theory

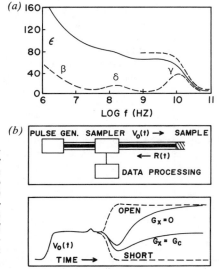

Figure 3.   (a) Dispersion regions in biopolymer solutions.   The β dispersion is attributed to biopolymer, the γ dispersion to solvent water, and the δ dispersion to bound water at the polymer surface. (b) Simplified schematic of apparatus for time domain reflection measurements. (c) Observed and reflected pulses for coaxial line terminated by open circuit, nonconducting dielectric, dielectric sample with conductance $G_x = G_c$, and short circuit.

approach a consequence of joint ion-dipole charge displacement
correlations in eq 6. Hubbard, Colonomos, and Wolynes ($\underline{34}$)have
evaluated these for a molecular model of the forces and find
that specific ion contributions are obtained. These are, however, not greatly different from the continuum result which is
also obtained in the limit of large ion sizes, and they showed
also that setting p' = p is necessary for consistency with the
Onsager reciprocal relations. For this discussion, it suffices
to use eq 16 with $\varepsilon_\infty << \varepsilon_s$, which in convenient units gives the
decrement in relative permittivity as

$$\Delta\varepsilon_s = -11.3p\ \tau_D(ps)\sigma_o(mho\ cm^{-1}) \tag{16}$$

The predicted decrement for an aqueous solution of con-
ductivity $\sigma_o = 10^{-2}$ mho cm^{-1} at 25C (corresponding to $\sim$ 0.1N NaCl)
is then $\Delta\varepsilon_s = -0.62$. Values of this order, but usually somewhat
larger, are observed for salt solutions, as summarized for example by Hasted ($\underline{27}$). Considerably larger decrements are expected for other solvents with longer relaxation times, which is
consistent with the larger decrements for methanol solutions
(with $\tau_D = 52$ ps) reported by Lestrade and coworkers ($\underline{28}$). A
rather spectacular example of large kinetic ion effects on permittivity is sulfuric acid with $\varepsilon_s = 95.0$, $\tau_D = 425$ ps, and an
intrinsic specific conductance $\sigma_o = 0.0104$ mho cm^{-1} at 25C.
Recent TDS results of D. G. Hall and the writer ($\underline{35}$),to be reported in detail elsewhere, show that addition of either H_2O or
SO_3 in small amounts sufficient to double the conductance is
accompanied by a decrement $\Delta\varepsilon_s = -33$, which agrees with the
theoretical prediction for p $\cong$ 2/3 to within a few percent.

The present evidence is thus that kinetic effects may account
for half or more of permittivity decreases of ionic solutions and
this may be an important factor in determing the amplitude of the
γ dispersion in conducting biopolymer solutions and lead to
revisions in estimated nature and amount of bound water. The
effect may also have some bearing on dielectric properties of
cell interiors and membranes if these have appreciable conductances. It would seem premature to attempt definitive answers to such questions until the relative importance of static
and kinetic effects in presumably simpler ionic solutions has
been better established experimentally in comparison with theory
which treats them self-consistently.

IV. Time Domain Measurements.

It is appropriate finally to say something about usefulness
of time domain methods for study of relaxation processes at megahertz to gigahertz frequencies. The need for improved precision
and more complete frequency coverage in this range has been
pointed out by several authors, as has the potential usefulness

of TDS methods for meeting it if the methods could be sufficiently refined. At the same time, serious doubts have been expressed about the possibilities when the systems of interest have
high ohmnic conductivities. Thus Suggett in his 1972 review of
time domain methods (35) concluded that "as yet, the measurement of ε* in the presence of appreciable conductivity, is a
hazardous affair: in this context the definition of 'appreciable
conductivity' is itself uncertain". Fortunately, this state of
affairs has since changed greatly by development of multiple
reflection methods which make measurements of ε* of very re-
spectable precision possible for solutions with σ as large as
0.03 mho cm^{-1}. Examples are measurements of ATP solutions by
Grant and co-workers (36),of whale myoglobin solutions reported
by Grant in the preceding paper, and of sulfuric acid solutions
by Hall and Cole (35)mentioned above. The analysis developed
by the writer (38) for evaluating admittance of an unknown
sample from the relation between incident and multiple reflected
pulses shows in a simple way what the possibilities and limitations for conducting systems are.

     The essential elements of time domain reflection methods,
shown schematically in Figure 3(b), are a generator of repeated
pulses with short rise time (ca 40 ps), a 50 ohm coaxial line
terminated by the sample of interest, and a fast sampling unit
between the generator and sample to sense, and convert to a
slower "stretched" time scale, the time dependence of the incident and reflected voltage pulses as they pass through the
sample with different time delays. From the records of these,
the incident pulse $V_o(t)$ and the multiple reflection pulse
$R(t)$ at the sample input can be obtained. Typical reflected
waves are shown schematically in Figure 3(c) for sample ter-
minations over the range from an open circuit to a non-conducting relaxing dielectric, a relaxing dielectric of "appreciable"
conductivity, and an ideal short circuit. The relation of the
Laplace transforms $v_o(i\omega)$ and $r(i\omega)$ of these pulse waveforms
to the complex input admittance $y_{in}(i\omega)$ of the sample termination is from transmission line theory given by

$$y_{in}(i\omega) = G_c \frac{v_o(i\omega) - r(i\omega)}{v_o(i\omega) + r(i\omega)} \tag{17}$$

where G_c is the characteristic conductance of the coaxial line
($= .020$ mho for 50 ohm line).

     The sample termination section or cell can be so simple
as the end of a coaxial line inner conductor in contact with
liquid filling a volume bound by the outer conductor or placed
between the end and a grounded plane terminating the outer
conductor. These and other arrangements have, again from
transmission line theory, an admittance $y_{in}(i\omega)$ related to

"total" specific sample conductance $\sigma_t^*(i\omega) = i\omega\varepsilon_t^* = \sigma_o + i\omega\varepsilon^*\varepsilon_o$ (where σ_o is the low frequency limiting conductance and ε_o is the permittivity of free space) by

$$y_{in}(i\omega) = i\omega G_c \frac{d}{c\varepsilon_o} \sigma_t^*(i\omega)/f(z^2) \tag{18}$$

where d is the length of coaxial line with equal electrostatic capacitance and c is the speed of light = 0.3000 mm/ps.

The function $f(z^2)$ with $z = i\omega(d/c)\sqrt{\varepsilon^*}$ accounts for propagation and multiple reflections in the sample length d as obtained from Maxwell's equation. Fortunately $f(z^2)$ can be expanded as a power series in z^2:

$$f(z^2) = 1 - a(\omega d/c)^2\varepsilon^* + 0(\omega d/c)^4 + \ldots \tag{19}$$

where the coefficient a depends on cell geometry and is 1/3 for a coaxial line section. Combining eq 17 and eq 18 gives the working formula

$$\frac{\sigma_t^*}{\varepsilon_o} = \frac{c}{d} \frac{v_o - r}{v_o + r} f(z^2). \tag{20}$$

Use of this formula or equivalent ones derived from it has proved to be both simple and effective in deriving values of σ_o and ε^* from numerical Laplace transforms of recorded pulse waveforms R(t), as discussed in detail elsewhere (38,39). The upper frequency limit for use with $f(z^2) \approx 1$ is typically 300 MHz to 1 GHz, somewhat below the quarter wavelength frequency (given by $(\omega d/c)\varepsilon^{*1/2} = \pi/2$ for coaxial line) at which the procedure becomes intractable, while use of the next term in the series expansion of $f(z^2)$ permits simple evaluation to several gigahertz for aqueous solutions in a cell with d = 0.7 mm. The formula 20 and its consequences shown in Figure 3(c) for the resultant reflection signals R(t) also show the limits imposed by sample conductance G_x. If this is 0.020 mho (= G_c), for example, the reflected signal is zero at long times and the differences at shorter times due to sample permittivity are confined to a range half that for a non-conducting sample with consequent reduction in sensitivity to ε^*. Higher conductances reduce this further until there is, obviously, no sensitivity at all for infinite conductance. In various measurements we have somewhat arbitrarily taken $G_x = G_c$ as an upper limit dictating cell design. For a cell with d = 0.7 mm, suitable for aqueous solutions, the corresponding maximum specific conductance σ_o for 50 percent loss in sensitivity is 0.040 mho cm^{-1}, permitting measurements for specific conductances higher than that of sea water for example.

These simple estimates of frequency and conductivity ranges usefully accessible by time domain methods are borne out by a variety of experimental results. Within such limits, the methods have the advantage that data at as many closely spaced frequencies as desired can be generated from transient records acquired by digital signal averaging for a few seconds at most, and are possibilities for further improvements by using difference techniques (39). Altogether, it seems fair to claim that time domain methods are often at least as useful as existing frequency domain techniques for conducting solutions at megahertz to gigahertz frequencies, and have some distinct advantages if one wants information over an extended range in considerable detail. Hopefully, the use of time domain methods will make measurements of "biologically fast" relaxation processes both easier and more precise than in the past.

Literature Cited

1. Grant, E. H.; Sheppard, R. J., South, G. P., "Dielectric Behaviour of Biological Molecules in Solution"; Oxford University Press: Oxford, 1978.

2. Davies, M., Ed., "Dielectric and Related Molecular Processes" Volume 1;The Chemical Society: London, 1972, p 163.

3. Kubo, R.,J. Phys. Soc. Japan, 1957, 12, 570.

4. Glarum, S. H., J. Chem. Phys., 1960, 33, 1371.

5. Cole, R. H., J. Chem. Phys., 1965, 42, 637.

6. Debye, P., "Polar Molecules"; Reinhold, New York, 1929.

7. Cohen, E. Jr., Edsall, J. T., Eds. "Proteins, Amino Acids, and Peptides"; Reinhold: New York, 1943, Chapter 22.

8. Perrin, F., J. Phys. Radium, 1934, 5, 497.

9. Shaw, T. M.; Jansen, E. F., Lineweaver, H., J. Chem. Phys., 1944, 12, 439.

10. Cole, K. S.; Cole, R. H. J. Chem. Phys., 1941, 9, 341.

11. Tung, M. S.; Molinari, R. J.; Cole, R. H.; Gibbs, J. H. Biopolymers, 1977, 16, 2653.

12. Berberian, J. G.; Cole, R. H. Rev. Sci. Inst. 1969, 40, 811.

13. McTague, J. P.; Gibbs, J. H., J. Chem. Phys., 1967, 44, 4295.

14. Takashima, S.; Biopolymers, 1966, 4, 6632.

15. Hauss, M.; Bernengo, J. C.; J. de Chimie Physique, 1975, 73, 724.

16. Sakamoto, M.; Kanda, H.; Hayakawa, R.; Wada, Y.; Biopolymers, 1976, 15, 879.

17. Shore, J. E.; Zwanzig, R. W.; J. Chem. Phys., 1975, 63, 5445.

18. Scher, H.; Montroll. E.; Phys. Rev. B. 1975, 12, 2455.

19. Ooosawa, F.;Biopolymers, 1970, 9, 677.

20. Van der Toux, F., Mandel, M.; Biophys. Chem., 1974, 2, 218.

21. Selegny, E., Ed. "Polyelectrolytes"; Reidel: Dordrecht, 1974; p 285.

22. Tung, M. S.; Molinari, R. J.; Cole, R. H.; Gibbs, J. H. Biopolymers, 1977, 16, 2653.

23. Scheider, W., Biophys. J., 1965, 5, 617.

24. South, G. P.; Grant, E. H. Biopolymers, 1973, 12, 1937.

25. O'Konski, C. T., Ed. "Molecular Electro-Optics, Parts 1 and 2"; Dekker: New York 1976.

26. Benoit, H.; Ann. Phys., 1951, 6, 561.

27. Hasted, J. B. "Aqueous Dielectrics"; Chapman and Hall, London, 1973; Chapters 5, 6, 7.

28. Davies, M., Ed. "Dielectric and Related Molecular Processes", Volume 2; The Chemical Society: London, 1975, p. 106.

29. Hubbard, J. B.; Onsager, L.; Van Beek, W. M.; Mandel, M. Proc. Nat. Acad. Sci., 74, 101 1977.

30. Hubbard, J. B.; Onsager, L. J. Chem. Phys., 1977, 67,4850.

31. Born, M. Z. Phys., 1920, 1, 221.

32. Zwanzig, R. W., J. Chem. Phys., 1963, 38, 1603.

33. Zwanzig, R. W., J. Chem. Phys., 1970, 52, 3625.

34. Hubbard, J. B.; Colonomos, P.; Wolynes, P. G., J. Chem.Phys.
     1979, 71, 2652.

35. Hall, D. G.; Cole, R. H., J. Chem. Phys., 1978, 68, 3942.

36. Reference (2), p 100.

37. Reference (1), p 119.

38. Cole, R.H., J. Chem. Phys., 1975, 79, 1469.

39. Cole, R. H.; Mashimo, S.; Winsor, P. J. Phys. Chem., 1980,
     84, 786.

RECEIVED October 31, 1980.

Spectroscopic Determination of the Low-Frequency Dynamics of Biological Polymers and Cells

L. GENZEL, F. KREMER, L. SANTO, and S. C. SHEN

Max-Planck-Institut für Festkörperforschung, 700 Stuttgart 80, West Germany

Raman Scattering

Low Frequency Scattering (<200 cm^{-1}). Raman scattering is known to be one of the most powerful spectroscopic methods owing to the use of the laser as the exciting source. Yet only a few investigations of low-frequency Raman scattering on dry films or crystals of homopolypeptides and of some proteins have been reported in recent years (1-6), probably because of the difficulties involved in the experimental techniques and the interpretation of the spectra. In the low-frequency region, one expects to see, in particular, skeletal torsional modes which involve displacements of larger parts of the biopolymer and which are, therefore, sensitive to the secondary and also tertiary structure. In solid samples one would have to distinguish furthermore between intra-molecular modes and more lattice-like intermolecular modes, the latter being affected by the degree of disorder in the sample. It is, therefore, not too astonishing that one finds mainly broad structures in the scattering spectrum. Some sharper Raman bands were observed in the 20–50 cm^{-1} region. However, these bands disappear when the biopolymer is dissolved in water (5), an effect which arises probably due to damping (6). Raman spectroscopy becomes increasingly difficult below 20 cm^{-1}, even if the iodine filter technique (7) is used. The reason for this difficulty is a scattering background originating either from unstructured water still present in the solid sample or from the lattice disorder mentioned above. It is unlikely that the background is simply related to the vibrational density of states, since this has been shown to decrease rapidly to lower frequencies, at least for the lighter polypeptides (8).

In aqueous solution, one is faced with the scattering of pure water (9), which is a strong scatterer below 200 cm^{-1} with some broad structure around 150 cm^{-1}. Since water scattering is not an instrumental artifact, one does not evade this problem in going from a double to a triple monochromator or by using the iodine filter technique. The rotating divided-cell technique (10)

0097-6156/81/0157-0083$05.00/0

has proved useful for certain types of samples. For these
measurements one half of the cell is filled with the solvent plus
sample and the other half with the pure solvent. The familiar
lock-in technique is then applied for instantaneous electronic
subtraction. Some precaution is necessary in applying this
technique if the sample shows luminescence. In a fixed cell,
luminescence may be largely quenched because of saturation due to
the strong laser illumination. In the rotating cell, this quenching could be suppressed. Solutions pose yet another problem for
Raman spectroscopy. The strong laser beam causes refractive-
index fluctuations in the liquid due to turbulences which in turn
cause additional noise in the spectrum. Capillary cells or rapid
flow systems (11) are therefore preferable to larger fixed cells.
A technique which reduces this noise is differential Raman
spectroscopy (12), yielding the derivative of the spectrum with
respect to time, and therefore to frequency. It is worth noting
a rather trivial, but nevertheless severe artifact occuring in
low-frequency Raman scattering on liquids, solutions or suspension
of cells. This is the occurrence of small particles (dust,
clumps of cells etc.). Due to convection in the liquid some of
these particles may move through the laser beam, causing a strong
Rayleigh scattered beam which enters the monochromator. This
can cause two effects. Firstly, a grating ghost of the monochromator may be enhanced if the grating is just positioned for
one of its ghosts. This may cause one to believe a sharp transient line of the bio-object has been observed. Secondly, the
rotational Raman lines of molecules in the air - especially N_2
and O_2 - can show up because the elastically scattered beam from
the particle travels through a large pathlength of air, from the
sample to the monochromator, corresponding to the properties of
a large gas cell.

High Frequency Scattering (> 200 cm^{-1}). Here the technique
is fully developed but sometimes not fully used. A change of the
laser wavelength or the additional observation of the anti-Stokes
spectrum is necessary to check whether luminescence of the sample
or plasma-lines of the laser are present. If the biological
sample has absorption bands in the visible, use can be made of
resonance Raman scattering. An example for this possibility is
the reported investigation of single-cellular algae (13) where
the chloroplasts yield some broad absorption bands in the visible
due to carotenoid- and chlorophyll-molecules. Dependent on which
parts of these bands the exciting laser is irradiating, one gets
a strong enhancement of the Raman lines of the corresponding molecules only. In this way an assignment of the Raman lines may
also be possible if the assignment in the visible spectrum is
known. It is worth noting in this connection that Raman scattering on living cells needs special caution because the strong, fo-
cussed laser beam will not be harmless to the cells, due to
bleaching of dyes, for instance. It is recommended, therefore, to

use a fast flow system (11) which exposes the cells for only a
few milliseconds to the laser radiation.

Brillouin Scattering

Brillouin scattering is a well developed spectroscopic tool today (14), especially for solid state physics in the very low frequency region (<1 cm^{-1}). For studying liquids, it has at least
the same difficulties as described above for low-frequency Raman
scattering. But for solid biological samples it might give very
useful information. A group in our institute, for instance, has
recently studied crystalline, oriented fibres of DNA (15). They
were able to measure the sound velocity of longitudinal phonons
in these DNA fibres, which turned out to be 3800 m/s in the highly dried state (A-conformation). The sound velocity decreased
to 1800 m/s, which is almost the value for water, if wet fibres
(probably B conformation) were used. The Brillouin scattering
was strong only for phonons travelling parallel to the DNA-axis,
whereas for phonon propagation perpendicular to this direction
the light scattering was weaker by about an order of magnitude.
This indicates a large anisotropy of the photoelastic response in
the oriented DNA fibres.

Sub-mm and mm Wave Spectroscopy

General Remarks. In the sub-mm range (10–100 cm^{-1}), as in
low-frequency Raman scattering, only a very limited number of investigations have been reported in recent years (3, 16–19). In
the mm range (1–10 cm^{-1}), almost nothing is known about the
spectroscopic behaviour of biomolecules or biological systems.
There are many reasons for this. There is first the strong
Debye-relaxation absorption of liquid water in the mm range (20).
Typically, a layer of 0.3 mm of water absorbs 80–90% of the
radiation. There is secondly the empirical fact, as we found,
that dry biopolymers absorb 10–1000 times less than water in the
mm region. Biomolecules in aqueous solution act, infact, more
as voids and cause, therefore, an overall reduction of the spectral absorption of water. To illustrate this, we have calculated, employing two models, the absorption of spherical molecules
having one dipole oscillator of a certain strength at 150 GHz,
and being dissolved in water with a volume concentration of 0.1
(Figure 1). In the first model, the molecule simply consists of
a homogeneous dielectric sphere. The second model was of the
Onsager-type, i.e. a spherical cavity of molecular size containing in its center a polarizable (non-rigid) point dipole. The
vacuum absorption coefficient and band-shape of the molecules
were assumed to be equal in both models. It is seen in Figure 1
that the resonance absorption of the molecules in solution can
hardly be detected, although the assumed oscillator strength is
probably by a factor of 10–100 larger than it is in reality.

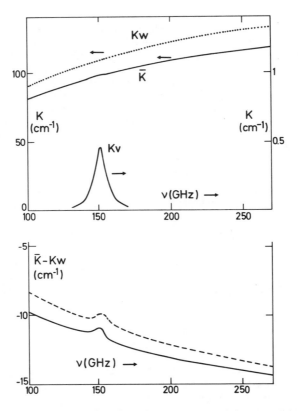

Figure 1. Model calculation of the absorption, centered at 150 GHz, of dipole oscillators in aqueous solution, 10% volume fraction.

(upper) (K_v) *Absorption coefficient of the oscillators in vacuum;* (K_w) *absorption coefficient of pure water;* ($\overline{K}$) *absorption coefficient of the aqueous solution.* (lower) ($\overline{K} - K_w$) *Differential absorption coefficient between solution and water;* (——) *dielectric sphere model;* (– – –) *Onsager-type model. (Explanation in text.)*

What is seen is the 10% overall reduction of the absorption of
the solution compared to that of the pure water. It is not surprising in view of this estimation that no one has found to date
specific absorption of water-dissolved biomolecules in the mm
range.

By going to the sub-mm range for the same problem one first
has to state that the water absorption is still larger than in
the mm range (21). The thickness of an aqueous solution must now
be less than 10 μm in order to get some radiation through. The
absorption of dry biopolymers, on the other hand, increases rapidly above 20 cm^{-1} (3, 16-19). We have measured a larger series
of poly-aminoacids and proteins between 20 and 500 cm^{-1} by means
of modern techniques of Fourier-transform-spectroscopy (22). The
two examples of lysozyme and myoglobin, shown in Figure 2, reveal
the rapid increase of absorption mentioned above. While globular
proteins only show rather broad spectral features we found in
poly-aminoacids, and also in denatured proteins, sharper bands
corresponding to dipole oscillators with strengths 0.01 to 0.05
and halfwidth of about 20 cm^{-1}. These results will be published
elsewhere. Using these findings and applying the same model calculations as for Figure 1, we come to the conclusion that it
might be possible to observe bands of dissolved biomolecules (see
Figure 3) although with great difficulty. At present, however,
all our sparse knowledge still stems from the spectroscopy of solid samples.

Quasi-Optical mm-Wave Techniques. Normally, in microwave
spectroscopy, one uses cavity resonators with a small number of
possible electromagnetic modes. An inserted sample must be small
enough in order to consider its influence on the filed distribution as a small perturbation. In the mm-range, however, this ca-
vity-perturbation technique becomes less and less applicable because of the small dimensions. In using waveguides instead of
resonators, one is faced with the problem of filling the wave-
guid homogeneously with a weakly absorbing sample over a larger
length.

As an alternative method, one can try instead to use quasi-
optical systems, for instance by placing the sample into a focus
in free space,which is accomplished by components like mirrors or
lenses (teflon, polyethylene) (23). Such a system suffers, however, severely from wavelength-dependent diffraction, interference and scattering, although it represents, in principle, a
broad-band system. It can be used quite successfully at a fixed
wavelength if only one parameter, like the temperature, is changed. A good technique now exists which can circumvent the above-
mentioned difficulties. It is the use of an untuned, oversized
cavity either in connectionwith tunable microwave sources
(klystrons, backward-wave oscillators, impatt diodes) or with a
Fourier-transform spectrometer (24-27). An approximately iso-
tropic and homogeneous field is generated in this cavity having

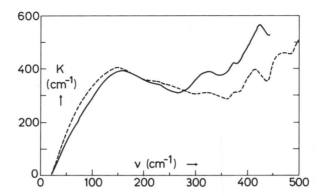

Figure 2. Measured far-infrared absorption coefficient of dry films of lysozyme (———) and myoglobin (– – –) cast from water solution. Accuracy of the absolute K values not better than 20%; spectral resolution, 1–2 cm^{-1}. The cast films were dried over P_2O_5 at room temperature for about 3 h.

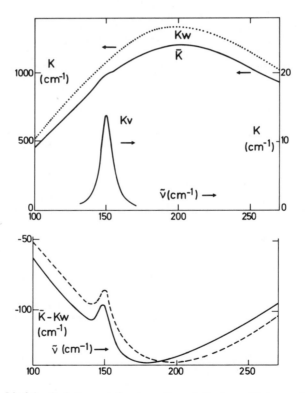

Figure 3. Model calculations of the absorption of dipole oscillators as in Figure 1. The oscillator, however, is now centered at 150 cm^{-1} in the far-infrared. For symbols see Figure 1.

highly reflecting walls, thus providing Q-values of the order of
10^5. Owing to the high degree of coherence of millimeter-wave
or far-infrared laser sources (28), a mode stirrer is necessary
in such case to produce a time-averaged field-homogeneity and
field-isotropy. A small fraction of the cavity field is coupled
out by a horn and measured by a detector. When a sample is inserted into the cavity, an energy loss is measured which is
caused only by the absorption, but not by the scattering, from
the sample.

The dimensions of this broad-band resonator must, of course,
bear a certain relation to the wavelength used. If the resonator is too large, too large a sample is necessary to obtain a
measurable energy loss. If the resonator is too small, on the
other hand, not enough modes are available and the sample would
strongly influence the mode pattern and hence also the output
coupling. A certain disadvantage of the untuned cavity technique is the difficulty of easily converting the measured energy
loss, due to a sample, to the absorption coefficient. This is
possible, however,for simple sample geometries, like slabs or
small spheres.

One of our first experiments with the oversized-cavity technique was the investigation of the temperature dependence of the
millimeter-wave absorption of cells like yeast (saccharomyces
cerevisiae) and monocellular algae (chlorella pyrenoidosa), in
the temperature range between -200°C and 0°C. For that purpose,
a highly concentrated (centrifuged) paste of these cells was produced. The amount of water outside the cells was thus small compared to that of the cell water, which amounts to about 80-85%
of the cell weight. The paste was placed in a liquid-nitrogen-
cooled cryostat made from fused silica, which is highly trans-
parent to radiation of the frequency range used (40-90 GHz). In
a reference experiment, the cells were replaced by a corresponding amount of pure ice, which in fact showed a negligible energy
loss until the temperature was raised to the melting point.
Since water has an absorption coefficient which is more than
three orders of magnitude higher than that of ice, a strong
energy loss suddenly occurs at 0°C. In view of the high water
content of cells one would expect for them a similar temperature
dependence of absorption. The samples of algae or yeast, however,
showed a completely different behavior in warming-up. As seen
in Figure 4, already at -100°C a measurable energy loss was found,
which continuously increased towards 0°C. The accuracy of these
measurements, as well as the above-mentioned difficulty for converting the data to absorption coefficients, do not yet allow one
to draw quantitative conclusions, especially above 0°C.

We remeasured, therefore, the cell-paste absorption by
using, in this case, a quasi-optical spectrometer (23). In order
to avoid wavelength-dependent diffraction of the sample, the millimeter-wave frequency was veried between 40 and 60 GHz, and the
average of the apparent transmission was measured. This averag-

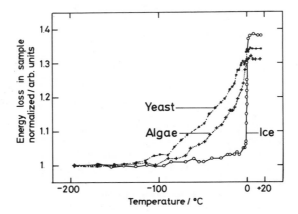

Figure 4.   Measured energy loss of pastes of yeast cells and of monocellular algae at 53 GHz as a function of temperature. The energy loss of ice is shown for comparison. All curves have been normalized to unity at −196°C. The measurements were performed with the untuned-cavity technique.

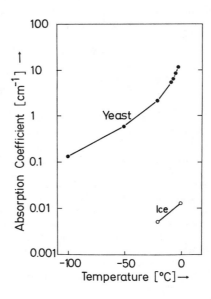

Figure 5.   Absorption coefficient of a paste of yeast cells vs. temperature. Two values of the absorption coefficient of ice are shown for comparison. The measurements were performed with a quasi-optical spectrometer.

ing was possible because of the small change of the sample absorption in that range. The result for yeast cells is shown in Figure 5, together with some data for the absorption coefficient of ice (20). The same experiment carried out at room temperature (~25°C) showed no appreciable difference between the cell-paste and a corresponding amount of water. Since the paste absorption-coefficient, determined at -1°C, is about 10 cm^{-1}, and since pure water at 0°C has an absorption coefficient between 50 cm^{-1} and 60 cm^{-1} (70 GHz), we conclude that at least 20% of the cell water behaves in an anomalous fashion below 0°C. This estimate is based on the highly probable assumption that the cell absorption is determined essentially by the water molecules and only negligibly by the other cell constituents. According to this view, the absorption mechanisms are Debye-like relaxation processes. Owing to the large inner surface of cells (29),a continuous distribution of relaxation times, which depends on the distance of layers of water molecules from surfaces and also on temperature, can be assumed. It should be mentioned that a similar behaviour as that shown here has been found for water in the capillaries of γ-alumina (30), in the same temperature interval and at 58 GHz. For a detailed discussion of the anomalous properties of cell-water determined by various other methods we refer to the literature (29).

Abstract

The paper deals with the experimental methods of Raman-scattering, Brillouin-scattering, sub-millimeter-wave and millimeter-wave spectroscopy, emphasizing the special problems arising with biomolecules and biological samples. Our discussion is mainly restricted to spectroscopy for the frequency region below 200 cm^{-1} where, in general, large parts of a biopolymer contribute to the eigenvector of a given vibrational mode. Various difficulties of such low-frequency spectroscopy are discussed, among which the presence of liquid water is perhaps the most serious. It is found that normal water has one to three orders of magnitude higher absorption in the millimeter-wave range than dry biopolymers. Also, the low-frequency Raman scattering is severely limited by the broad scattering of water. Several techniques for reducing these difficulties are discussed. Also described is a new method for measurement of the low-frequency absorption in cases where the sample exists in form of crystallites or fibres and where scattering normally dominates the extinction.

Literature Cited

1. Fanconi, B.; Tomlinson, B; Nafie, L.A.; Small, W.; Peticolas, W.L., *J. Chem. Phys.* 1969, 51, 3993.

2. Small, E.W.; Fanconi, B.; Peticolas, W.L.; J. Chem. Phys. 1970, 52, 4369.

3. Fanconi, B. Biopolymers 1973, 12, 2759.

4. Brown, K.G.; Erfurth, S.C.; Small, E.W.; Peticolas, W.L. Proc. Natl. Acad. Sci. USA 1972, 69, 1467.

5. Genzel, L.; Keilmann, F.; Martin, T.P.; Winterling, G.; Yacoby, Y.; Fröhlich, H.; Makinen, M.W. Biopolymers 1976, 15 219.

6. Peticolas, W.L.; in "Methods in Enzymology" Vol. 61, Part H; Hirs, C.H.W.; Timasheff, S.N., Eds.; Academic Press, New York 1979.

7. Peticolas, W.L.; Hibler, G.W.; Lippert, J.L.; Peterlin, A; Olf, H. Appl. Phys. Lett. 1971, 18, 87.

8. Gupta, V.D.; Trevino, S.; Boutin, H. J. Chem. Phys. 1968, 48, 3008.

9. "Water", Vol. 1, Chapter 5, p. 159; Franks, F., Ed.; Plenum Press, New York 1972.

10. Keifer, W.; Bernstein, H.J. Appl. Spectrosc. 1971, 25, 500.

11. Drissler, F.; Hügele, W.; Schmid, D.; Wolf, H.C. Z. Naturforsch. 1977, 32a, 88.

12. Yacoby, Y.; Linz, A. Phys. Rev. 1974, B9, 2723.

13. Drissler, F. Phys. Lett. 1980, 77A, 207.

14. Sandercock, J. Phys. Rev. Lett. 1972, 28, 237.

15. Maret, G.; Oldenbourg, R.; Winterling, G.; Dransfeld, K.; Rupprecht, A. Colloid and Polymer Science 1979, 257, 1017.

16. Buontempo, U,; Careri, G.; Fasella, P.; Ferraro, A. Biopolymers 1971, 10, 2377.

17. Chirgadze, Y.N.; Ovsepyan, A.M. Biopolymers 1973, 12, 637.

18. Shotts, W.J.; Sievers, A.J. Biopolymers 1974, 13, 2593.

19. Ataha, M.; Tanaka, S. Biopolymers 1979, 18, 507.

20. Ray, P.S. Appl. Optics 1972, 11, 1836.

21. Afsar, M.N.; Hasted, J.B. Infrared Physics 1978, 18, 835.

22. Genzel, L.; Sakai, K. J. Opt. Soc. Am. 1977, 67, 871.

23. Chandrasekhar, H.R.; Genzel, L. Z. Physick 1979, B35, 211.

24. Lamb Jr., W.E. Phys. Rev. 1946, 70, 308.

25. Gebbie, H.A.; Bohlander, R.A. Appl. Optics 1972, 11, 723.

26. Llewellyn-Jones, D.T.; Knight, R.J.; Moffat, P.H.; Gebbie, H.A. private communication.

27. Kremer, F.; Izatt, J.R.; to be published.

28. Yamanaka, M. The Review of Laser Engineering (Japan), 1976, 3, 253.

29. Clegg, J.S. in "Cell-Associated Water"; Drost-Hansen, W.; Clegge, J.S.; Eds.; Acadmeic Press, 1979, pp. 363-413.

30. Dransfeld, K.; Frisch, H.L. Wood, E.A. J. Chem. Phys. 1962, 36, 15574.

RECEIVED October 31, 1980.

Long-Range Forces in DNA

W. N. MEI, M. KOHLI, L. L. VAN ZANDT, and E. W. PROHOFSKY

Department of Physics, Purdue University, West Lafayette, IN 47907

Recently Maret et al. (1) have observed the longitudinal acoustic mode in oriented DNA fibres and films in a Brillouin scattering experiment. They observed the largest acoustic velocity for the driest samples, smallest for wet samples and at all times the observed velocity was larger than that for water itself. We have assumed that the velocities for propagation parallel to the helix axis are characteristic of acoustic modes in the DNA double helix and have used these values along with previously refined valence force field parameters (2,3) to fit the non-bonded force constants for the double helix.

Empirical Force Constants

We have chosen simple empirical forms for these non-bonded force constants. We have considered short range forces which could be characterized by a potential

$$V_s = B_s r^{-6} \tag{1}$$

and long range forces characterized by

$$V_L = B_L r^{-1} . \tag{2}$$

The force constants are defined in terms of the potentials as

$$V = \Sigma_{ij} \, f_{ij} (\Delta r_{ij})^2 \tag{3}$$

where f_{ij} is the force constant between the i-th and the j-th atom, r_{ij} is the distance between the i-th and j-th atom and the force is assumed parallel to r_{ij}. The sum runs over all atoms not in the same base pair. The form of the force constants then are

$$f_{ij} = (\frac{\beta}{r_{ij}})^n \tag{4}$$

0097-6156/81/0157-0095$05.00/0

where n = 8 for short range forces and n = 3 for long range forces. Some calculations were carried out for an intermediate case of n = 6.

The force constants characterized in this manner mimic Van der Waals forces for the short range interaction and electrostatic interactions for the long range forces. The sign of the interaction is always such that the interaction stiffens the helix without regard for the actual sign of the unbalanced charge. This is, of course, a crude approximation but is about all that can be done considering that the fitting is done to one number – the longitudinal velocity. Nonetheless we believe that some interesting conclusions can be drawn from these calculations.

Methods

Values of force constants for bonded interactions previously refined for poly(dG)·poly(dC) (2,3) were projected onto a mass weighted cartesian coordinate frame by properly constructed B matrices (4). The force constants defined in Eq. (4) were also projected onto the mass weighted cartesian frame for various values of β. These two contributions were added to give the combined force constant matrix. This was diagonalized for a value of θ = 4.5°. The parameter θ is the phase shift in displacement from one unit cell (i.e. base pair unit) to the next. This value of θ is in the linear region of the dispersion. The eigenvalues were the squared frequencies of the vibrational modes. The eigenvectors were checked to determine which solution corresponded to the longitudinal acoustic mode. The acoustic modes are known from group theory to have ν = 0 at θ = 0. The slope of the mode was then easily determined from the two known values and known linear relationship.

The sonic velocity is determined from this slope by the equation:

$$\mathbf{v} = 2\pi p c_o \left(\frac{\Delta\nu}{\Delta\theta}\right)_{\theta \to 0} \tag{5}$$

where c_o is the velocity of light, p is the pitch of the double helix and $\left(\frac{\Delta\nu}{\Delta\theta}\right)_{\theta \to 0}$ is the slope of the acoustic band near zero in cm^{-1}/radian.

Results A Conformation

We found it unrealistic to try to fit the longitudinal acoustic velocity to short range forces for A conformation polydG·poly dC. A value of β = 2.64 gave a velocity $\mathbf{v}_\ell$ = 1094 m/s. This value of β would imply the average near neighbor nonbonded force constant is $\approx$ 1.0 md/Å. Fitting the observed value (1) of 2600 m/s would require even larger individual force constants. This would require Van der Waals force constants larger than typical bonded compressional force constants. We concluded that long range forces were necessary to explain the large velocity measured in such a loosely wound helix. The value of the longitudinal velocity as a function of long range strength (i.e. $n = 3$)β is plotted in Fig. 1 as curve #3. In this calculation eleven base-pairs on either side of the central base pair were included in the long range interactions. The observed velocity is fit for $\beta = 0.53$.

The value of the velocity for $\beta = 0$ is very small. This calculation at $\beta = 0$ did include reasonable values for torsion force constants. The nonbonded interactions are essential to fit observed velocities.

A further calculation was performed increasing the number of base pairs included in the long range interaction. Significant changes in velocity occurred when adding additional base pairs out to 40 base pairs. The contribution from base pairs 41-100 was less than a few percent. This range is discussed more fully in another paper ($\underline{5}$). The value of β for this more accurate calculation which matches the observed velocity is $\beta = 0.44$. The largest near neighbor force constant based on $\beta = 0.44$ is $(f_{ij})_{max} = 5.6 \times 10^{-3}$ md/Å. One can compare this to estimates of electrostatic interactions which range up to 7.5×10^{-2} md/Å ($\underline{4}$).

Results B Conformation

It is not as unreasonable to fit the acoustic velocity for B conformation in polydG·polydC to a short range nonbonded interaction. This occurs because the stacking in B conformation is more compact and short range forces can more effectively stiffen the helix. In addition the velocity is less for these more hydrated samples. We have chosen to fit the velocity $v_\ell = 1800$ m/s as characteristic of B conformation ($\underline{1}$).

The calculations of v vs. β are the same for this section except that the B matrix transformations to mass weighted cartesian coordinates are appropriate to the B structure ($\underline{4}$). Figure 1 also shows the velocity vs. β for long and short range forces for B conformation. This calculation included 10 base pair neighbors on either side. Curve #1 is for short range $n = 8$ and $\beta = 2$ gives the desired velocity. Curve #2 is for the intermediate case of $n = 6$. The value $\beta = 1.68$ fits the desired velocity in this case. The value of the largest f_{ij} for $\beta = 1.68$ is $f_{ij} = 0.015$ md/Å which is of the order of torsional constants and roughly 1% of the value associated with bonded stretch force constants. This value is however likely still large for Van der Waal interactions.

The long range $n = 3$ calculation is shown in Fig. 1 as curve #4. The value of $\beta = 0.3$ fits the desired velocity. We have calculated the velocity for polydA·polydT and a similar value of β gives the same velocity. The result seems independent of base content and justifies our fitting polymers to experimental data taken on natural DNA.

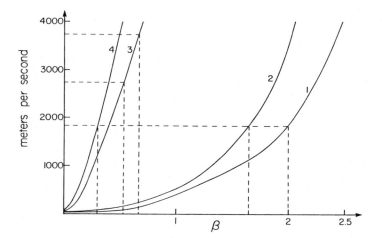

Figure 1.   Velocity of longitudinal acoustic mode of poly(dG)·poly (dC) as a function of nonbonded strength parameter β. Various curves as listed in text.

We have also carried out a longer range interaction in B conformation and find that the effect of base pairs out to 30 base pairs away is still significant in this case. The corrected value of β for longer range is β = 0.26. More detail is given in another paper (5). The value of β for long range forces gives rise to a near neighbor f_{ij} = 6.9 x 10^{-4} md/Å.

Discussion

Based on the above calculation it seems necessary to include long range nonbonded interactions in double helical DNA to be able to fit observed longitudinal acoustic velocities. Certainly these long range forces are dominant in A conformation, where their effect can be felt out to 40 base pairs. It seems likely that long range forces are also dominant in B conformation where their range is significant to 30 base pairs. Weak short range forces may be present but their effect can't be separated as yet since only one experimental parameter exists which is useful in refining nonbonded interactions (4,5). A more specific atom interaction model rather than the empirical averaged model presented here is also as yet not justified by available data.

One can investigate the magnitude of the change in effective dielectric constant which would have to occur to explain the observed changes in acoustic velocity based on the assumption that the non bonded forces were primarily determined by electrostatic interactions. If one assumes that the unbalanced charge on the various atoms is not affected by the hydration process then changes in β result only from changes in atom spacing and changes in dielectric constant. The changes in atom spacing is determined in our calculations by choosing the conformation. The changes in β can then be related with these assumptions to changes in dielectric constant. The value β = 0.44 which was determined for the intermediate hydration samples assumed in A conformation can be transformed to the value β = 0.26 determined for the wettest samples assumed in B conformation by an eleven fold increase in dielectric constant. Since the dielectric constant of bulk water is 80 this does not seem to be an unreasonable result.

One can extend this estimation of dielectric change to that needed to explain the entire range of velocities observed by Maret et al.[1] The very driest samples had a velocity of 3700 m/s and the wettest a velocity of 1800 m/s. If we assume the driest in A conformation and the wettest in B conformation, this entire range requires a change in dielectric constant by a factor of twenty.

We have made classical calculations of the effect of water surrounding a helix on the acoustic velocity (5). The effects seem small at frequencies of 5GHz and higher which were found in the Brillouin scattering results. In our recent calculations the lowest optical mode occurs at ≃ 150 GHz in B conformation and is much higher for A conformation.

Acknowledgements

This work was supported in part by: Air Force contract F33615-78-0617, FDA grant FD 00949, NSF grant DMR 78-20602 and NIH grant GM 24443.

Literature Cited

1. Maret, G., Oldenbrourg, R. Winterling, G., Dransfeld, K. and Rupprecht, A. Colloid and Polymer Science, 1979, 257, 339-340.

2. Lu, K.C., Prohofsky, E.W., and Van Zandt, L.L. Biopolymers, 1977, 16, 2491-2506.

3. Tsuboi, M., Tokahashi, S. and Harada, I. Physico-Chemical Properties of Nucleic Acids Vol. 2, Duchesne, J. Ed. Academic, N.Y., 1973, 91-145.

4. Eyster, J.M. and Prohofsky, E.W. Biopolymers, 1974, 13, 2505-2526.

5. Mei, W.N., Kohli, M., Prohofsky, E.W., Van Zandt, L.L. Submitted for publication.

RECEIVED October 31, 1980.

Calculated Microwave Absorption by Double-Helical DNA

M. KOHLI, W. N. MEI, L. L. VAN ZANDT, and E. W. PROHOFSKY

Department of Physics, Purdue University, West Lafayette, IN 47907

The direct absorption of moderate to low frequency, non-ionizing, electromagnetic radiation - microwaves - by DNA polymer molecules is a potential source of biological effects. As an introductory study of this question, we have evaluated the absorption of isolated homopolymer straight chains of poly dG-poly dC. For some absorption processes we have also investigated some effects of a surrounding aqueous medium.

The effect of absorbing a microwave photon by a molecule is to excite one of the fundamental normal modes of the molecular vibration. On a long polymer chain these normal modes correspond to traveling waves of varying wavelengths and corresponding frequencies as well as different relative motions of the atoms within a monomeric unit. It is convenient to group together the modes of similar monomeric atomic displacements into bands of modes. Within a band, the modes are individually specified by a wavelength parameter, θ. θ varies in small but discrete steps from 0 to $\pm \pi$; each different value of θ corresponds to a different number of half wavelengths on the total chain length.

On a very long chain, θ values corresponding to very few half wavelengths (i.e., long wavelengths) label motion in which the atoms of neighboring monomers execute very nearly the same motions simultaneously. At infinite wavelength, the motions of neighboring monomers are exactly identical. The simplest case of this kind of motion occurs when the chain as a whole is uniformly translated, or rotated about the central axis. Since no relative atomic positions are changed in this type of displacement, no restoring forces between atoms arise from it. Viewed as a type of normal mode motion, these displacements have zero force constants and therefore zero frequency. Also, the bands of normal modes in which they are grouped will all be of relatively low frequency.

The structure of the lowest frequency vibrational bands of a helical chain is shown in Figure 1. The two zero frequency modes at $\theta = 0$ correspond to rotation and translation along the central helical axis. Translations perpendicular to the helical axis are described by the modes at $\theta = \pm 36°$, the helix pitch angle; that these occur at $\pm 36°$ instead of 0 is a consequence of the twist in the structure.

The curves in figure 1 are in fact our computed structure of normal mode frequencies of poly(dG)-poly(dC) double helix (1). Modes near $\theta = 0$ have characteristic motions corresponding to gentle twisting of the chain (i.e., overall rotation of the chain by different amounts in separated regions) and gentle compression (overall translation by different amounts in separated regions.) The modes near $\theta = \pm 36°$ correspond to transverse displacements by differing amounts in separated regions. This motion is best describable as a bending of the chain. For modes further removed from $\theta = \pm 36°$, a certain amount of shearing motion accompanies the bending.

In a long wavelength torsional or compressional motion, the displacement of the molecule requires relatively little motion of the surrounding solvent; in the course of the motion, each portion of the molecule is carried into a volume previously occupied by another portion of the molecule. In contrast to this, the transverse displacement "bending" modes require that surrounding water be displaced; the molecule moves into and out of, spaces formerly occupied by solvent.

We have used the known elastic properties of bulk water at long wavelengths to calculate the correction to the normal mode frequencies of the transverse displacements. Damping and associated frequency pulling by water viscosity has been left out of all modes. The altered frequencies of the transverse modes are displayed in figure 1 and contrasted with the frequencies of the bending molecule in vacuo. Similar calculations on the longitudinal mode show that the frequency of that mode is not changed by the coupling of the molecule with the medium.

Methods

The double helix has unbalanced charge on many atoms. The displacements associated with vibrational modes generate oscillating dipole moments. These moments are constructed from our eigenvector displacements and models of atomic net charge taken from the literature (2, 3). These dipole moment matrix elements have been calculated (4).

The Einstein coefficient of absorption of radiation for the longitudinal (along the z axis) and the transverse (perpendicular to the z axis) electromagnetic fields can be obtained from these matrix elements and are given by

$$B_L = \frac{8\pi^3}{h^2} \left| \langle \mu_{\ell\theta}^L \rangle \right|^2 \qquad (1)$$

$$B_T = \frac{8\pi^3}{h^2} \left| \langle \mu_{\ell\theta}^T \rangle \right|^2 \qquad (2)$$

where ℓ refers to a particular band.

These coefficients can be evaluated for any biopolymer by taking an arbitrary chain length and determining the allowed values of frequencies for any set of boundary conditions. In our calculations we have assumed that the ends of the chain are fixed and we determine the frequency of the modes that permit an odd number of half wavelengths to be present on the chain. The eigenvectors for these frequencies are determined from the dispersion curves for an infinite chain. To make these calculations more compatible with experiment we have determined the absorption cross section which can be related to the Einstein coefficient by the following expression

$$a(\nu) = \frac{\kappa_\nu}{N_o} = \frac{h}{c} B S(\nu) . \qquad (3)$$

Here k_ν is the absorption coefficient at frequency ν, N_o is the number of absorbing centres per cubic centimeter, ν is the frequency of absorption, and $S(\nu)$ is the line shape function. For our estimates we shall assume that the line shape is Lorentzian having half width δ_L. If one evaluates the absorption cross section when the absorption is maximum the above expression takes the form

$$a_{max}(\nu) = \frac{1}{\pi} \frac{h}{c} \frac{\nu_{max}}{\delta_L} B . \qquad (4)$$

The significance of the above theoretical estimates of the absorption cross section lies in comparing the absorption of the incoming radiation by the biopolymer with that of the surrounding medium (water). The absorption cross section for water in the microwave frequency range can be obtained from the dielectric dispersion data (5) by using the following expression

$$a(\nu) = \frac{\alpha(\nu)}{N_1} = \frac{1}{N_1} \frac{2\pi\varepsilon''\nu}{nc} , \qquad (5)$$

where ε'' is the imaginary part of the dielectric constant at the frequency ν, n is the refractive index at the same frequency, and N_1 the number of molecules of water per cubic centimetre.

In our model the absorption is a maximum when a sonic half wavelength is equal to the length of the finite helix. The absorption approaches zero for helix length equal to a whole wavelength. The absorption is large again for $(3/2)\lambda = L$ etc. We plot the envelope of these absorption peaks (per base pair) for the acoustic modes as a function of frequency from Eq. (4) in Fig. 2 for helix segments of 51 and 451 base pairs in length. The figure shows the absorption for all the acoustic modes. We have assumed a line width of 10% for use in Eq. (4). Larger line widths cannot effect the result by more than order of magnitude.

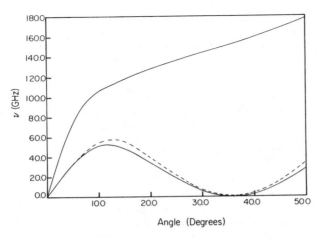

Figure 1.   Calculated frequency vs. phase shift θ dispersion curves for the two lowest bands in poly(dG)·poly(dC) in B conformation based on recent refinements.

The more steeply rising curve is the longitudinal or compression mode. The less steep curve at θ = 0 is the torsional mode. The quadratic curves at θ = 36 are beam bending modes. The dashed curve is the dispersion obtained after taking into account the coupling to water.

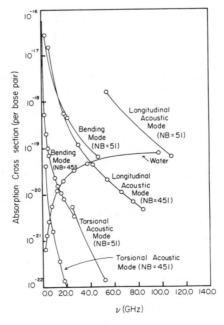

Figure 2.   Absorption cross section per base pair vs. frequency for the longitudinal, torsional, and bending acoustic modes for chains of poly(dG)·poly(dC) B conformation of lengths 51 and 451 base pairs. The absorption of a similar mass of water is shown also.

The absorption by water in this same frequency range is also displayed for comparison. The values for water come from Eq. (5) making use of experimental observations (5). The values in Fig. 2 have been scaled to the absorption of a mass of water comparable to the mass of a unit cell of DNA. The curves represent a comparison of absorption per equal mass of material.

The compressional and torsional modes couple to an E field polarized parallel to the helix axis, the bending mode couples to a transverse polarized wave. In the previous paper (1) we showed that water does affect the bending modes but that the effect is fairly small over most of the band. We have used our eigenvectors from the diagonalization of the DNA helix without explicit water interactions in calculating the dipole moment for the bending modes used in the absorption calculation. We have, however, used the dispersion curve corrected for water effects in determining the frequency of the absorption. For values of θ that are close to Ψ the two branches of the dispersion curve that originate at $\theta = \Psi$ will be symmetrical. Ψ is the pitch angle of the helix. Therefore for the same $(\theta - \psi)$ differences above and below ψ the frequencies will be the same. The eigenvectors corresponding to these values of θ do not differ significantly, therefore in our estimate of the absorption cross section we have a sum over the two frequencies originating from the portions of the dispersion curve for theta values greater than and less than ψ.

Discussion

In an experimental situation DNA segments can be of various lengths, all finite, and would have resonant modes such as described above. The choice of 51 and 451 base pairs comes from an attempt to estimate some size segments that may be able to resonate in chromatin. DNA in chromatin is wrapped into nucleosomes with short sections connecting the nucleosomes (6). The segments connecting nucleosomes are of the order of 50 base pairs in length. It may be that this strand of DNA could resonantly absorb radiation acting something like a segment pinned at both ends.

The nucleosomes themselves contain DNA wrapped around a core. The circumference of the DNA in this situation is roughly 100 base pairs. In this circular geometry one would couple to full wavelengths rather than half wavelengths. Again the absorption of a 100 base pair circle would be very similar to that of a 50 base pair segment. The 51 base pair segment calculation could relate to DNA absorption in vivo in advanced cells. The longer segment was included to indicate how the absorption does depend on the length of the segment undergoing coherent oscillation.

The largest resonances of the shorter segment occur at $\approx$ 50 GHz for the longitudinal mode, $\approx$ 25 GHz for the torsional mode and at $\approx$ 3.2 GHz for the bending mode. Recent calculations (7)

indicate that the bending mode is very strongly damped by surrounding water and we expect this mode to be broad and overdamped.
Energy absorbed by this mode would very rapidly be distributed to
the surrounding water.

We believe that the longitudinal and torsional mode are not
critically damped for frequencies above one GHz. These absorp-
tions may be of importance. Large scale motion of nucleosomes
and of the fibres made of coils of nucleosomes (6) would certainly oscillate below one GHz and likely be overdamped.

Acknowledgements

This work supported in part by Air Force Contrast F33615-
78-0617 and FDA grant FD 00949.

Literature Cited

1. Mei, W. N., Kohli, M.,Prohofsky, E. W.,Van Zandt, L. L.,
    submitted for publication.

2. Renugopalakrishnan, U., Biopolymers, 1971, 10, 1159-1170.

3. Stamatiadou, M.N., Swissler, T.J., Rabinowitz, J.R., Rein, R.
    Biopolymers (1972), 11, 1217-1234.

4. Kohli, M., Mei, W.N., Prohofsky, E. W., Van Zandt, L. L.
    submitted for publication.

5. Hasted, J. B.,"Water": A Comprehensive Treatise, 1972, 1,
    Franks, F., ed., Plenum Press, New York - London, Ch. 7 pp.
    255-305.

6. Bradbury, E. M. Federation Proceedings, Federation of
    American Societies for Experimental Biology, 1980, 39, 1650.

7. Van Zandt, L. L. to be published.

RECEIVED October 31, 1980.

DIELECTRIC AND SPECTROSCOPIC PROPERTIES OF MEMBRANE SYSTEMS AND BIOLOGICAL TISSUE

Dielectric Properties of Biological Tissue and Biophysical Mechanisms of Electromagnetic-Field Interaction

H. P. SCHWAN

Department of Bioengineering/D3, University of Pennsylvania, Philadelphia, PA 19104

The propagation of electromagnetic waves in tissues is de-termined by their electrical properties. In addition, these properties tell us much about the mechanism of interaction of electromagnetic fields with various biological systems, including biopolymers, membranes, and cells. Our present-day knowledge of the electrical properties is rather advanced (1), and I shall first summarize the state of our present knowledge of such prop-erties. Then I shall draw some conclusions about possible mechanisms which may or may not give cause to subtle nonthermal effects. No consideration will be given to magnetic properties since the latter are, for our purposes, identical to those of free space.

Electrical Properties

We will summarize the two electrical properties which define the electrical characteristics, namely, the dielectric constant relative to free space ε and the conductivity σ. Both properties change with temperature and strongly with frequency. As a matter of fact, as the frequency increases from a few Hertz to gigahertz, the dielectric constant decreases from several million to only a few units. Concurrently, the conductivity increases from a few mMho/cm to nearly a thousand.

Figure 1 indicates the dielectric behavior of practically all tissues. Two remarkable features are apparent: exceedingly high dielectric constants at low frequencies and three clearly separated relaxation regions α, β, γ of the dielectric constant at low, medium, and very high frequencies. Each of these re-laxation regions is in its simplest form characterized by equa-tions of the Debye type

$$\varepsilon = \varepsilon_\infty + \frac{\varepsilon_o - \varepsilon_\infty}{1 + x^2} \quad ; \quad \varepsilon = \sigma_o + (\sigma_\infty - \sigma_o)\,\frac{x^2}{1 + x^2} \qquad (1)$$

where x is a multiple of the frequency and the constants are

0097-6156/81/0157-0109$05.75/0

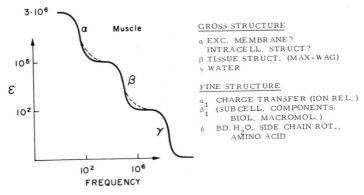

Plenum Publishing Company

Figure 1.   Frequency dependence of the dielectric constant of muscle tissue (61).
Dominant contributions are responsible for the α, β, and γ dispersions. They include
for the α-effect, apparent membrane property changes as described in the text; for the
β-effect, tissue structure (Maxwell–Wagner effect); and for the γ-effect, polarity of the
water molecule (Debye effect). Fine structural effects are responsible for deviations as
indicated by the dashed lines. These include contributions from subcellular organelles,
proteins, and counterion relaxation effects (see text).

determined by the values at the beginning and the end of the dis-
person change. However, biological variability may cause the
actual data to change with frequency somewhat more smoothly than
indicated by the equations.

TABLE I

Electrical Relaxation Mechanism *(61)*

Inhomogeneous Structure	β
(Maxwell-Wagner)	
Permanent Dipole Rotation	γ,β tail
(Debye)	
Subcellular Organelles	α
(Maxwell-Wagner)	
Counterion Relaxation	α

(See Text)

Plenum Publishing Company

Three categories of relaxation effects are listed as they contribute to gross and fine structure relaxational effects. They
include induced dipole effects (Maxwell-Wagner and counterion)
and permanent dipole effects (Debye).

The separation of the relaxation regions greatly aids in the
identification of the underlying mechanism. The mechanisms responsible for these three relaxation regions are indicated in
Table I. Inhomogeneous structure is responsible for the β-
dispersion, i.e., the polarization resulting from the charging
of interfaces, i.e., membranes through intra- and extracellular
fluids (Maxwell-Wagner effect). A typical example is presented
in Figure 2 in the form of an impedance locus. The dielectric
properties of muscle tissue are seen to closely conform to a
suppressed circle, i.e., to a Cole-Cole distribution function
of relaxation times. A small second circle at low frequencies
represents the α-dispersion effect. Rotation of molecules
having a permanent dipole moment such as water and proteins is
responsible for the γ-dispersion (water) and a small addition
to the tail of the β-dispersion resulting from a corresponding
β_1-dispersion of proteins. The tissue proteins only slightly
elevate the high frequency tail of the tissue's β-dispersion
since the addition of the β_1-effect caused by tissue proteins
is small compared to the Maxwell-Wagner effect and since it
occurs at somewhat higher frequencies. Another contribution to

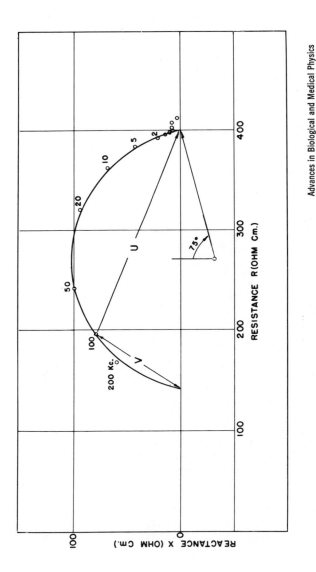

Figure 2. Dielectric properties of muscle in the impedance plane, with reactance X plotted against resistance R and the impedance Z = R + jX (1). The large circle results from the β-dispersion and the small one from the α-dispersion. The plot does not include the γ-dispersion.

the β-dispersion is caused by smaller subcellular structures, such as mitochondria, cell nuclei, and other subcellular organelles. Since these structures are smaller in size than the surrounding cell, their relaxation frequency is higher, but their total dielectric increment smaller. They, therefore, contribute another addition to the tail of the β-dispersion (β_1).

The γ-dispersion is solely due to water and its relaxational behavior near about 20 GHz. A minor additional relaxation (δ) between β and γ-dispersion is caused in part by rotation of amino acids, partial rotation of charged side groups of proteins, and the relaxation of protein bound water which occurs somewhere between 300 and 2000 MHz.

The α-dispersion is presently the least clarified. Intracellular structures, such as the tubular apparatus in muscle cells, which connect with the outer cell membranes, could be responsible in all such tissues which contain such cell structures. Relaxation of counterions about the charged cellular surface is another mechanism suggested by us. Last, but not least, relaxational behavior of membranes per se, such as reported recently for the giant squid axon membrane, can account for it (2). The relative contribution of the various mechanisms varies, no doubt, from one case to another and needs further elaboration.

No attempt is made to summarize conductivity data. Conductivity increases similarly in several major steps symmetrical to the changes of the dielectric constant. These changes are in accord with the theoretical demand that the ratio of capacitance and conductance changes for each relaxation mechanism is given by its time constant, or, in the case of distributions of time constants, by an appropriate average time constant and the Kramers-Kronig relations.

Table II indicates the variability of the characteristic frequencies for the various mechanisms α, β, γ and δ from one biological object to another. For example, blood cells display

TABLE II

Range of Characteristic Frequencies Observed with
Biological Material for α-, β- and γ-dispersion Effects

Dispersion	Frequency Range (Hz)
α	$1 - 10^4$
β	$10^4 - 10^8$
δ	$10^8 - 10^9$
γ	$2 \cdot 10^9$

a weak α-dispersion centered at about 2 KHz, while muscle displays a very strong one near 0.1 KHz. The β-dispersion of blood
is near 3 MHz, that of muscle tissue near 0.1 MHz. Clearly
there is considerable variation depending on cellular size and
other factors. There may not be as strong a variation in the δ-
case as there is for the α- and β-dispersion frequencies. The
γ-dispersion, however, is always sharply defined at the same
frequency range.

TABLE III (61)

Biology Components and Relaxation Mechanisms They Display

Electrolytes	γ
Biological macromolecules	
amino acids	δ + γ
proteins	β + δ + γ
nucleic acids	α + β + δ + γ
Cells, free of protein	β + γ
charged	α + β + γ
with excitable membranes	α + β + γ

Plenum Publishing Company

    Table III attempts to summarize at what level of biological
complexity the various mechanisms occur. Electrolytes display
only the γ-dispersion characteristic of water. Biological macromolecules in water add to the water's γ-dispersion a δ-
dispersion. It is caused by bound water and rotating side groups
in the case of proteins, and by rotation of the total molecule
in the case of the amino acids; and, in particular, proteins and
nucleic acids add further dispersions in the β and α-range as
indicated. Suspensions of cells free of protein would display
a Maxwell-Wagner β-dispersion and the γ-dispersion of water.
If they contain protein, an additional comparatively weak β-
dispersion due to the polarity of protein is added and a δ-
dispersion. If the cells carry a net charge, an α-mechanism due
to counterion relaxation is added; and if their membranes relax
on their own, as some excitable membranes do, an additional α-
mechanism may appear.
    Evidence in support for the mechanism outlined above may be
summarized as follows.

A. Water and Tissue Water. The dielectric properties of
pure water have been well established from dc up to microwave
frequencies, approaching the infrared (3). For all practical
purposes they are characterized by a single relaxation process
centered near 20 GHz at room temperature. Static and infinite
frequency permittivity values are, at room temperature, close to
78 and 5, respectively. Hence, the microwave conductivity increase predicted by Eq. (1) is close to 0.8 mho/cm above 20 GHz,
much larger than typical low-frequency conductivities of biological fluids which are about 0.01 mho/cm. The dielectric properties of water are independent of field strength up to fields of
the order 100 kV/cm.

The dielectric properties of electrolytes are almost identical to those of water with the addition of a σ_o term in Eq. (1)
due to the ionic conductance of the dissolved ion species. The
static dielectric permittivity of electrolytes of usual physiological strength (0.15 N) is about two units lower than that of
pure water (4), a negligible change.

Three dielectric parameters are characteristic of the electrical and viscous properties of tissue water: a) the conductance of ions in water, b) the relaxation frequency f_c, and
c) the static dielectric permittivity ε_o observed at $f \ll f_c =$
20 GHz. A detailed study of the internal conductivity of erythrocytes revealed the intracellular ionic mobility to be identical
with that of ions in dilute electrolyte solutions if appropriate
allowance is made for internal friction with suspended macromolecules (5). Tissue conductivities near 100 or 200 MHz, sufficiently high that cell membranes do not affect tissue electrical
properties, are comparable to the conductivity of blood and to
somewhat similar protein suspensions in electrolytes of physiological strength. Hence, it appears that the mobility of ions
in the tissue fluids is not noticeably different from their
mobility in water.

Characteristic frequencies may be found from dielectric permittivity data or, even better, from conductivity data. The
earlier data by Herrick et al. (6) suggest that there is no
apparent difference between the relaxation frequency of tissue
water and that of the pure liquid (7). However, these data extend only to 8.5 GHz, one-third the relaxation frequency of
pure water at 37°C (25 GHz), so small discrepancies might not
have been uncovered. We have recently completed measurements on
muscle at 37°C and 1°C (where the pure water relaxation frequency
is 9 GHz), up to 17 GHz. The dielectric properties of the tissue
above 1 GHz show a Debye relaxation at the expected frequency of
9 GHz (8) (Figure 3). The static dielectric constant of tissue
water as determined at 100 MHz compares with that of free water
if allowance is made for the fraction occupied by biological
macromolecules and their small amount of bound water (1, 9).
Thus, from all points considered, tissue water appears to be
identical with normal water.

B. <u>Protein Solutions</u>. The dielectric properties of proteins and nucleic acids have been extensively reviewed (10, 11).
Protein solutions exhibit three major dispersion ranges. One
occurs at RF's and is believed to arise from molecular rotation
in the applied electric field. Typical characteristic frequencies range from about 1 to 10 MHz, depending on the protein size.
Dipole moments are of the order of 200-500 Debyes and low-frequency increments of dielectric permittivity vary between 1 and 10
units/g protein/100 ml of solution. The high-frequency dielectric permittivity of this dispersion is lower than that of water
because of the low dielectric permittivity of the protein leading
to a high-frequency decrement of the order of 1 unit/g protein/
100 ml. This RF dispersion is quite noticeable in pure protein
solutions, but in tissues and cell suspensions it contributes
only slightly to the large β dispersion found in these materials.

At microwave frequencies the dielectric properties of tissues are dominated by the water relaxation centered near 20 GHz.
The magnitude of this water dispersion in tissues is typically
diminished by some 20 dielectric units due to the proteins which
displace a corresponding volume of water.

Between these two readily noticeable dispersions is a small
one, termed the δ-dispersion by Grant. It was first noted for
hemoglobin (12) and then carefully examined for hemoglobin (13)
and albumin (14). This dispersion is characterized by a fairly
broad spectrum of characteristic frequencies extending from some
hundred to some thousand MHz. Its magnitude is considerably
smaller than that of the other two dispersions and it is thought
to be caused by a corresponding dispersion of the protein bound
water and/or partial rotation of polar subgroups.

Grant (15) and Schwan (16) have recently pointed out that
the conductivity of protein bound water is higher than that of
water and electrolytes in the frequency range from ~500 to ~2000
MHz. Grant has suggested that this might establish a local
interaction mechanism of some biological significance.

Dielectric saturation for proteins can be predicted from
the Langevin equation and occurs in the range of 10 to 100 kv/cm.
Indeed, onset of saturation has been experimentally observed in
PBLG (poly-γ-benzyl-L-glutamate) at 50 kV/cm (17), which is in
good agreement with the Langevin estimate. Any irreversible
changes in protein structure that accompany its rotational responses to an electrical field are unlikely to occur at field
levels smaller than required for complete orientation, i.e.,
dielectric saturation. The thermal energy kT (where k is the
Boltmann constant, and T the absolute temperature) is in this
case greater than the product μE (where μ is the dipole moment,
and E the field strength), representing the change in potential
energy that occurs with rotation. Thus, changes in protein
structure caused by nonsaturating electric fields would probably
occur spontaneously in the absence of any exciting field at
normal temperatures.

Illinger (18) has discussed the possibilities of vibrational and torsional substructural effects at microwave or millimeter
wave frequencies. A calculation of internal vibrations in an
alanine dipeptide in water, using a molecular dynamics approach,
has been presented recently by Rossky and Karplus (19). In this
model, the lowest frequency internal oscillations which occur
(dihedral angle torsions at 1500 GHz) are strongly damped. Con-
ceivably, large proteins might exhibit lower frequency internal
vibrations. But we would expect that any macromolecular vibration which displaces the surrounding water will be overdamped by
the water medium, which is quite lossy at frequencies below 100
GHz. However, a detailed analysis of the response of such a
resonator surrounded by a lossy medium has not yet been applied
to this case. Illinger has not discussed the field strengths required to saturate submolecular vibrational transitions. But the
Langevin equation predicts that saturation for smaller polar
units requires higher field strength values (20). Thus, we would
expect that biologically critical field strengths are, for the
various modes suggested by Illinger, probably well above the
levels required by the Langevin equation for the complete rotational orientation of the total molecules.

In summary, the dielectric properties of proteins and biopolymers have been investigated extensively. For the rotational
process the field saturation levels are rather high; for internal
vibrational and torsional responses, perhaps even higher; and for
nonlinear RF responses due to counterion movement and chemical
relaxation, the levels are unknown, but probably also high. In
all these processes reversible polarizations occur in competition with large thermal energies and irreversible changes are
not expected at field strength levels of the order of a few volts
per centimeter.

C. Membranes. Membranes are responsible for the dielectric
properties of tissues and cell suspensions at RF's, as demonstrated by studies involving cell suspensions. Yeast, blood, bacteria, pleuropneumonia-like organisms, vesicles, and cellular organelles have been extensively investigated by many investigators, including Fricke (21), Cole (22), and Schwan (1). This
work has led to a detailed understanding of the role of cell
membranes in the polarization processes of biological media in
the RF range, which was facilitated by the relatively simple
geometrical shapes which cells in suspensions possess. The
principal mechanism for dielectric polarization at RF's and
below is the accumulation of charges at membranes from extra-
and intracellular fluids. For spherical particles the following
expressions were derived (1):

$$\varepsilon_o - \varepsilon_\infty = \frac{9}{4\varepsilon_r} \frac{\rho R C_m}{[1 + R G_m (\rho_i + \tfrac{1}{2}\rho_a)]^2} \rightarrow \frac{9}{4\varepsilon_r} \rho R C_m \qquad (2)$$

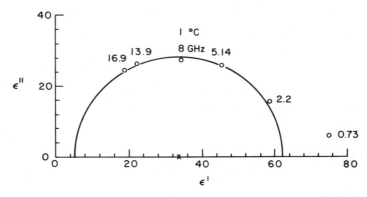

Biophysical Journal

Figure 3.   Dielectric properties of barnacle muscle in the microwave frequency range are presented in the complex dielectric constant plane (8).

ε' and $\varepsilon'' = \sigma/\omega\varepsilon_r$ are the components of the complex dielectric constant $\varepsilon^* = \varepsilon' - j\varepsilon''$. The frequency at the peak of the circle is the characteristic frequency of the dispersion and identical with that of normal water, demonstrating the indentity of tissue water in normal water from a dielectric point of view.

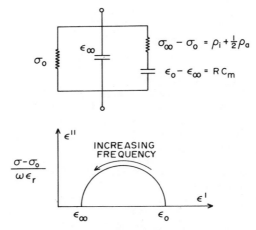

Proceedings of the Institute of Electrical and Electronic Engineers

Figure 4.   Equivalent circuit for the β-dispersion of a cell suspension and corresponding plot in the complex dielectric constant plane (9)

$$\sigma_o = \sigma_a \left[1 - 1.5\rho \frac{1 + RG_m(\rho_i - \rho_a)}{1 + RG_m(\rho_i + \frac{1}{2}\rho_a)} \right] \rightarrow \sigma_a(1-1.5\rho) \tag{3}$$

$$\sigma_\infty = \sigma_a \left[1 + 3\rho \frac{\sigma_i - \sigma_a}{\sigma_i + 2\sigma_a} \right] \tag{4}$$

for the limit values of the simple dispersion which characterizes the frequency dependence. The time constant is

$$\tau = \frac{RC_m}{2\frac{\sigma_a\sigma_i}{\sigma_i + 2\sigma_a} + RG_m} \rightarrow RC_m \ (\rho_i + 0.5 \ \rho_a) \ . \tag{5}$$

In these equations C_m and G_m are capacitance and conductance per cm^2 of the cell membrane, R is the cell radius, ρ the cellular volume fraction, $\sigma_i = 1/\rho_i$, and $\sigma_a = 1/\rho_a$ are the conductivities of the cell interior and suspending medium. The equations apply for small volume fractions ρ and assume that the radius of the cell is very large compared with the membrane thickness. More elaborate closed form expressions have been developed for cases when these assumptions are no longer valid (23, 24) and an exact representation of the suspension dielectric properties as a sum of two dispersions is available (25). If, as is usually the case, the membrane conductance is sufficiently low, equations (2)-(5) reduce to the simple forms to the right of the arrows.

A physical insight into eqs. (2)-(5) is gained by considering the equivalent circuit shown in Figure 4, which displays the same frequency response defined in eqs. (2)-(5). The membrane capacitance per unit area C_m appears in series with the access impedances ρ_i and $\rho_a/2$, while the term σ_a (1-1.5ρ) provides for the conductance of the shunting extracellular fluid. Hence the time constant τ which determines the frequency where the impedances $1/\omega C_m R$ and $(\rho_i + \rho_a/2)$ are equal is given by eq. (5). Using typical values of σ_i, $\sigma_a \sim 0.01$ mho/cm, $C_m = 1$ µF/cm^2, R = 10 µm and $\rho = 0.5$, with eqs. (2)-(5), we see that the dispersion must occur at RF's and its magnitude $\varepsilon_o - \varepsilon_\infty$ is exceptionally high.

From experimental dispersion curves and, hence, values of the four quantities σ_o, σ_∞, $(\varepsilon_o - \varepsilon_\infty)$, and τ, the three quantities C_m, σ_i, and σ_a can be determined with an additional equation available to check for internal consistency. Values for extracelluar and intracellular resistivities thus obtained agree well with independent measurements. Dispersions disappear as expected after destroying the cell membranes, and their characteristic frequencies are readily shifted to higher or lower frequencies

by experimentally changing intracellular or extracellular ionic
strengths. This gives confidence in the model, whose validity
is now generally accepted.

This work led to the important conclusion that the capacitance of all biological membranes, including cellular membranes
and those of subcellular organelles, such as mitochondria, is of
the order of 1 $\mu F/cm^2$. This value is apparently independent of
frequency in the total RF range; at low audio frequencies, capacitance values increase with decreasing frequencies due to additional relaxation mechanisms in or near the membranes (1, 26).
These mechanisms will not be discussed here and have been summarized elsewhere (1, 26).

From the membrane capacitance, we can estimate values for
the transmembrane potentials induced by microwave fields. At
frequencies well above the characteristic frequency (a few MHz),
the membrane capacitance impedance becomes very small by comparison with the cell access impedance ($\rho_i + \rho_a/2$) and the membrane
behaves electrically like a short circuit. Since intracellular
and extracellular conductivities are comparable, the average
current density through the tissue is comparable to that in the
membrane. For an in situ field of 1 V/cm (induced by an external
microwave field flux of about 10 mW/cm^2) the current density i
through the membrane is about 10 mA/cm^2 since typical resistivities of tissues are of the order of 100 Ω-cm at microwave frequencies. Thus the evoked membrane potential $\Delta V = i/j\omega C_m$ is
about 0.5 μV at 3 GHz and diminishes with increasing frequency.
This value is 1000 times lower than potentials recognized as
being biologically significant. Action potentials can be triggered by potentials of about 10 mV across the membrane, but (dc)
transmembrane potentials somewhat below 1 mV have been recognized
as being important (27).

If $f<<f_c$, the total potential difference applied across the
cell is developed across the membrane capacitance. In this
limit, the induced membrane potential ΔV across a spherical cell
is $\Delta V = 1.5$ ER, where E represents the applied external field.
Thus the cell samples the external field strength over its dimensions and delivers this integrated voltage to the membranes,
which is a few mV at these low frequencies for cells larger than
10 μm and external fields of about 1 V/cm. These transmembrane
potentials can be biologically significant.

Membrane Interactions

Table IV attempts to summarize information relevant to electrical fields and their effects on biological membranes. Membrane destruction can be achieved with low frequency alternating
fields of the order of some hundred millivolts across the membrane, as later described. The propagation of action potentials
along nerves is initiated or interfered with by pulses or low
frequency potentials of roughly 10 mV across the membrane. Cor-

TABLE IV

Electrical Field Effects on Membranes

	ΔV_M		E, in situ	
Membrane Destruction	100 - 300	mV		
Action Potential (Excitation)	10	mV	1	V/cm
Subtle Effects	0.1 - 1	mV		
Extraordinary Sensitivities				
A. Related to membranes	0.1	μV	0.01	μV/cm
B. Possibly not related to membranes	< 1	nV	0.1	μV/cm
Microwave Sensitivities (1 GHz)	1	μV*	1	V/cm

*From ΔV_M = 1.5 ER

Summary of various field effects on membranes (some established, some proposed). ΔV_M is the field induced membrane
potential, E corresponding field strength in situ. E and
ΔV_M are interrelated by ΔV_M = 1.5 ER (for spherical cells).

responding current densities and field strength values in tissues and the medium external to the affected cell are of the order of 1 mA/cm^2 and 1 V/cm ($\underline{28}$, $\underline{29}$, $\underline{30}$).

In recent years some extraordinary sensitivities have been reported. Electrosensitive species such as rays and sharks detect fields of intensities as low as 0.01 µV/cm. In order to achieve these sensitivities, they sample the field over considerable distances with the aid of special organs, the Ampullae Lorenzini, and operate over a small frequency range extending from dc to only a few Herz ($\underline{29}$, $\underline{31}$). Some other reports also indicate effects due to ELF fields of the order of V/cm in air on timing responses and calcium efflux ($\underline{32}$, $\underline{33}$). Corresponding in situ fields would be of the order of 0.1 µV/cm as listed in the table and corresponding fields across membranes below 1 nV. It is, however, not yet obvious if the reported effects are caused by membrane processes; hence, the reduction of external fields to in situ fields and then membrane potentials, is not necessarily sensible. A more detailed discussion of this topic is given by Schwan ($\underline{30}$) and Bawin and Adey ($\underline{32}$) and the detailed report of the National Academy of Sciences - National Research Council on the Biological Effects of Electric and Magnetic Fields ($\underline{29}$).

Microwave sensitivities of the order of 1 V/cm in situ have been frequently reported and correspond to external flux values of the order of 1 to 10 mW/cm^2. (See, for example, the recent text by Baranski and Czerski ($\underline{34}$).) Some suspect that these sensitivities correspond to direct interactions with the central nervous system. However, it is straightforward to translate in situ field levels to corresponding membrane potentials and these are at levels of the order of 1 µV or less, depending on microwave frequency as discussed by Schwan ($\underline{30}$). The implications of these calculations have been challenged ($\underline{34}$, $\underline{35}$) by the argument that we do not yet know how the brain processes information. But the writer finds it difficult to see how this rather general and no doubt valid statement pertains to his calculation of microwave-induced membrane potentials. At microwave frequencies field strength levels in membranes and in situ field levels are comparable within one order of magnitude. This must be so since in situ currents readily pass the membranes and enter the cell interior as well as the interior of subcellular organisms ($\underline{1}$). Moreover, dielectric constants of membranes (about 10) and cellular fluids (about 60 or less, depending on frequency) are similar in magnitude ($\underline{1}$). Hence, the membrane potential is simply the product of in situ field strength and membrane thickness of about 10^{-6} cm. This simple argument does not depend on any particular model.

It may be argued that the microwave-induced membrane potential of about 1 µV is comparable and even higher than the perception level across the end-epithelium of the Ampullae of Lorenzini. However, it should be realized that the high sensitivity of this end-organ is only achieved over a narrow bandpath range

of some Hertz. If microwave sensitivities existed over such narrow bandpath ranges, they would be hardly noticeable experimentally.

It also should be noted that the sensitivities of excitable
cells to electric fields decrease rapidly as the electric stimulus is applied for time periods decreasingly short in comparison
to the refractory period of the order of 1 msec. Hence,
quotation of reported low frequency membrane sensitivities as
done by Frey (35) carries no implication with regard to sensitivities claimed at microwave frequencies correspond to time
periods of the order of 1 nsec, which is a million times smaller
than the refractory period. More recently, it has been postulated (36) that microwave fields may well be perceived, provided
they are modulated with frequencies below 10 or 20 Hz. This
would be possible in principle if induced in situ fields and currents could be rectified with some degree of efficiency so that
microwave fields would generate detectable low frequency currents. No evidence for such a mechanism has been demonstrated so
far at the membrane level.

TABLE V

Biological Thresholds

Cardiology	$0.03 - 10 \ mA/cm^2$
Electrosleep and Electrical Anesthesia	$10 - 100 \ mA$
Electro-hazards:	
Sensation	1 mA
"Let Go"	10 mA
Fibrillation	100 mA
Biophysics and Axonology	$1 \ mA/cm^2$
$\Delta V_M = 1.5 \ ER$	$(10 \ \mu, \ 1 \ mV)$
$\Delta V_M = R \cdot J \ (mA/cm^2)$	

Current density thresholds noticed in various disciplines.

In Table V available evidence on the threshold of biological
excitation phenomena is summarized for various fields. In cardi-
ology, extended experience exists with pacemakers and threshold
values range about $0.1-10 \ mA/cm^2$, depending on electrode size and

other parameters (37). In electrohypnosis, electrosleep and electrical anesthesia total currents applied are about 10 to 100 mA.
Corresponding current densities in the brain may be estimated
based on the work by Driscoll (38). For a total current applied
to the head of 1 mA, internal brain current densities (38) are of
the order of 10 $\mu A/cm^2$. Hence, 10–100 mA total current corresponds to brain tissue current densities of the order of 0.1–1 mA/
cm^2. Very extended work (28) has been carried out on electrical
hazards caused by low frequency potentials applied to the human
body. The values quoted in the table as thresholds for sensation,
"let go" current, and fibrillation are all consistent (28) with a
current density of about 1 mA/cm^2. Thus, membrane potentials in
the mV range as discussed above are consistent with the experience
gained with pacemakers, and the effects on brain tissue and in the
electrical hazards field.

Field Generated Force Effects

Electric fields can directly interact with matter and create
forces that can act on molecules as well as on cellular and larger
structures. Most of these interactions are reversible and do not
necessarily have demonstrable biological effects. An example is
the movement of ions in an ac field, which is inconsequential,
provided that the field is weak enough to prevent undue heating
from molecular collisions (e.g., below about 1 V/cm, corresponding
to 1 mA/cm^2 in a physiological medium). Another example is the
orientation of polar macromolecules. For field strength values of
interest here, only a very partial preferential orientation with
the field results. Complete orientation and consequent dielectric
saturation requires field strengths of thousands of volts per centimeter. (Changes of this magnitude do occur in membranes on depolarization. Hence, field-induced orientation and changes in
orientation of membrane molecules appear possible. Corresponding
tissue current densities would be in milliamperes per square centimeter, as discussed above.)
Electric fields can interact just as well with nonpolar cells
and organelles in the absence of any net charge. These "ponderomotive" forces are well known and understood. Any system exposed
to an electric field will tend to minimize its electric potential
energy by appropriate rearrangement. This statement is equally
true for dc and ac fields, because the potential energy is a function of the square of the field strength. Inasmuch as the induced
dipole moment of a cell or large particle depends on both the
square of field strength and the volume, it is not surprising that
the threshold field to overcome thermal agitation is proportional
to $R^{-1.5}$, where R is the effective radius of the particle. Experimental evidence confirms the principle; threshold field values
for responses of 10 μm cells are about 10 V/cm. But for 10 nm
macromolecules, they are about 10 kV/cm and comparable with the
fields needed for complete orientation, owing to the existence of
a typical dipole moment of about 10 or 100 debyes.

Table VI summarizes observed manifestations of field-generated forces. The field effects may manifest themselves as an orientation of particles in the direction of the field or perpendicular to it; or, "pearl chain" formation, i.e., the alignment of particles in the field direction may occur. This has long been considered a mysterious demonstration of microwave induced biological effects. Deformation or destruction of cells can be achieved with fields. The movement of cells in inhomogeneous electrical fields can be affected.

Zimmerman et al. (39) have observed the destruction of red cells and ghost formation. Neumann and Rosenheck (40) studied the effects of fields on chromaffin vesicles. Friend et al. (41) as well as Goodman (42, 43), studied the effects of fields on fairly large cellular organisms. Orientation effects have been observed by Teixerira-Pinto et al (44), by Sher (45), and by Novak (46). Pohl (47) developed "dielectrophoresis" as a tool of separating cells in inhomogeneous fields. And Elul et al. (48) observed cell destruction phenomena and cell shape changes. No attempt is made here to summarize the total literature on this topic and additional discussions have been presented elsewhere (36, 49). Some of these field-generated force effects can be very startling and dramatic, especially near the tip of small electrodes. Of a similar nature is the movement of magnetotactic bacteria recently reported by Blakemore (50) in magnetic fields of fairly low intensity. Apparently, these bacteria are equipped with magnetic properties and are therefore significantly oriented by the magnetic field and motivated to move in the field direction.

Experimental and theoretical evidence indicates that pulsed fields cannot have greater effects than continuous fields of the same average power (51). Hence, modulation is not expected to have special effects.

TABLE VI

Field Generated Forces

Orientation

"Pearl Chain" Formation

Deformation

Movement

Destruction

Summary of various mechanisms caused by field generated forces

Field forces due to the induced dipole moment of the field
have been listed as evidence of nonthermal action of electric
fields on biologic systems. However, the effects require fairly
large field strengths, frequently above those that give rise to
heating or stimulation of excitable tissues. The field forces
also depend on the electric properties of the particle considered
and its environment.

A more detailed derivation of the dielectrophoretic force in
lossy dielectric media has been given by Sher (52) and is based
in turn on a derivation of the potential electric energy of a
lossy dielectric body given by Schwarz (53).

All sorts of biological particles of different effective
complex dielectric constants behave similarly in an electrolyte
medium. Figure 5 illustrates this fact. Neumann and Rosenheck's
(40) results on chromaffin vesicles are combined with E. coli
data obtained by Sher and erythrocyte data obtained by Sher and
silicon particles (full circles), also by Sher (45). The total
material fits convincingly the solid line of slope -1.5 which
is demanded by the theoretical requirement that particle volume
must be inversely related to the square of the threshold field
strength mentioned above and discussed in greater detail elsewhere (Schwan and Sher (54)).

The dashed curves in Figure 5 pertain to another model. It
is assumed that the threshold of a cellular response or destruction is reached when the induced membrane potential reaches the
dielectric breakthrough level. This level may well be in the
range of 0.1 to 1 V across the membrane, corresponding to membrane field strength levels from 100 KV/cm to one million V/cm.
The inverse relationship of the threshold field level in the
medium with the particle diameter follows from the equation
ΔV_M = 1.5 ER already quoted in Table IV. The dashed curves establish threshold particle relationships somewhat similar to
those resulting from a consideration of field-generated forces.
Hence, it may at times be difficult to separate biological effects due to field-generated forces from those due to induced
high membrane potentials.

In general, available evidence and present understanding
indicate that significant effects with field-evoked forces require field strength values above 1 V/cm in the medium, unless
cellular dimensions are well above 100 μm.

Possibility of Weak Nonthermal Interactions

The considerations presented above do not suggest any weak
nonthermal mechanism by which biological systems could react to
low-intensity microwave fields. It requires fields of the order
of a few kV/cm to orient long biopolymers, and probably still
higher fields to excite internal vibrations or produce submolecular orientation. External fields acting on biopolymers must
further overcome strong local fields, which are 1.5 kV/cm at a

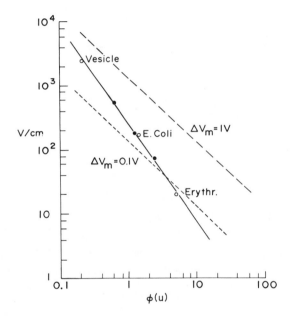

Figure 5.   *Threshold field strength values as a function of particle size (49).*

(———) *Field-generated force effects; (– – –) damage resulting from membrane breakdown at the quoted membrane potentials of 0.1 and 1 V; (○) results obtained with biological cells; and (●) data with silicone particles. The data fit the theoretical demand indicated by (———) and appear to be insensitive to the dielectric properties of the particles.*

distance of 100 Angstroms from a monovalent ion and 1.8 kV/cm at
the same distance from a hemoglobin molecule. Microwave frequencies are well above those corresponding to significant rotational
diffusion times, excluding orientational effects. Transmembrane
potentials induced by typical nonthermal microwave fields are
vanishingly small relative to potentials required for stimulation
and compare with membrane noise. Field induced force effects are
unlikely to be significant on a single molecular or cellular
level, since the threshold field strengths necessary to overcome
thermal disturbances are too high (49).

However, some principles emerge regarding possible mechanisms of weak microwave interaction, if such a concept exists.
Field force effects become more probable as the volume of the
exposed particle increases (49). Transmembrane potentials become
larger for a given in situ field strength as the cell size is increased. Finally, molecules can become significantly reoriented
by the field if $\mu E \geq kT$, (where μ is the dipole moment, E the
field strength, k is the Boltzman constant, and T is the absolute
temperature). Thus larger physical dimensions or larger permanent or induced dipole moments are more likely to respond to weak
fields.

The large dimensions necessary for biological responses to
weak microwave fields might be achieved by a cooperative reaction
of a number of cells or macromolecules to the microwave stimulus,
which increases the effective size of the structure and corres-
pondingly reduces the threshold that is required for an effect.
Adey suggested that such cooperativity might be induced in the
counterions loosely bound near membrane surfaces which contain
a loose frame work of charged polysaccharides (32).

Froehlich has suggested (55, 56) that giant dipole moments
may be formed during enzyme substrate reactions and that the
corresponding dielectric absorption processes might be highly
resonant and nonlinear, and likely to channel energy into lower
frequency modes of vibration. He also considered the membrane
as a likely site of resonant electromagnetic (EM) interactions,
and derived an estimate of the resonant frequencies from the
velocity of sound and the membrane thickness to be of the order
of 100 GHz. Acceleration and deceleration of a variety of biological responses which suggest resonances have been reported by
Webb (57), Devyatkov (58), and, more recently, by Grundler et al.
(59) in the millimeter frequency range. But some of these
studies have been criticized on technical grounds, and the Rus-
sian work, only summarized in 1974, has not yet been published
in detail. Gandhi has conducted continuous dielectric spectroscopy measurements at millimeter-wave frequencies with no indica-
tions of any resonance processes (60). He also found no effects
of millimeter-wave radiation on a variety of cellular processes
which were not attributable to sample heating. But the resonance
phenomena reported by Grundler and Keilmann and postulated by
Froehlich may only involve a minor fraction of the total cellular

entity and, hence, not demonstrate itself strongly enough to be
observed in the bulk dielectric data.

Abstract

The dielectric properties of tissues and cell suspensions
will be summarized for the total frequency range from a few Hz
to 20 GHz. Three pronounced relaxation regions at ELF, RF and
MW frequencies are due to counterion relaxation and membrane in-
vaginations, to Maxwell-Wagner effects, and to the frequency dependent properties of normal water at microwave frequencies.
Superimposed on these major dispersions are fine structure effects caused by cellular organelles, protein bound water, polar
tissue proteins, and side chain rotation.

Insight into the biophysical mechanism of EM-field interactions is gained from the understanding of these dielectric
properties. At ELF frequencies cells sample the external field
over their dimensions and apply the resulting potential to the
membranes with cut-off frequencies extending up to the RF range.
Tissue water appears to be identical in its dielectric properties
with normal water, except for a small fraction of protein bound
water. Field effects on large biopolymers are indicated only at
field values above 10 kV/cm, but field induced dipole effects on
large cells are possible at considerably lower values. More
subtle field interactions with biological matter require either
cooperative interactions or very large dipole moments so far not
yet identified.

Literature Cited

1.   Schwan, H.P. Adv. Biol. Med. Phys., 1957, 5, 147. Academic
     Press: New York.
2.   Takashima, S.; Schwan, H.P. J. Membr. Biol., 1974, 17, 51.
3.   Afsar, M.N.; Hasted, J.B. J. Opt. Soc. Amer., 1977, 67, 902.
4.   Hasted, J.B. "Aqueous Dielectrics"; Chapman and Hall:
     London, England.
5.   Pauly, H.; Schwan, H.P. Biophys. J., 1966, 6, 621.
6.   Herrick. J.F.; Jelatis, D.G.; Lee, G.M. Fed. Proc., 1950,
     9, 60.
7.   Schwan, H.P.; Foster, K.R. Biophys. J., 1977, 17, 193.
8.   Foster, K.R.; Schepps, J.L.; Schwan, H.P. Biophys. J., 1980,
     29, 271.
9.   Schwan, H.P.; Foster, K.R. Proc. IEEE, 1980, 68, 104.
10. Takashima, S. "Dielectric Properties of Proteins. I. Di-
     electric Relaxation." In: Leach, J.S., Ed. "Physical Prin-
     ciples and Techniques of Protein Chemistry"; Academic Press:
     New York, 1969.
11. Takashima, S.; Minikata, A. "Dielectric Behavior of Biologi-
     cal Macromolecules." In: "Digest of Dielectric Literature";
     National Research Council: Wash., DC, V. 37, 1975, p. 602.

12. Schwan, H.P. Ann. N.Y. Acad. Sci., 1965, 125, 344.
13. Pennock, B.E.; Schwan, H.P. J. Phys. Chem., 1969, 73, 2600.
14. Grant, E.H.; Keefe, S.E.; Takashima, S. J. Phys. Chem., 1968, 72, 4373.
15. Grant, E.H. "Determination of Bound Water in Biological Materials." In: Proc. Workshop Physical Bases of Electromagnetic Interactions with Biological Systems, University of Maryland, 1979, p. 113.
16. Schwan, H.P. "Classical Theory of Microwave Interactions with Biological Systems." In: Proc. Workshop Physical Bases of Electromagnetic Interactions with Biological Systems, University of Maryland, 1977, p. 90.
17. Jones, G.P.; Gregson, M.; Davies, M. Chem. Phys. Lett., 1969, 4, 33.
18. Illinger, K.H. "Millimeter-wave and Far-infrared Absorption in Biological Systems." In: Taylor, L.S.; Cheung, A.Y., Eds., "The Physical Basis of Electromagnetic Interactions with Biological Systems, Proc. Workshop"; University of Maryland, 1977, p. 43.
19. Rosskey, P.J.; Karplus, M. J. Amer. Chem. Soc., 1979, 101, 1913.
20. Froehlich, H. "Theory of Dielectrics"; Oxford University Press: Oxford, England, 1949.
21. Fricke, H. Phys. Rev., 1923, 21, 708.
22. Cole, K.S. "Membranes, Ions and Impulses"; University of California Press: Berkeley, Ca., 1972.
23. Schwan, H.P.; Morowitz, H.J. Biophys. J., 1962, 2, 395.
24. Schwan, H.P.; Takashima, S.; Miyamoto, V.K.; Stoeckenius, W. Biophys. J., 1970, 10, 1102.
25. Pauly, H.; Schwan, H.P. Z. Naturforsch., 1959, 14b, 125.
26. Schwan, H.P. J. Cell Compar. Phys., 1965, 66, 5.
27. Schmitt, F.O.; Dev, P.; Smith, B.H. Science, 1976, 193, 114.
28. Schwan, H.P. NWL Tech. Report, TR-2713, U.S. Naval Weapons Lab.: Dahlgren, Va., 1972.
29. "Biological Effects of Electric and Magnetic Fields Associated with Proposed Project Seafarer"; National Academy of Sciences-National Research Council: Wash., DC, 1977.
30. Schwan, H.P. IEEE Trans., 1971, MTT-19, 146.
31. Kalmijn, A.J. Nature, 1966, 212, 1232.
32. Bawin, S.M.; Adey, W.R. Proc. Nat. Acad. Sci. USA, 1976, 73, 1999.
33. Gavalas-Medici, R.; Day-Magdaleno, S.R. Nature, 1976, 261, 265.
34. Baranski, S.; Czerski, P. "Biological Effects of Microwaves"; Dowden, Hutchinson and Ross., Inc.: Stroudsburg, Pa. 1976.
35. Frey, A.H. IEEE Trans., 1971, MTT-19, 153.
36. Bawin, S.M.; Adey, W.R. Neurosci. Res. Prog. Bull., 1977, 15, 1.
37. Roy, O.Z.; Scott, J.R.; Park, G.C. IEEE Trans., 1976, BME-23, 45.

38. Driscoll, D.A. "An Investigation of a Theoretical Model of
     the Human Head with Application to Current Flow Calculations
     and EEG Interpretation"; Ph.D. Thesis, University of Vermont,
     1970.
39. Zimmerman, U.; Pilwat, G.; Riemann, R. Biophys. J., 1974,
     14, 881.
40. Neumann, E.; Rosenheck, K. J. Memb. Biol., 1972, 10, 279.
41. Friend, A.W.; Finch, E.D.; Schwan, H.P. Science, 1974, 187,
     357.
42. Goodman, E.M.; Greenebaum, B.; Marron, M.T. "Effects of
     Extremely Low Frequency Electromagnetic Fields on Growth
     and Differentiation of Physarum polycephalum"; Technical
     Report Phase I (Continuous Wave), University of Wisconsin,
     1975.
43. Goodman, E.M.; Greenebaum, B.; Marron, M.T. "Effects of
     Extremely Low Frequency Electromagnetic Fields on Physarum
     polycephalum"; Technical Report, Office of Naval Research,
     Contract N-00014-76-C-0180, Univ. of Wisconsin, 1976.
44. Teixeira-Pinto, A.A.; Nejelski, L.L.; Cutler, J.L.; Heller,
     J.H. Exp. Cell Res., 1960, 20, 548.
45. Sher, L.L. Ph.D. Thesis, "Mechanical Effects of AC Fields
     on Particles Dispersed in a Liquid: Biological Implica-
     tions"; University of Pennsylvania: Philadelphia, Pa. 1963.
46. Novak, B.; Bentrup, F.W. Biophysik, 1973, 9, 253.
47. Pohl, H.A. J. Biol. Phys., 1973, 1, 1.
48. Elul, R. J. Physiol., 1967, 189, 351.
49. Schwan, H.P. Ann. N.Y. Acad. Sci., 1977, 303, 198.
50. Blakemore, R. Science, 1975, 190, 377.
51. Sher, L.D.; Kresch, E.; Schwan, H.P. Biophys. J., 1970,
     10, 970.
52. Sher, L.D. Nature, 1968, 220, 695.
53. Schwarz, G. J. Chem. Phys., 1963, 39, 2387.
54. Schwan, H.P.; Sher, L.D. J. Electrochem. Soc., 1969, 116, 170.
55. Froehlich, H. Proc. Nat. Acad. Sci. USA, 1975, 72, 4211.
56. Froehlich, H. Coll. Phen., 1973, 1, 101.
57. Webb, S.J.; Booth, A.D. Science, 1971, 174, 72.
58. Devyatkov, N.D. Sov. Phys. USPEKHI, 1974, 16, 568 (Transl.).
59. Grundler, W.; Keilmann, F.; Froehlich, H. Phys. Lett., 1977,
     62A, 463.
60. Gandhi, O.P.; Hagmann, M.J.; Riazi, A.; Hill, D.W.; Partlow,
     L.M. "Millimeter Wave and Raman Spectra of Living Cells -
     Some Problems and Results"; presented at the Workshop on
     Mechanisms of Microwave Biological Effects, University of
     Maryland, May 14-16, 1979.
61. Schwan, H.P. "Dielectric Properties of Biological Materials
     and Interaction of Microwave Fields at the Cellular and
     Molecular Level"; In: Michaelson, S.M.; Miller, M.W., Eds.
     "Fundamental and Applied Aspects of Nonionizing Radiation";
     Plenum Publ. Co.: New York, 1975.

RECEIVED October 31, 1980.

Frequency Response of Membrane Components in Nerve Axon

SHIRO TAKASHIMA

Department of Bioengineering/D2, University of Pennsylvania, Philadelphia, PA 19104

The mechanism of nerve excitation is well documented phenomenologically by the Hodgkin-Huxley equation (1,2,3). According to this empirical formulation, the nerve impulse is generated by two types of non-linear currents, i.e., inward sodium
and outward potassium currents. The magnitudes of these currents
are controlled by the membrane potential, indicating that there
are voltage sensing mechanisms somewhere in the membrane. First
of all, the bulk of nerve membranes is hydrophobic. Therefore,
for the charged sodium and potassium ions to flow across the
membrane, there must be special regions in the membrane which
have polar groups projecting into them. These polar regions
have been called ionic channels. They are highly specific and
there are two types of channels, one for sodium and another for
potassium ions. These channels are normally closed at the
resting state and, therefore, no ions can flow through them.
However, when electrical stimuli are applied, the field
is detected by the voltage sensor which, in turn, sends a
command to the gate to open. It is still debatable whether
there is a voltage sensor which is separate from the channel
gate itself. Nevertheless, the field sensing device, including
the gate or gating particles, must be a group of charged particles or a group of molecules having dipole moments. If the
gating particle is a charged molecule, the opening of gates
must be an electrophoretic movement of these charges. If the
gate is a group of dipole moments, the opening of channels must
be an orientation of these dipolar species. Of these, dipole
orientation has been preferred by neurophysiologists as the
possible mechanism of channel opening. In any case, the opening
of channels is initiated by the change of the field in the membrane and the rate of the opening is controlled by the frequency
response or relaxation time of gating particles.
Of the two different types of ionic channels, the opening
of sodium channels is considered as the first step of nerve
excitation. The opening of potassium channels is a delayed response and lags behind that of sodium channels. There are

0097-6156/81/0157-0133$05.00/0

roughly two ways to investigate the mechanism of channel opening. One method is to study the gating current in the time domain and the other is to measure voltage dependent membrane capacitance in the frequency domain. Measurements of gating currents in the time domain have been done by several groups (4-9). The magnitude of the gating current is small and is of the order of 20-40 $\mu A/cm^2$. Because of their small magnitude, both sodium and potassium currents must be either reduced or blocked by various means, including use of tetrodotoxin (TTX). Based on the analyses done by these people, the gating current is believed to be due to sodium channels rather than potassium channels. The gating current due to potassium channels was reported by Armstrong (10) recently. The time constant of the gating current is approximately 80 to 110 μsec and is almost independent of membrane potentials. Therefore, the opening of sodium channels is a slow process having a frequency response of a few kilo-hertz.

The other experiments, i.e., frequency domain measurements of membrane capacitance and its voltage dependence, have been done by various investigators (11-18). The rationale behind these experiments is the following. If there are dipolar particles in the membrane and if they are capable of orienting in response to applied fields, this movement must manifest itself as a frequency dependent membrane capacitance, the indication of the presence of relaxation processes. Therefore, the initial step in this series of experiments is to establish the membrane capacitance in a wide frequency range and confirm the presence of frequency dependent capacitance. Secondly, if application of an external voltage causes dislocation of gating particles from resting position to open position, this must manifest itself in the change in the magnitude of capacitance and its frequency dependence. Since time domain measurements indicate the existence of gating currents, i.e., essentially a capacitive current, membrane capacitance must change upon application of electrical pulses.

As is well known, biological membranes consist of two major components, i.e., lipids and proteins. Although the progress in the research on membrane proteins is very slow, investigators are beginning to find that there are a variety of proteins in biological membranes having molecular weights ranging from 20,000 to 300,000. Moreover, even the lipid part is not uniform and monodisperse. There are several different types of lipids in biological membranes which form a bilayer structure. Under these circumstances, it is wise to start the investigation of membrane impedance by using simple systems rather than complex natural membranes. Artificial lipid membranes, which resemble biological membranes except for the absence of proteins, are readily available these days (19,20). Their physical and electrical characteristics are well documented and these membranes are quite suitable for the study of membrane capacitance and its frequency dispersion.

Membrane Capacitance of Artificial Membranes

The techniques used to form lipid bilayer membranes are discussed by Mueller and Rudin (19) in detail. In their methods, lipids are dissolved in alkane solvents and the solution is painted to an aperture on the wall of a teflon cup. The entire cup is immersed in an electrolyte solution such as NaCl or KCl. The thickness of the membrane, which is multi-layered at the beginning, will reduce with time and finally a bilayer membrane is formed with a thickness of 30 to 60A depending upon the length of non-polar tails of lipid molecules. Some solvents such as n-decane are miscible with lipids and form mixed membranes. However, some other solvents, such as hexadecane, separate from lipid molecules when membranes are formed. Either solvent molecules form micro-lenses on the surface of the membrane or they accumulate in the torus region at the edge. In either case, the presence of solvent molecules produces certain errors. However, as will be discussed later, use of hexadecane is much better than n-decane for our purpose. Thus, our experiments were all carried out using hexadecane as the solvent. Although we used several lipids, such as oxidized cholesterol, sphingomyelin and egg-lecithin, we will illustrate only the results obtained with egg-lecithin and hexadecane.

Membrane capacitance and conductance were measured using the Wayne-Kerr admittance bridge and measurements were made between 100 Hz and 20 KHz using a PAR lock-in amplifier model 124. One of the results obtained is shown in Figure 1. The dotted curve shown in this figure indicates measured values at high frequencies and the downward slope arises from the presence of electrolyte solutions between the membrane and electrodes. The error due to series resistance was already discussed in detail by Takashima and Schwan (15). The solid line is obtained after the correction for this error using the method described previously.

First of all, the capacitance of lecithin-hexadecane membrane is about 0.62 $\mu F/cm^2$. This value is smaller than the capacitance of biological membranes, i.e., 1 $\mu F/cm^2$. The difference is perhaps partially due to the absence of proteins in artificial membranes. In addition, it is known that the presence of solvents decreases the values of membrane capacitance. For example, membranes formed by the Montal-Mueller Method (21), which are believed to be free of solvents, have a capacitance of 0.7 $\mu F/cm^2$ (22). Thus, the capacitance of bilayer membranes shown in this figure may be in error by about 0.1 $\mu F/cm^2$ because of the presence of solvent molecules. However, it is more important to note that membrane capacitance is independent of frequency, which provides unequivocal evidence that there is no relaxation process in lipid membranes in this frequency range. Coster and Smith (23) reported that they observed a frequency dispersion of membrane capacitance of artificial layers at very

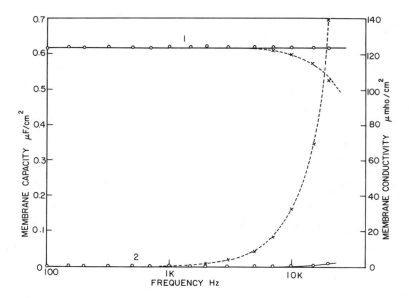

Figure 1.   Membrane capacitance and conductance of lecithin bilayers. Curve 1:
*membrane capacitance ((−− × −−) measured values at high frequencies before
correction for series resistance); Curve 2: membrane conductance ((−− × −−)
measured conductances without correction for series resistance).*

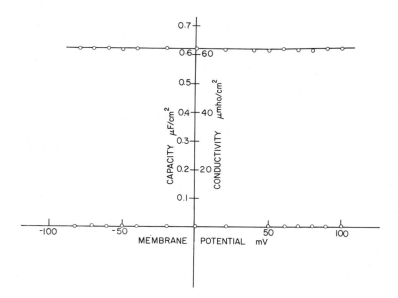

Figure 2.   Membrane capacitance (Curve 1) and conductance (Curve 2) at different
membrane potentials

low frequencies below 10 Hz. However, the meaning of this dispersion is not clearly known and it may have been due to the presence of solvent molecules which tend to form some type of boundaries within the membrane. The characteristic frequencies of sodium and potassium currents are of the order of 200 Hz to 3 KHz. As has been discussed, lipid bilayers do not exhibit any relaxation processes in this frequency range, indicating that lipid molecules may not play an important role in the permeation of ions through ionic channels.

The voltage dependence of lipid bilayer capacitance has been studied by White and Thompson (24). They noted that the presence of n-decane in these membranes gives rise to a false voltage dependence of membrane capacitance. On the other hand, Latorre et al. (25), using solvent-free membranes, demonstrated that the capacitance of these membranes is only negligibly dependent on external voltages. Unlike the experiments by White and Thompson, we used hexadecane instead of n-decane as the solvent. The capacitances of lecithin bilayers at various membrane potentials are shown in Figure 2. Clearly, membrane capacitance is independent of applied potentials, indicating that 1) the presence of hexadecane does not produce a voltage dependent capacitance and 2) the membrane capacitance of lecithin bilayers is itself independent of external potential. As stated before, hexadecane does not form mixed membranes with lecithin and they are spatially separated when the membrane is formed. This may be the reason why hexadecane does not produce the artifact as n-decane does. In any event, these observations clearly indicate that lecithin bilayer does not exhibit a frequency dependent capacitance between 100 Hz and 20 KHz and externally applied potentials have no effect on the membrane capacitance.

Membrane Capacitance of Nerve Membrane

Giant axons from squid have a large diameter ranging from 300 to 700 μm. Because of this large size, we are able to insert metal electrodes directly into the axon and measure capacitance and conductance across the membrane. This is the most unequivocal method to measure transmembrane capacitance and is far better than the use of external electrodes as done previously by Cole and Curtis (11). In spite of the simplicity and ease of this technique, there are still a few unsolved problems which will be discussed later. Figure 3 shows one of the exemplary results of nerve membrane capacitance and conductance measurements. Comparison of this result with the one shown in Figure 2 readily demonstrates that there are considerable differences between these two sets of curves.

First of all, membrane capacitance of nerves has a negative frequency dependence below 300 Hz, namely capacitance increases with frequency in this region. This is a behavior which cannot be explained by a simple RC circuit and indicates the presence

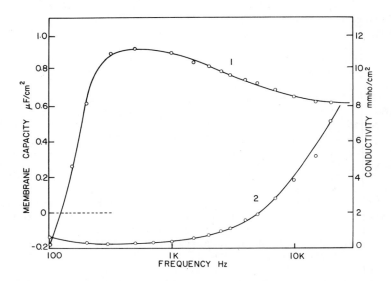

Figure 3.   Membrane capacity (Curve 1) and conductivity (Curve 2) of squid giant axon at various frequencies. Note anomalous behavior at low frequencies.

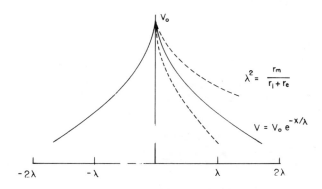

Figure 4.   Schematic of the field distribution at various distances from the point of current injection: λ is the space constant, r_m, r_i, and r_e are membrane resistance and resistances of internal and external media, respectively. The dimension of r_m is ohm cm; those of r_i and r_e are ohms.

of an inductive element in the membrane (26). Membrane capacitance reaches a peak value of 1 $\mu F/cm^2$ between 300 Hz and 1 KHz.
This is the value of capacitance which has been accepted univer-
sally for most biological membranes (26,27). Above this frequency, membrane capacitance dereases from 1 $\mu F/cm^2$ to approximately 0.6 $\mu F/cm^2$ between 1 and 20 KHz. This gradual decrease
may be, at least partially, due to a real dispersion of membrane
capacitance. However, there is disturbing evidence that a portion of this frequency dependent capacitance is due to a fringe
effect at the tip of the internal axial electrode.

Suppose one injects a current at one point of the membrane,
and monitors the voltage along the x-coordinate of the axon. The
peak voltage values will decay exponentially along the fiber as
shown in Figure 4. Thus,

$$V(x) = V(0) \exp - \left| x/\lambda \right|$$

where $V(0)$ and $V(x)$ are the peak voltages at x and 0. λ is the
space constant and is given by:

$$\lambda^2 = \frac{r_m}{r_1 + r_2} \qquad (1)$$

where r_m, r_1, and r_2 are membrane resistance and resistances of
internal and external media of the axon.

If the voltage at the tip of the internal electrode is
$V(0)$, the field will taper off according to eq. (1), giving rise
to an axial component in addition to the radial distribution of
the field. Therefore, the magnitude of the fringe capacitance
depends on the space constant, which in turn is a function of
membrane resistance r_m. Furthermore, the space constant is
known to depend on frequency (28) and decreases with increasing
frequencies. Thus, the stray capacitance due to fringe effect
decreases as the frequency increases. Accordingly, the presence
of fringe effect at the tip of the internal electrode produces a
frequency dependent capacitance. The frequency dependence of
membrane capacitance as shown in Figure 4 is, therefore, at least
partially due to the fringe effect at the tip of the internal
electrode. In order to reduce the relative contribution of stray
capacitance, we use a long internal electrode with a length of
27 qm. As shown in Figure 5, the membrane capacitance per unit
area is shown at various lengths of the internal electrode. For
example, if the length of the internal electrode is 5 mm (Point
1), the membrane capacity per unit area becomes as large as
2 $\mu F/cm^2$ due to the presence of a relatively large stray capacitance. However, if the length of the internal electrode is 27mm,
the capacitance per unit area decreases to 0.9 $\mu F/cm^2$ because
the stray capacitance contributes a relatively small value.

Since the results shown in Figure 4 were obtained with a

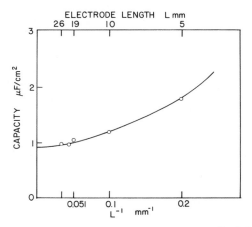

Figure 5.   Membrane capacity per unit area of squid giant axon as a function of the length of the electrodes (29) ((upper scale) electrode length in mm; (lower scale) inverse of length in mm⁻¹)

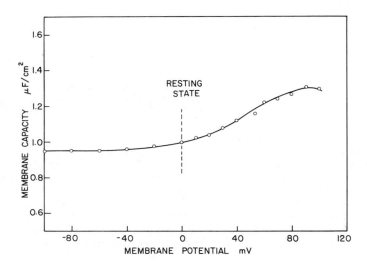

Figure 6.   Membrane capacitance of squid giant axon at various membrane potentials. Membrane potential was shifted by injecting currents. The abscissa shows actual potential across the membrane in mV.

long internal electrode (27 mm), the relative contribution of
stray capacitance is small. It may be safe, therefore, to conclude that the frequency dependence of measured capacitance is
due to a real dispersion of membrane capacitance. Once the frequency dependence of membrane capacitance is established, the
time constant or characteristic frequency of the relaxation
within the membrane can be easily determined. As can be seen,
the center frequency is about 3 KHz, which gives rise to a time
constant of 53 μsec.

The origin of the frequency dependent membrane capacitance
is not well understood, although it is likely to be due to membrane proteins. However, there are a variety of proteinous components in the membrane and most of them are not directly related
to ionic channels. Therefore, it is virtually impossible to
physically separate the capacitance due to gating proteins from
capacitances due to other proteins. However, if the frequency
dependent capacitance is related to gate proteins, the capacitance must change with an increase or decrease in the membrane
potential. It is known that ionic channels are not tightly
closed at the resting state (membrane potential near −60 mV).
Only when the membrane potential is reduced to −120 mV, are all.
ionic channels nearly completely closed, and the membrane becomes
really passive. Under these circumstances, the membrane will be
tightly packed and proteins as well as lipids will be locked
into a tightly constrained state leading to a small capacitance.
Figure 6 shows the membrane capacitances at various potentials.
As one can see, the membrane capacitance at −60 mV (resting
state) is 0.95 μF/cm^2, while hyper-polarized membrane has an
even smaller capacitance. On the other hand, ionic channels
open with depolarization, i.e., channel proteins become relatively free to rotate because of removal of the negative bias
voltage. Therefore, the membrane capacitance must increase with
depolarizing potentials if the contribution of gating proteins
to membrane capacitance is significant. As shown in this figure, clearly the membrane capacitance increases when the membrane
potential decreases from −60 mV to smaller values. It is important to note that the increase in capacitance reaches a peak
value at a potential of +20 mV. This is the value of the membrane potential when sodium channels are almost wide open.
Beyond this value, the magnitude of sodium current begins to
decrease. The peak value of membrane capacitance around 20–30
mV clearly reflects the behavior of sodium channels.

From these observations, it became apparent that the frequency dependent capacitance must be due, at least partially,
to gating particles, and, in particular, to those of sodium
channels. If the capacitance change shown in Figure 6 is indeed
due to sodium channels, then the change must be affected by TTX,
which is known to block sodium channels selectively. Figure 7
shows the membrane capacitance at various potentials. As can
be seen, TTX effectively eliminates the voltage dependence of

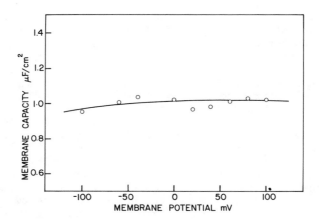

Figure 7.   Membrane capacitance of squid giant axon at various membrane potentials. The external medium contained 3×10^{-7}M TTX in order to block the sodium current.

the membrane potential, offering unequivocal evidence that the
voltage dependent capacitance is due to sodium channels.

From these observations, we can draw the following conclusions. 1) The membrane capacitance of nerve axon is dependent
upon frequency, indicating the presence of a relaxation process
in the membrane even at rest. 2) The membrane capacitance decreases with hyperpolarization, when the membrane has a tightly
packed structure. 3) The membrane capacitance increases with
depolarization, when ionic channels are wide open. 4) The
voltage dependent capacitance is due to sodium channels.

It is well known that both sodium and potassium currents
through nerve membranes are slow processes having a frequency
response of a few kilo-hertz or less. However, there are at
least two possibilities behind this observation. 1) The frequency response of channels is fast, but ionic currents are
diffusion limited. That is, the rate of channel opening is fast,
but diffusion of ions is slow and rate limiting. 2) Opening and
closing of ionic channels are intrinsically slow and rate
limiting. Case (1) suggests the presence of fast components in
nerve membrane. In this case, high frequency perturbation may
interfere with the excitation mechanism. However, as has been
discussed, the characteristic frequency of channel proteins is
in the range of a few kilo-hertz. Under these circumstances,
opening or closing of ionic channels may be the rate limiting
step in the nerve excitation. In this case, external high frequency fields will have no effect on nerve excitation unless they
cause substantial retardation of ionic movements.

These considerations lead us to a conclusion that nerve excitation is a very slow process and the membrane does not contain elements which has a frequency response of MHz or GHz. The
only molecular species which may have such a frequency response
are water molecules. However, the role of water in nerve excitation is totally unknown and does not offer, at present, any evidence for the possible mechanism of interaction between microwaves and nerve membranes.

The author is supported by ONR N00076-C-0642. The author
is indebted to Dr. H. P. Schwan for his valuable suggestions.

Abstract

The frequency response of various chemical constituents of
nerve membrane was studied. Biological membranes in general
consist of lipids and proteins. Firstly, impedance characteristics of artificial lipid bilayer membranes are examined using
lecithin-hexadecane preparations. It was observed that the
capacitance of plain lipid membranes was independent of frequency
between 100 Hz and 20 KHz. Moreover, application of external
voltages has no effect up to 200 mV. Secondly, membrane capacitance and conductance of nerve axon were investigated. There are
three components in nerve membranes, i.e., conductance, capaci-

tance and inductance. Of these, inductive elements are known to
arise from K$^+$ current. The remaining components, capacitance
and conductance, have a characteristic frequency of 2-3 KHz, indicating the presence of structures which undergo a relaxation in
this frequency range. Furthermore, the capacitance of nerve membrane depends on membrane potential, increasing with depolarization and decreasing with hyperpolarization. Therefore, the
frequency dependent capacitance may be due to dipolar components
in or near ionic channels. These observations clearly show that
the components which are related to nerve excitation have a frequency response of a few kilohertz. Therefore, it us unlikely
that high frequency fields of MHz or GHz interfere with these
slow processes.

Literature Cited

1. Hodgkin, A.L. and Huxley, A.F. J. Physiol., 1952, 117, 500.
2. Adelman, W.L. "Biophysics and Physiology of Excitable Mem-
    branes"; Van Nostrand-Reinhold: New York, 1971.
3. Plonsey, R. "Bioelectric Phenomena"; McGraw-Hill Publ. Co.:
    New York, 1969.
4. Armstrong, A.M. and Bezanilla, F. Nature, 1973, 242, 459.
5. Bezanilla, F. and Armstrong, A.M. Science, 1974, 183, 753.
6. Keynes, R.D. and Rojas, E. J. Physiol., 1974, 239, 393.
7. Keynes, R.D. and Rojas, E. J. Physiol., 1976, 255, 157.
8. Meves, H. J. Physiol., 1974, 243, 847.
9. Nonner, W., Rojas, E. and Stampfli, R. Pflugers Arch. Ges.
    Physiol., 1975, 354, 1.
10. Gilly, W.R. and Armstrong, A.M. Biophys. J., 1980, 29, 485.
11. Cole, K.S. and Curtis, H. J. Gen. Physiol., 1941, 22, 649.
12. Cole, K.K. and Curtis, H. J. Gen. Physiol., 1941, 25, 29.
13. Taylor, R.E. J. Cell. Comp. Physiol., 1965, 66, 21.
14. Matsumoto, N., Inoue, I. and Kishimoto, U. Japanese J.
    Physiol., 1970, 20, 516.
15. Takashima, S. and Schwan, H.P. J. Membrane Biol., 1974, 17,
    51.
16. Takashima, S. J. Membrane Biol., 1976, 27, 21.
17. Takashima, S., Yantorno, R. and Novack, R. Biochim. Biophys.
    Acta, 1977, 469, 74.
18. Fishman, H.M., Moore, L.E. and Poussart, D.J.M. Biophys. J.,
    1977, 19, 177.
19. Mueller, P., Rudin, D.O., Tien, H.T. and Westcott, W.C.
    Nature (London), 1962, 194, 979.
20. Mueller, P. and Rudin, D.O. "Lab-Tech. in Membrane Bio-
    physics"; Passaw, H. and Stampfli, R., Eds., Springer-Verlag:
    Berlin, 1969.
21. Montal, M. and Mueller, P. Proc. Natl. Acad. Sci. USA, 1972,
    69, 3561.
22. White, S. Biochim. Biophys. Acta, 1968, 196, 354.

23. Coster, H.G.L. and Smith, J.R.   Biochim. Biophys. Acta,
     1964, 373, 151.
24. White, S. and Thompson, T.E.   Biochim. Biophys. Acta, 1973,
     323, 7.
25. Alvarez, O. and Latorre, R.   Biophys. J., 1978, 21, 1.
26. Cole, K.S.   "Membrane, Ions and Impulses"; University of
     California Press: Berkeley, Ca., 1968.
27. Schwan, H.P.   "Electrical Properties of Tissues and Cell
     Suspensions"; Advances in Biol. and Med. Phys.; Lawrence,
     J.H. and Tobias, C.A., Eds., Academic Press: New York, 1957.
28. Tasaki, I. and Hagiwara, S.   Am. J. Physiol., 1957, 188,
     423.
29. Takashima, S. and Yantorno, R. In "Electrical Properties of
     Biological Polymers, Water, and Membranes"; Takashima, S.,
     Ed.; N.Y. Acad. Sci.: New York, 1977, 309.

RECEIVED October 31, 1980.

A Perturbation Model for Electromagnetic-Field Interaction with Excitable Cellular Membranes

CHARLES A. CAIN

Department of Electrical Engineering, Bioacoustics Research Laboratory,
University of Illinois at Urbana–Champaign, Urbana, IL 61801

Voltage sensitive ion channels for Na^+, K^+, and Ca^{++} in the lipid bilayer membrane of excitable cells are protein macromolecules with several intraconvertible conformations, one of which is open and the others closed or nonconducting. Charged or dipolar components of the channel protein (or protein complex) move in response to perturbation of the membrane electric field and act as voltage sensors which trigger "gating" or conformational substates resulting in the channel being either open or closed. Graded changes in membrane conductance is the result of the average behavior of a large number of channels which open or close stochastically in response to changes in the electric field within the lipid bilayer and background thermal agitation.

Some ion channels are exquisitely sensitive to small perturbations in the membrane electrostatic field. Moreover, the probability of a channel being in a given state is a highly nonlinear function of the applied electric field. Because of these nonlinearities, it will be shown that an alternating (AC) electric field might bias the probability of the channel being in a given state. The possibility that the voltage sensing charges (or dipoles) incur a steady or DC displacement in an alternating electric field is the basis for the theory discussed herein. The model predicts that an AC field of sufficient magnitude will affect the average conductance of the membrane to particular ion species. The resulting biological effect would depend on the magnitude of the conductance changes and the physiological function of the affected channel.

A model, based on a perturbation analysis of the highly successful empirical formulation of Hodgkin and Huxley (1), has been developed which makes predictions of the effect of oscillating fields on a particular nerve membrane system (2). In the present paper, a theoretical model will be presented along with some of the predicted effects of AC electric fields on the Hodgkin-Huxley (HH) model of squid axon membranes.

0097-6156/81/0157-0147$05.00/0

Theory

A Channel Model. Consider a two state <u>voltage</u> <u>sensor</u> for an ionic channel illustrated diagramatically as

$$
A \underset{\xrightarrow{\hspace{2cm} b(V) \hspace{0.5cm}}}{\xleftarrow{\hspace{2cm} a(V) \hspace{2cm}}} B
$$

(closed)   b(V)   (open)

where rate constants a(V) and b(V) are functions of membrane potential. Assume Q(V) is the equivalent charge carried across the membrane when a voltage sensor moves (rotates?) from A to B. Let η_o be the occupancy of state B [fraction of voltage sensitive dipoles or charged groups in the open state] and let η_c be the occupancy of state A. If pressure and temperature remain unchanged, an equilibrium constant defined as $K = \eta_c/\eta_o$ will be a function only of membrane potential. From first principles of thermodynamics [e.g., see Schwarz (3)]:

$$\frac{d \ln(K)}{dV} = \frac{Q(V)}{kT} \tag{1}.$$

Assume for simplicity that Q(V) = constant = Ze where e is the elementary charge and Z is a positive number. Integrating Eq. (1) then gives

$$K = \frac{\eta_c}{\eta_o} = \exp[Ze(V-\overline{V})/kT]$$

where $\overline{V}$ is the membrane potential at which K = 1 [or $\eta_c = \eta_o$]. This is immediately recognizable as the Boltzmann relation. Moreover, since $\eta_o + \eta_c = 1$, then

$$\eta_o(V) = \frac{1}{1 + \exp[-Ze(V-\overline{V})/kT]} \tag{2}$$

and

$$\eta_c(V) = \frac{1}{1 + \exp[+Ze(V-\overline{V})/kT]} \tag{3}.$$

Thus, the fraction of voltage sensors in a given state can be calculated if the membrane potential is known.

Now, assume the actual opening and closing of the 2-state channel is a first order process such that

$$
A \underset{\xrightarrow{\hspace{2cm} \beta(V) \hspace{0.5cm}}}{\xleftarrow{\hspace{2cm} \alpha(V) \hspace{2cm}}} B
$$

channel   β(V)   channel
open   open

where the rate constants $\alpha(V)$ and $\beta(V)$ depend on the state of the
voltage sensor as follows:

$$\beta(V) = k_1 \eta_o \tag{5}$$

and

$$\alpha(V) = k_2 \eta_o \tag{6}.$$

The constants k_1 and k_2 reflect an assumed direct proportionality
of the rate constants for opening and closing the <u>channel</u> on the
occupancies of the "open" and "closed" states respectively of the
<u>voltage sensor</u>.
    Let p be the fraction of the channels (<u>not</u> voltage sensors)
in the open state. For a first order process, p is the solution
of the differential equation

$$\frac{dp}{dt} = \beta(V) [1-p] - \alpha(V)p \tag{7}.$$

The rate constants α and β determine both the rate of change and
final steady-state value of p. The steady state value of p after
a step input is

$$p_\infty = \frac{\beta(V)}{\alpha(V) + \beta(V)} \tag{8}$$

where p reaches p_∞ exponentially with time constant

$$\tau_p = \frac{1}{\alpha(V) + \beta(V)} \tag{9}.$$

    The preceding model provides the basis for a discussion of
how AC electric fields might interact with a voltage sensitive
ion channel in such a way as to bias the conductance of the channel in a particular direction. In what follows, the basic assumption made is that the voltage sensing process is considerably
faster then the physical opening and closing of the channel. With
this assumption, an AC field which might affect the voltage sensing process would cause a much slower change in channel conductance.

    <u>Sensitivity to an AC Field.</u> Assume the membrane potential
V is replaced by

$$V(t) = V_o + V_m \cos\omega_o t \tag{10}$$

where V_o is the DC membrane potential and V_m is the peak amplitude
of the alternating component of applied membrane potential [see
Barnes and Hu (4) or MacGregor (5)].

If the channel opens or closes with a time constant τ_p and the voltage sensor has a relaxation time τ_{vs}, then assume $\tau_p \gg \tau_{vs}$ and $1/\tau_p \ll \omega_o \leq 1/\tau_{vs}$. If this relationship holds, then η_o, the fraction of voltage sensors in the open state, is given by

$$\eta_o(\omega t) = \cfrac{1}{1 + \exp[\cfrac{-Ze(V_o - \overline{V} + V_m \cos\omega_o t)}{kT}]} \qquad (11).$$

Note that $\eta_o(\omega t)$ is a periodic non-negative function which has an average value given by

$$\overline{\eta}_o = \frac{1}{2\pi} \int_0^{2\pi} \eta_o(\omega t)\,d\omega t \qquad (12).$$

Because of the nonlinear form of Eq. (11), an AC field will cause the average or DC value of $\eta_o(\omega t)$ to shift in a particular direction depending on the unperturbed value of η_o.

Based on the above argument, it is clear that a change in the average value of η_o (or η_c) will bias the rate of opening or closing of a particular channel because of Eqs. (5) and (6). The change in state of the channel will then progress at a rate slower than the voltage sensing processes which triggered the change.

Modified Hodgkin-Huxley Model. In the HH model, the membrane current I, written as a function of V is expressed by the system of coupled equations given in Table I. In these equations V is the displacement of membrane potential from the resting value (depolarization negative). Constants C_M, $\overline{g}_k$, $\overline{g}_{Na}$, $\overline{g}_1$, V_K, V_{Na}, and V_1 are explained in detail in (1). In Table I, $\overline{g}_K n^4$ and $\overline{g}_{Na} m^3 h$ are the potassium and sodium conductances, respectively. The dimensionless dynamical quantities m, n, and h are solutions of the given first order differential equations and vary between zero and unity after a change in membrane potential. The α and β rate constants are assumed to depend only on the instantaneous value of membrane potential.

Note that the equations in Table I have a similar mathematical structure as the much simpler 2-state channel model developed earlier in this paper. One major difference should be emphasized; namely, that the rate constants of the model depend on the physical movement of charge so are not instantaneous functions of membrane potential as assumed in the HH model. However, if the voltage sensing process is sufficiently faster than the dynamics of channel opening and closing, then the assumption of an instantaneous dependence of α's and β's on V is reasonable (see Discussion).

Some Numerical Results. Figure 1 is a plot of the

TABLE I. The Hodgkin–Huxley equations which describe
the relationship between total membrane current I and
transmembrane potential V in the squid giant axon
[see (1)].

$$I = C_M \frac{dV}{dt} + \bar{g}_K n^4 (V - V_K) + \bar{g}_{Na} m^3 h(V - V_{Na}) + \bar{g}_1 (V - V_1)$$

where

$$dn/dt = \alpha_n (1 - n) - \beta_n n$$

$$dm/dt = \alpha_m (1 - m) - \beta_m m$$

$$dh/dt = \alpha_h (1 - h) - \beta_h h$$

and

$$\alpha_n = 0.01(V + 10)/(\exp \frac{V + 10}{10} - 1)$$

$$\beta_n = 0.125 \exp(V/80)$$

$$\alpha_m = 0.1(V + 25)/(\exp \frac{V + 25}{10} - 1)$$

$$\beta_m = 4 \exp(V/18)$$

$$\alpha_h = 0.07 \exp(V/20)$$

$$\beta_h = 1/(\exp \frac{V + 30}{10} + 1)$$

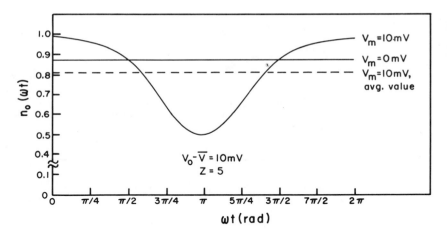

Figure 1.   Instantaneous values of $\eta_o(\omega t)$ when $V_o - \overline{V} = 10$ mV and V_m is 0 mV or 10 mV. $\overline{\eta}_o$, the average value of $\eta_o(\omega t)$ when $V_m = 10$ mV, is shown.

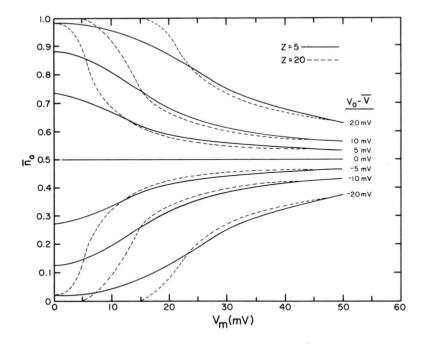

Figure 2.   Average value of $\eta_o(\omega t)$, $\overline{\eta}_o$, as a function of V_m for different values of Z and $V_o - \overline{V}$ ((———) $Z = 5$; (– – –) $Z = 20$)

probability $\eta_o(\omega t)$ of a voltage sensor being in state B (open)
over a full period of the applied alternating membrane potential
of angular frequency ω and peak amplitude V_m of 10 mV. Equation
(11) is evaluated at room temperature [290K where kT/e = 25 mV]
with Z = 5 and at a DC membrane potential 10 mV more positive
than $\overline{V}$ [$V_o - \overline{V} = 10$]. If $V_m = 0$, the probability η_o that the
voltage sensor is in the open state is 0.881 under these condi-
tions. The variation in this probability for nonzero values of
V_m is not symmetric about the unperturbed value of η_o, e.g., the
average value of $\eta_o(\omega t)$, $\overline{\eta}_o$, is 0.808 when $V_m = 10$ as shown with
the dashed line in Fig. 1. Thus an applied AC potential results
in a decrease in the average probability of the voltage sensor
being open.

    Figure 2 shows the changes in $\overline{\eta}_o$ as a function of V_m for
five different values of $V_o - \overline{V}$ with Z = 5 and Z = 20. A graph
of $\overline{\eta}_c$ using the same parameters would look identical to Fig. 2
except that curves for negative values of $V_o - \overline{V}$ would appear at
the top of the drawing. Note that, as one would expect, higher
values of Z result in both steeper changes in η_o with increasing
V_m and a lower threshold for changes to occur. Estimated values
of Z for actual membrane channels range from 3 to 20 (see Discussion).

    A plot of $\overline{\eta}_o$ and $\overline{\eta}_c$ as a function of $V_o - \overline{V}$ with V_m as a
parameter is given in Fig. 3. Thus, an AC field biases the aver-
age occupancy of a particular state of the voltage sensor in a
direction depending on the unpreturbed value of η_o or η_c. Since
the rate constants $\beta(V)$ and $\alpha(V)$ associated with opening and closing of the channel were assumed to be proportional to η_o and η_c,
the respective occupancies of the "open" and "closed" state of the
voltage sensor, then an AC field results in a steady shift in
these rate constants. This would result in a change in the probability of the channel being open for a given DC membrane potential. This effect is the basis for the HH perturbation model
which follows.

    Using the same argument implicit in Eqs. (11) and (12), the
average values of the α and β rate constants of the HH equations
(Table I) will be shifted in an AC field in a way qualitatively
similar to the DC shifts of Fig. 3 [see (2)]. Since the α and β
rate constants determine both the rate of change in m, n, and h
and the final steady state value of these quantities, an AC
field-induced bias of the rate constants will affect g_K and g_{Na}
as well as the membrane potential V [see (2)]. Such an effect
is shown in Fig. 4 where a 10 ms pulsed AC component of membrane
electric field is applied to the model. The change in g_K, g_{Na},
and V in response to the pulse can be obtained by numerically
solving the HH equations (Table I) with initial conditions being
the resting state values for V, m, n, and h. The AC field is
assumed to be applied uniformly along the axon so that dV/dx = 0.
After each iteration through the modified HH equations, new
estimates for the average values of the $\alpha(\omega t)$'s and $\alpha(\omega t)$'s are
obtained numerically.

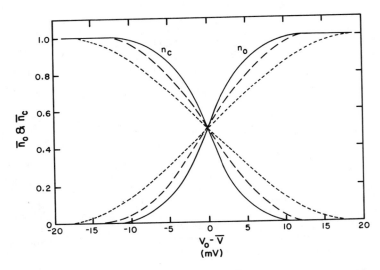

Figure 3.   *Plot of $\overline{\eta}_o$ and $\overline{\eta}_c$ as a function of $V_o - \overline{V}$ for different values of V_m with Z = 10 ((———) $V_m = 0\ mV$; (– – –) $V_m = 5\ mV$; (- - - - -) $V_m = 10\ mV$)*

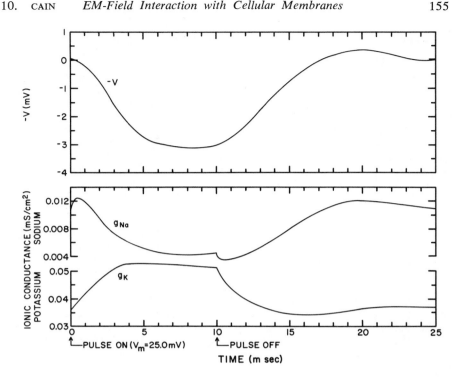

Figure 4.   Solutions of the modified HH equations (see text) with a pulsed alter-nating component of membrane potential. Computed response is for a 10-ms pulse with $V_m = 25$ mV.

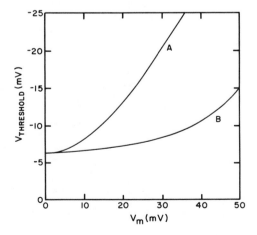

Figure 5.   Threshold depolarization for generating an action potential as a function of V_m. Threshold voltages were determined from the modified HH model. Trace A: V_m applied over interval $-\infty < t < \infty$; .Trace B: V_m applied over interval $0 < t < 10$ ms. Stimulus applied at $t = 0$.

Since an applied AC field produces a steady-state decrease in g_{Na} and an increase in g_K (see Fig. 4), it has a hyperpolarizing or inhibitory effect on the axon. This is illustrated in Fig. 5 where the threshold depolarization required to generate an action potential is plotted vs V_m, the applied AC field. Note that even a pulsed field of 10 ms applied simultaneously with the excitatory depolarization will raise the threshold potential significantly. It should be noted that the effect of an AC field depends on the details of the particular model and is not necessarily inhibitory. It is interesting, however, that an inhibitory effect is opposite to that which would be produced by heating so perhaps could be more readily recognizable experimentally.

Discussion

As pointed out by Hodgkin and Huxley, the extreme steepness of the relation between ionic conductance and membrane potential in the squid giant axon implies the presence in the membrane of polar molecules having large charges or dipole moments (1). In order to explain their experimental results, the equivalent number of electronic charges Z carried across the membrane when a voltage sensor goes from the closed to the open state must be about 6 for activation of the Na^+ channel (1,6). Moreover, at an appropriate static membrane potential, it was determined experimentally that $g_{Na} \propto \exp[v/4.17]$ where v is the displacement from the membrane potential. Thus, a 4 mV depolarization will cause an e-fold increase in sodium conductance. If the voltage sensor is assumed to be a dipole, then the above proportionality becomes $g_{Na} \propto \exp[\mu v/kTd]$ where μ is the dipole moment of the voltage sensor and d is the distance over which v is dropped. If v = 4 mV causes an e-fold change in g_{Na} and d $\simeq$ 100Å (membrane thickness), then at room temperature kT $\simeq 40(10^{-22})$J so that $\mu \simeq 10^{-26}$ C.m. or about 3000 Debye. This is a rather extraordinary dipole moment since μ for an average protein is at least an order of magnitude less, e.g., $\mu \simeq$ 300 D for hemoglobin. When one considers that the voltage sensor most probably occupies a small fraction of the volume of the protein complex comprising the channel, these estimates of the dipole moment of the voltage sensor are even more interesting.

For the simple 2-state channel model discussed earlier, values of Z from 3 to 20 result in estimated dipole moments of the voltage sensor from 1400 to 9600 D respectively. These values of Z span the range of values estimated in the literature for different voltage sensitive ionic channels (6). One consequence of these large values of μ is that it is possible for the electrical energy of interaction between the dipole and the field to be greater than the thermal energy kT at relatively small perturbations in the membrane field (less than 1 mV for some channels). Induced AC fields in membranes from RF or microwave irradiation have been estimated to be this large in some models (4,5).

A key assumption in the theoretical discussion given earlier is that a voltage sensing process exists with a relaxation time (or distribution of times) faster than the fastest time constant for ionic conductance changes. The fastest conductance changes in the squid axon, with time constant τ_m on the order of 100 µs, involve opening of the Na^+ channel or sodium activation ([1]). A voltage sensor with a minimum relaxation time of 100 µs would not respond, in the sense discussed herein, to AC fields of frequency greater than $(2\pi\tau_m)^{-1}$ or about 2 kHz.

Pickard and Rosenbaum, based on several physical arguments, place the upper frequency for possible interaction with the voltage sensors solidly in the microwave region ([7]). On the other hand, in squid ([8],[9],[10]) and a number of other preparations ([11]-[15]), one can detect small asymmetrical displacement currents in response to step changes in membrane potential which, based on a number of lines of evidence ([6]) appear to be associated in some way with the gating process itself. Moreover, in the squid axon Rojas and Keynes ([16]) and Keynes and Rojas ([17]) were able to show that the relaxation time constant of this "gating current" was very nearly τ_m over a broad range of membrane potentials. However, it is not clear whether the measured charge movements are due to reorientation of the voltage sensors directly or to displacement currents attributable to larger protein conformational changes ("gating") triggered by perturbation of the voltage sensors by the applied field. If the latter case is true, this suggests that voltage sensing and ion gating are two separate processes each of which may have different characteristic relaxation times or distribution of times. The assumption of two separate processes is inherent in the 2-state model discussed herein.

Due to certain behaviors anomalous to the HH model obtained from some preparations in voltage clamp experiments ([18],[19]), a number of models have been proposed whereby Na^+ activation and inactivation are coupled into a multistate sequence rather than proceeding independently as suggested by HH m^3h dynamics. For example, consider the following kinetic scheme suggested by Goldman and Hahin ([20])

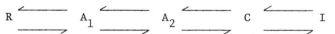

$$R \quad A_1 \quad A_2 \quad C \quad I$$

where R, C, and I are the resting, conducting, and inactivated states respectively and A_1 and A_2 are activated but non-conducting states. In a simulation based on this scheme, it was necessary for one relaxation time to be at least an order of magnitude faster than τ_m in order to fit the time course of sodium conductance during steps in potential ([20]). This kinetic scheme has other interesting consequences. Due to the sequential nature of this model, only one voltage sensor is required as opposed to separate sensors implied for the h and m processes in the HH

model. Furthermore, transition through either or both of the
A states in the above kinetic scheme may directly involve voltage
sensing, a separate process from actual channel gating.
   In another kinetic model suggested by Jakobsson, the conducting state is preceded by an "excited state" which is entered with
a rate constant proportional to the time derivative of membrane
potential (19). Thus, membrane potential perturbations which are
rapid can result in very small relaxation times. This model very
successfully predicts a wide range of voltage clamp data which
are well described by the HH equations as well as behavior anomalous to the HH model which have been seen experimentally. Furthermore, a very rapid initial process may be a necessary condition for any kinetic model to fit some experimental voltage clamp
data which is anomalous to the HH model (E. Jakobsson, personal
communication). Thus, although relaxation times faster than τ_m
relating to channel gating have not been detected experimentally
in asymmetrical displacement current experiments, there are theoretical reasons for expecting that such rapid processes do occur.
   Research on the bioeffects of nerve and muscle exposure to
electromagnetic fields has resulted in a literature filled with
contradicting phenomenology. Thus, a number of researchers have
published evidence which supports (21,22,23,24) or does not support (25,26,27,28) the hypothesis that AC fields can affect excitable cells by nonthermal mechanisms. With few exceptions,
little attention has been given to possible underlying mechanisms
of interaction. It is hoped that this paper will help to provide
a rational basis for design of experiments based on specific
hypotheses which can be tested in the laboratory.

Literature Cited

1. Hodgkin, A. L.; Huxley, A. F. A quantitative description of
    membrane current and its application to conduction and ex-
    citation in nerve. J. Physiol. 1952, 117, 500-544.
2. Cain, C. A. A theoretical basis for microwave and RF field
    effects on excitable cellular membranes, IEEE Trans. Micro-
    wave Theory Tech. 1980, MTT-28, 142-147.
3. Schwarz, G. On dielectric relaxation due to chemical rate
    processes. J. Phys. Chem. 1967, 71, 4021-4030.
4. Barnes, F. S.; Hu, C. H. Model for some nonthermal effects
    of radio and microwave fields on biological membranes. IEEE
    Trans. Microwave Theory Tech. 1977, MTT-25, 742-746.
5. MacGregor, R. J. A possible mechanism for the influence of
    electromagnetic radiation on neuroelectric potentials. IEEE
    Trans. Microwave Theory Tech. 1979, MTT-27, 914-921.
6. Almers, W. Gating currents and charge movements in excitable
    membrane. Rev. Physiol. Biochem. Pharmacol. 1978, 82, 97-190.
7. Pickard, W. F.; Rosenbaum, F. J. Biological effects of micro-
    waves at the membrane level: two possible athermal electro-
    physiological mechanisms and a proposed experimental test.

Math. Biosci. 1978, 39, 235–253.

8. Armstrong, C. M.; Bezanilla, F. Charge movement associated with the opening and closing of the activation gates of the Na channels. J. Gen. Physiol. 1974, 63, 533–552.

9. Keynes, R. D.; Rojas, E. Kinetics and steady state properties of the charged system controlling sodium conductance in the squid giant axon. J. Physiol. 1974, 239, 393–434.

10. Meves, H. The effect of holding potential on the asymmetry currents in squid giant axons. J. Physiol. 1974, 243, 847–867.

11. Neumcke, B.; Nonner, W.; Stämpfli, R. Asymmetrical displacement current and its relation with the activation of sodium current in the membrane of frog myelinated nerve. Pflügers Arch. 1976, 363, 193–203.

12. Schneider, M. F.; Chandler, W. K. Voltage-dependent charge movement in skeletal muscle: a possible step in excitation-contraction coupling. Nature 1973, 242, 244–246.

13. Almers, W.; Best, P. M. Effects of tetracaine on displacement currents and contraction in frog skeletal muscle. J. Physiol. 1976, 262, 583–611.

14. Rudy, B. Sodium gating currents in *Myxicola* giant axons. Proc. Roy. Soc. Lond. (Biol.) 1976, 193, 469–475.

15. Adams, D. J.; Gage, P. W. Gating currents associated with sodium and calcium currents in an *Aplysia* neuron. Science 1975, 192, 783–784.

16. Rojas, E; Keynes, R. D. On the relation between displacement currents and activation of the sodium conductance in the squid giant axon. Phil. Trans. R. Soc. 1975, 270, 459–482.

17. Keynes, R. D.; Rojas, E. The temporal and steady-state relationships between activation of the sodium conductance and movement of the gating particles in the squid giant axon. J. Physiol. 1976, 255, 157–190.

18. Goldman, L. Kinetics of channel gating in excitable membrane. Q. Rev. Biophys. 1976, 9, 491–526.

19. Jakobsson, E. A fully coupled transient excited state model for the sodium channel. J. Math. Biology 1978, 5, 121–142.

20. Goldman, L.; Hahin, R. Initial conditions and the kinetics of the sodium conductance in *Myxicola* giant axons. J. Gen. Physiol. 1978, 72, 879–898.

21. Frey, A. H.; Seifert, E. Pulse modulated UHF energy illumination of the heart associated with change in heart rate. Life Sci. 1968, 7, 505–512.

22. Bawin, S. M.; Kaczmarek, L. K.; Adey, W. R. Effects of modulated VHF fields on the central nervous system. Ann. NY Acad. Sci. 1975, 247, 74–81.

23. Tinney, C. E.; Lords, J. L.; Durney, C. H. Rate effects in isolated turtle hearts induced by microwave irradiation. IEEE Trans. Microwave Theory Tech. 1976, MTT-24, 18–24.

24. Seaman, R. L; Wachtel, H. Slow and rapid responses to CW and pulsed microwave radiation by individual *Aplysia* pacemakers. J. Microwave Power 1978, 13, 77–86.
25. Clapman, R. M.; Cain, C. A. Absence of heart-rate effects in isolated frog heart irradiated with pulse modulated microwave energy. J. Microwave Power 1975, 10, 411–419.
26. Liu, L. M.; Rosenbaum, F. J.; Pickard, W. F. The insensitivity of frog heart to pulse modulated microwave energy. J. Microwave Power 1976, 11, 225–232.
27. Chou, C. K.; Guy, A. W. Effect of 2450 MHz microwave fields on peripheral nerves. Dig. Tech. Papers (IEEE Int. Microwave Symp., Boulder, CO), 1973, 318–320.
28. Courtney, K. R.; Lin, J. C.; Guy, A. W.; Chou, C. K. Microwave effect on rabbit superior cervical ganglion. IEEE Trans. Micrwoave Theory Tech. 1975, MTT-23, 809–813.

RECEIVED October 31, 1980.

DIELECTRIC AND SPECTROSCOPIC PROPERTIES OF NONEQUILIBRIUM SYSTEMS

11

Developmental Bioelectricity

PETER J. ORTOLEVA

Department of Chemistry, Indiana University, Bloomington, IN 47405

An ever increasing body of experimental data has pointed
out the importance of the effect of imposed and autonomous
electric fields on developing living systems. Here we
bring together a number of recent theoretical advances which may
unravel the nature of these effects in a number of physico-
chemical and biological systems with special attention to effects
on biopattern formation and signal propagation.

Overview

Patterning in biological and physico-chemical systems
typically involves the spatial variation of ionic concentrations.
It should thus not be surprising that interesting electric
effects arise in such systems. We show here that the situation
in these systems is very rich in important and surprising
developmental phenomena as has been realized historically in
isolated studies dating from the last century and more generally
since the 1940's ($\underline{8}$, $\underline{28}$, $\underline{53}$, $\underline{54}$).
Experiments on the effects of autonomous and imposed elec-
tric fields in biomorphogenesis have been done on many systems
including seaweed eggs, plant roots, nerve and muscle in
culture, Cecropia oöcyte-nurse cell cyncytae, amphibian and
rodent limb regeneration and wound healing and regeneration in
man ($\underline{8}$, $\underline{28}$, $\underline{53}$, $\underline{54}$). It is clear from these experiments that a
number of different effects come into play in the various
systems. In the near future this field should lead to a number
of important theoretical and experimental advances in elucidating
the detailed mechanisms of developmental biology. One main goal
of these studies must be to determine to what degree the electrical effects play a key role in the developmental process
rather than being a consequence of some other more fundamental
pattern forming process.

The effects to be discussed here fall into two categories--
autonomous and induced. In the former case it is shown that
biological systems are capable of spontaneously creating their
own electric fields and currents and use them to guide the
course of development and associated breaking of symmetry. The
second group of effects occurs when electric fields (or other
symmetry breaking imposed influences) are applied to a developing or signal propagating system. Important effects also occur
in association with the interplay of autonomous and imposed
effects. The very interesting effects due to high frequency
imposed fields are not covered here but are reviewed in Refs.
53 and 54.

   Self-Organizing Bioelectricity. Since Turing (1) many
authors have discussed the idea that a reaction-diffusion system
can spontaneously form patterns in a manner suggestive of some
aspects of biomorphogenesis. Turing's idea is that a system
involving reaction and diffusion could become unstable to small
deviations in composition that were of lower symmetry (i.e. more
highly patterned) than the initial state of the system. This
was conjectured to be the underlying mechanism whereby biological systems could self-organize to increasingly higher states of
order. However, these studies have not provided a framework for
a quantitative theory of biomorphogenesis in analogy to the role
played by the Hodgkin-Huxley (HH) theory (2) of nerve propagation. The key factor in developing the HH theory was the existence of a relatively simple model experimental system, the
squid giant axon. The many experiments on this system allowed
for the formulation of a phenomonology that can explain many
quantitative aspects of axonal signal propagation. In the
section on cellular electrophysiological self-organization we
shall discuss theoretical work (3-7) on the spontaneous generation of electrochemical patterns in single cells and in particular in the early development of the seaweed Fucus (4, 8).
It appears that, because of the relative simplicity of this
system, these calculations lead to the first morphogenetic
theory capable of making quantitative predictions on the development of biological patterns.
   In typical situations of biological development the system
is under a situation of changing control parameters (such as
permeabilities or energy stores). This can mask the existence
of a Turing pattern formation phenomenon. In the popular view
of Turing's theory, much has been made of the theory of bifurcations which assume that system parameters change slowly or not
at all (28). However, in Fucus for example, it is found that
permeabilities change on a time scale similar to or even shorter
than that of the growth of small fluctuations from the unpatterned state. To deal with this we introduce a theory of
dynamical self-organization which develops evolution equations
for the growing pattern under the influence of changing

conditions. This theory, based on a time dependent Ginzburg-Landau (TDGL) type formalism, is sketched below for a single cell system.

Autonomous phenomena in multicellular systems are considered in the section on bioelectric patterning in cell aggregates. A mathematical model is considered which describes the cell aggregate via macroscopic variables--concentrations and voltage. Cells are "smeared out" to formulate the theory in terms of continuum variables. A nonlinear integral operator is introduced to model the intercellular transport that corrects the cruder diffusion-like terms usually assumed. This transport term is explicitly related to the properties of cell membranes.

Effects of Applied Fields. External electric fields are known experimentally to profoundly effect the course of development in single cells and multicellular systems ($\underline{8}$, $\underline{28}$, $\underline{53}$, $\underline{54}$). This is examined in the section on cells in external gradients in the context of single cell effects. A bioelectric theory of applied field effects in multicellular aggregates is presented in a section on bioelectric patterning in cell aggregates. In both the single and multicellular cases, the response to external fields under certain "critical conditions" is shown to exhibit "hyperpolarizability" such that the system reacts strongly to the external field but in a manner determined profoundly by its internal dynamics. This hyperpolarizability can be "adaptive," allowing the system to be programmed to take advantage of external gradients, or "accidental," demonstrating a large response to an external field that is not an environmental requirement or feature of normal development. Applied field phenomena may be broken up into those leading to "imperfect bifurcations" and those involving induction of new phenomena. An imperfect bifurcation ($\underline{20}$) is a situation wherein a small imperfection or applied field breaks the symmetry of the system and thereby breaks the symmetry in the state diagram for the system. The induction phenomena arise because the application of a sufficiently large field can actually change the dynamics so much that distinctly new phenomena, not present in the field free medium, can arise.

Signal propagation in bioelectric and physico-chemical (Zhabotinskii, $\underline{9}$) systems are often accompanied by ionic species gradients. This is shown in signal propagation under imposed electric fields to allow the use of these fields to not only effect this propagation but also lead to the induction of distinctly new phenomena ($\underline{10}$-$\underline{14}$).

Cellular Electrophysiological Self-Organization

It has been shown experimentally ($\underline{8}$) for some single cell systems, notably the fertilized _Fucus_ egg, that at a certain stage of development transcellular ionic currents spontaneously

arise. In <u>Fucus</u> these currents and associated electric fields
are established despite the absence of any apparent initial asym-
metry--the <u>Fucus</u> egg starts out spherically symmetric--and can
develop in the absence of any externally imposed gradients. Thus
we ($\underline{3}$-$\underline{7}$, $\underline{14}$) envision this early developmental event in <u>Fucus</u> as
a symmetry breaking instability as suggested by the Turing theory
($\underline{1}$). In this section we emphasize the self-organizing aspects of
certain cellular phenomena and their theoretical description.

Although the theory presented here is in the spirit of
Turing's hypothesis, it differs significantly from Turing's morphogenetic model in that (1) the importance of electrical effects
on ionic transport and (2) the key role of the membrane in cellular processes are accounted for.

Formulation. Consider the cell of interest to be bounded by
an outer membrane specified by the set of points $\vec{r}$ such that
$S(\vec{r}) = 0$, see Fig. 1. In the cell interior the concentrations of
the N mobile species $\underline{c} = \{c_1, c_2, \ldots c_N\}$ evolve according to ($\underline{4}$, $\underline{5}$)

$$[\underline{I} + \underline{\Lambda}(\underline{c})]\frac{\partial c}{\partial t} = -\vec{\nabla} \cdot \vec{\underline{J}} + \underline{R}(\underline{c}). \tag{1}$$

We have assumed that the mobile species take part in rapid attachment $\rightleftarrows$ detachment (chromatographic) processes with (for simplicity) a single type of fixed site of total concentration Y_T. The
empty site is at concentration Y and the site occupied with an
i-molecule is at concentration Y_i^O ($\sum_{i=0}^{N} Y_i = Y_T$). Assuming the
attachment kinetics are rapid, the site concentrations are at
the equilibrium values $Y_i^{eq}(\underline{c})$ and hence follow the instantaneous
value of $\underline{c}$. The matrix $\Lambda_{ij}(\underline{c})$ is given by

$$\Lambda_{ij}(\underline{c}) = \partial Y_i^{eq}/\partial c_j. \tag{2}$$

The fluxes $\vec{\underline{J}}$ are found to have the form

$$\vec{\underline{J}} = -\underline{D}(\underline{c})\vec{\nabla}\underline{c} - \underline{M}(\underline{c})\underline{c}\vec{\nabla}V \tag{3}$$

where $\underline{D}(\underline{c})$ and $\underline{M}(\underline{c})$ are effective diffusion and mobility matrices
modified by the presence of the fixed sites ($\underline{5}$). The rates of
the nonchromatographic reaction are denoted $\underline{R}(\underline{c})$.

The cell communicates with the external world through the
outer membrane at $S(\vec{r}) = 0$. This interaction is represented
mathematically via the boundary conditions, namely

$$-\hat{n} \cdot \vec{\underline{J}} = \underline{J}^M, \text{ at } S(\vec{r}) = 0, \hat{n} = \vec{\nabla}S/|\vec{\nabla}S|, \tag{4}$$

where we neglect the membrane flux of the mobile species along
the membrane. The transmembrane flux J_i^M of mobile species i is
taken to be positive if directed into the cell. $\underline{J}^M$ accounts
for both active and passive processes. We focus on slow
processes of development here so that time delays associated with
transmembrane fluxes are neglected.

The presence of ionic species at biological ionic strengths imposes the condition of charge neutrality. In the presence of the chromatographic effects accounted for in (1) we have

$$\sum_{i=1}^{N} z_i [c_i + Y_i^{eq}(\underline{c})] + y_o Y_T = 0 \qquad (5)$$

where z_i and y_o are the valences of mobile species i and the empty fixed site respectively.

The outer cell membrane contains molecules such as pumps or carrier species which profoundly effect the transmembrane fluxes $\underline{J}^M$ of the mobile species. Since these membrane bound molecules often have charged groups they may be moved by voltage gradients along the outer membrane (15). These two factors allow for important feedback effects which can (3-8), as we shall see, lead to cellular electrophysiological self-organization. Thus we introduce a set of species bound to the outer membrane with concentrations $\Gamma(\xi_2, \xi_3, t)$ that depend on a set of curvilinear coordinates ξ_2, ξ_3 specifying a location on the outer membrane. If we neglect reactions changing the concentration of these species then Γ is taken to satisfy

$$\frac{\partial \underline{\Gamma}}{\partial t} = -\vec{\nabla}_s \cdot \vec{\underline{j}} \qquad (6)$$

$$\vec{\underline{j}} = -\underline{\underline{d}} \vec{\nabla}_s \underline{\Gamma} - \underline{\mu}^i \underline{\Gamma} \vec{\nabla}_s v^i - \underline{\mu}^e \underline{\Gamma} \vec{\nabla}_s v^e. \qquad (7)$$

Here $\vec{\nabla}_s$ is a gradient operator along the surface $S(\vec{r}) = 0$ defining the outer membrane. The electric fields $-\vec{\nabla}_s v^i$ and $-\vec{\nabla}_s v^e$ along the outer membrane, at the membrane i and e interface respectively (see Fig. 1) may both act on the membrane bound species; the ultimate result depends on the sign of the charged ends of these molecules sticking out into the i or e regions. This interplay is reflected via the last two terms in (7) where $\underline{\mu}^i$ and $\underline{\mu}^e$ represent a diagonal matrix of mobilities $\underline{\mu}$ multiplied by a diagonal matrice $\underline{z}^{i,e}$ whose diagonal elements $z_{\alpha\alpha}^i$ and $z_{\alpha\alpha}^e$ are the valences of the i and e charged end of membrane species α.

Quasi-Steady State Ca^{2+} Mediated Membrane Feedback Models.
An extensive literature exists to point out the active role of Ca^{2+} in many biological processes (17). Jaffe has suggested that this might indeed be of relevance to Fucus development (8). We now show how a number of physical properties of Ca^{2+} strongly suggest such a role and that these factors lead the way to a number of approximations that yield a simple intuitive model for the spontaneous generation of cellular electrophysiological patterns.

The model we shall derive focuses on the important role of the outer membrane. We first assume that the slowest process in the developmental scenario is the migration of membrane bound molecules along the membrane. This is manifest in the fact that

the transport coefficients $\underline{d}$, $\underline{\mu}^{i,e}$ in (7) are small for the large
molecules which we shall assume to most dramatically effect the
transmembrane fluxes $\underline{J}^M$. Because of this time scale separation,
the bulk processes adiabatically follow the instantaneous value
of $\Gamma(\underline{\xi}, \underline{\xi}, t)$ and hence by introducing an appropriate smallness
parameter we can arrive, via the usual arguments, to quasi-steady
state bulk equations; (1) becomes

$$\vec{\nabla} \cdot \vec{\underline{J}} = \underline{R} \tag{8}$$

and $(4, 5)$ are unchanged.

Transport in the outside medium, typically seawater as for
developing Fucus, is relatively fast and may even be aided by
stirring. Thus from an evolutionary perspective we do not expect
that biological self-organization for free single cells should
typically depend strongly on the development of external gradients
for spontaneous pattern formation. The large transport coeffi-
cients $\underline{D}$ and $\underline{M}$ for the external world will tend to repress deviations from uniformity and hence we assume the external problem to
be linearizable. Assuming $\underline{R}$ in the external world is zero (8)
becomes $\underline{D}\vec{\nabla}^2\delta\underline{c} + \underline{M}c^h\vec{\nabla}^2\delta V = 0$ where superscript "h" denotes the
average culture medium value, $\delta\underline{c} = \underline{c} - \underline{c}^h$ and $\delta V = V - V^h$. Since
$\underline{D}$ is invertible and charge neutrality in the outside world (free
of chromatographic effects) yields
$\sum_{i=1}^{N} z_i \delta c_i = 0$ we see that $\vec{\nabla}^2 \delta V = 0$ outside. But the transmembrane
flux is relatively slow compared to the bulk flux in e. Hence to
lowest order in the smallness of the ratio of the $\underline{J}^M$ transport
coefficients to those of $\underline{D}$ and $\underline{M}$ we see that the normal derivative
$\partial(\underline{D}\delta\underline{c} + \underline{M}c^h\delta V)/\partial n$ vanishes. Again since $\underline{D}$ is invertible this can
be used to show that $\partial\delta V/\partial n = 0$ and $\partial\delta\underline{c}/\partial n = 0$. Thus $\delta\underline{c}$ and δV
are found to be small in the outside world since the solution of
the problem $\vec{\nabla}^2\phi = 0$, $\partial\phi/\partial n = 0$ has the unique solution $\phi = 0$
identically if it is zero at any one point. Thus we shall assume
that $\underline{c}$ and V in e are fixed at their bath values $\underline{c}^\infty$, $V^\infty \equiv 0$ where
we take the convention that the voltage is defined to be zero at
infinity. (These assumptions will be relaxed later in the context
of the effects of externally applied electric fields.)

An intuitive and mathematically elegant reduced model arises
if we assume that the main nonlinear feedback is due to the mobile
membrane bound species affecting the distribution of ions which
modifies the voltage and hence feeds back into the $\underline{\Gamma}$ equation. If
we retain only the linear response of the bulk to the deviation of
$\underline{\Gamma}$ from its uniformally distributed value the problem may be
reduced to a closed equation for $\underline{\Gamma}$ as follows. For simplicity
here we neglect the effect of reactions, $\underline{R} = \underline{0}$, in the cell interior for the ionic species of interest $(Na^+, K^+, Ca^{2+}, Cl^-,$
etc.), retaining the chromatographic reactions only. The uni-
form state $\underline{c}^h$, $\Delta V^h \equiv V^{ih} - V^{eh}$ is given by solving $\underline{J}^M(\underline{c}^h, \underline{c}^\infty, \Delta V^h,$
$\underline{\Gamma}^h) = 0$ with (5) where superscripts i, e indicate that quantities

are evaluated at the interface between i or e and the outer membrane. For the homogeneous state they therefore indicate their constant values in the relevant domain. Small deviations $\delta\underline{c}$ and δV from the homogeneous state then obey Laplace's equation

$$\nabla^2\delta\underline{c} = 0, \quad \nabla^2\delta V = 0, \quad s(\vec{r}) < 0. \qquad (9)$$

The linearized boundary conditions take the form

$$\underline{\underline{D}}\frac{\partial\delta\underline{c}}{\partial n} + \underline{\underline{M}}\underline{c}^h\frac{\partial\delta V}{\partial n} = \underline{\underline{C}}\delta\underline{c} + \underline{\mathcal{V}}\delta\Delta V + \underline{\underline{\mathcal{B}}}\delta\underline{\Gamma}, \quad s(\vec{r}) = 0, \quad (10)$$

where

$$\left.\begin{array}{l} C_{ij} = \partial J_i^M/\partial c_j \\[2mm] \mathcal{V}_i = \partial J_i^M/\partial\Delta V \\[2mm] \mathcal{B}_{i\alpha} = \partial J_i^M/\partial\Gamma_\alpha \end{array}\right\} \quad \left.\begin{array}{l} i,j = 1, 2,\ldots N \\[2mm] \alpha = 1, 2,\ldots B \end{array}\right\} s(\vec{r}) = 0 \quad (11)$$

for a system of N mobile bulk and B membrane bound species. The charge neutrality condition

$$\sum_{j=1}^{N}\zeta_j\delta c_j = 0, \quad \zeta_j \equiv z_j + \sum_{k=1}^{N}z_k\frac{\partial Y_k^{eq}}{\partial c_j} \qquad (12)$$

completes the theory. All quantities in the expressions for $\underline{\underline{C}}$, $\underline{\mathcal{V}}$, $\underline{\underline{\mathcal{B}}}$ and $\underline{\zeta}$ are evaluated at the uniform state $\underline{c}^h$, V^h, $\underline{\Gamma}^h$.

One of the special features of Ca^{2+} is that it tends to bind rather strongly to many fixed sites; hence, since $[Ca^{2+}]$ is small it is easy to show that $\partial Y_{Ca^{2+}}^{eq}/\partial[Ca^{2+}]$ is large. This tends to repress $\delta[Ca^{2+}]$ because of its amplified electrical effect (through $\zeta_{Ca^{2+}}$ in (12)). Since $[Ca^{2+}]^h$ and $\delta[Ca^{2+}]$ are small, it is instructive to assume for the moment that (11) for Ca^{2+} becomes

$$\sum_{i\neq Ca^{2+}}^{N}C_{Ca~i}\delta c_i + \mathcal{V}_{Ca^{2+}}\delta V + \sum_{\alpha=1}^{B}\mathcal{B}_{Ca^{2+}~\alpha}\delta\Gamma_\alpha = 0. \qquad (13)$$

For species like Na^+, K^+ and Cl^- the transport coefficients in the cell interior are essentially those in seawater and hence the RHS of (10) is negligible. This implies that $\partial\delta c_i/\partial n = -D_i^{-1}M_i c_i^h\partial\delta V/\partial n$ for these species (assuming diagonal diffusion for simplicity). For cells of general ellipsoidal geometry (that includes spheres, cylinders, etc. as special cases) it is easy to show that for the above mentioned species the boundary condition implies $\delta c_i = -(M_i c_i^h/D_i)\delta V$. Hence combining this with (13) the voltage deviation δV inside the cell becomes

$$\delta V = \sum_{\alpha=1}^{B}Q_\alpha\delta\Gamma_\alpha \qquad (14)$$

where

$$Q_\alpha = -\mathscr{Y}_{Ca^{2+},\alpha} / [\mathscr{V}_{Ca^{2+}} - \sum_{i \neq Ca^{2+}} (M_i c_i^h / D_i) C_{Ca^{2+}i}]. \quad (15)$$

Thus with (6), taking $\underline{\underline{d}}$ and $\underline{\mu}^i$ to be constant and repressing the superscript i on $\underline{\mu}^i$, we get

$$\frac{\partial \Gamma}{\partial t} = \underline{\underline{d}} \vec{\nabla}_s^2 \Gamma + \vec{\nabla}_s \cdot [\underline{\mu} \Gamma \vec{\nabla}_s \sum_{\alpha=1}^{B} Q_\alpha \Gamma_\alpha], \quad (16)$$

a closed equation in Γ.

To illustrate the behavior of the model let us consider the case of one species bound to the membrane, $B = 1$. Then small deviations $\delta\Gamma$ from the uniform state Γ^h satisfy

$$\frac{\partial \delta\Gamma}{\partial t} = u \vec{\nabla}_s^2 \delta\Gamma, \quad u \equiv d + \mu Q \Gamma^h. \quad (17)$$

From this it is clear that asymmetric perturbations will grow if $u < 0$ and the membrane bound species would be expected to self-organize in a patterned distribution on the membrane. For this to occur we see that Q, a measure of the feedback strength, must be sufficiently large (and $\mu Q < 0$).

This simple picture breaks down in a number of situations. If the perturbations vary sufficiently rapidly in space then the $\partial [Ca^{2+}]/\partial n$ term, dropped from (13), becomes important and stabilizes these short length scale perturbations. Mathematically we find (5-7, 19) that this effect manifests itself in the fact that Q in (15) has a much more complex structure; Q is an integral operator that acts to diminish the effect of short length scale perturbations.

Focusing attention on the case of spherical geometry, patterns arise in association with the spherical harmonics $Y_{\ell m}(\theta,\phi)$ (where θ,ϕ are the usual polar coordinate angles). Conditions in the environment and in the cell interior can thus determine the ℓ-symmetry of the emergent pattern. This suggests that under certain conditions such a system might have some difficulty in discriminating which ℓ-symmetry pattern to acquire. In fact in Fucus where $\ell = 1$ is the normal situation, $\ell = 2$ (double rhizoid leading to double root system) patterns are sometimes observed. Thus this "birth defect" could be due to decreased Ca^{2+} intra-cellular effective transport coefficients caused, for example, by an overabundance of Ca^{2+} binding sites. Decreased $[Ca^{2+}]$ in the medium might also be expected to favor multi-rhizoidism for similar reasons.

A complete analysis of a Ca^{2+} type model for the early development of Fucus has been carried out (5-7). It was found that early developmental phenomena can be quantitatively described using available Fucus transport and fixed Ca^{2+} binding site data obtained experimentally. An important feature of this type of calculation is that it provides a framework with which one may integrate a wide range of complex experimental data and sort out which experiments are most crucial. Many detailed

comparisons of the theory and experiment are found in Ref. 5
where the instability of the spherically symmetric state of the
Fucus egg is studied. Both in the theory and the experiments the
instability is found to occur less than an hour after fertilization. Also, spontaneously growing transcellular ionic currents,
as shown schematically in Fig. 2, are found to arise.

   Nonlinear Aspects of Cellular Self-Organization. A linear
stability analysis like that carried out in the previous section can give much insight into the conditions needed for pattern formation and the symmetry of the emerging structure, but
it cannot determine the amplitude of the structure. The latter
requires a nonlinear analysis. The nonlinear analysis also
yields information about the stability of the emerging patterns
to small perturbations and sometimes rules out patterns that
appear to be possible from the linear stability analysis. It has
been shown by a number of authors that if conditions are not too
far from the point of onset of instability, then the emergent
structure can be analyzed via bifurcation theory (18). The main
idea of this approach is to formulate the equations in such a way
as to just balance the tendency towards linearized (exponential)
growth of a perturbation with the dominant nonlinear term in a
small amplitude expansion. (Actually this is termed a "normal"
bifurcation; for an "inverted" bifurcation the tendency towards
decay of the perturbation according to the linearized dynamics
is balanced off by the dominant nonlinear growth process.)
Bifurcation analysis has been applied to the Fucus problem and
details are to be found in Ref. 7 for the full equations and in a
reduced quasistatic model in Ref. 19.

   It is shown in Ref. 19 that, if we assume that the bulk
dynamics adiabatically follows the evolution of the membrane
bound species and does so in linear response to them, (16) gets
replaced by (assuming a single relevant membrane species, B = 1,
for simplicity)

$$\frac{\partial \Gamma}{\partial t} = d\vec{\nabla}_s \cdot [\vec{\nabla}_s \Gamma + \lambda \Gamma \vec{\nabla}_s \mathcal{K}\Gamma].$$ (18)

Here λ is a parameter and $\mathcal{K}$ is a linear integral operator such
that

$$\mathcal{K}\Gamma \equiv \int d\omega \mathcal{K}(\xi_2,\xi_3|\xi_2',\xi_3')\Gamma(\xi_2',\xi_3',t).$$ (19)

Physically $\vec{\nabla}_s \mathcal{K}(\Gamma-\Gamma^h)$ is (modulo constants) the net electrical
force on the Γ molecule along the membrane as induced by an inhomogeneous distribution of Γ over the cell surface. In (18)
ξ_2,ξ_3 are curvilinear coordinates specifying points on the cell
surface and $d\omega$ is an area element on the cell surface. The
kernel K may be explicitly related to the membrane flux (linearized around the symmetric state) and the transport coefficients
in i and e and is discussed further below and in Ref. 19.

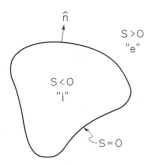

Figure 1. Schematic of geometry of a single cell bounded by a membrane defined by the mathematical surface $S(\vec{r}) = 0$.

The cell interior, Region "i" ($S < 0$), interacts with the environment, Region "e" ($S > 0$), via the membrane ($S = 0$). The same notation is also used for the case where the above object represents a cell mass.

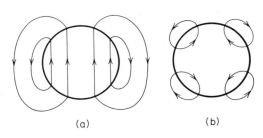

            (a)   (b)

Figure 2. Self-organized ionic current loops found both experimentally and theoretically in the single-cell state early development of the egg of the seaweed Fucus.

Patterns (a) and (b) correspond to $l = 1, 2$ pattern symmetries, respectively. The $l = 1$ pattern is the normal course of development for Fucus *and is the primary developmental event that sets the direction and sense of the later development that allows for the (leaf, stem) — (root) differentiation. The $l = 2$ patterns also are observed experimentally as occasional "birth defects" where two roots germinate.*

Steady state solutions of (18) are easily obtained because for simplicity here Γ is assumed not changed due to any chemical reaction. Hence the flux of Γ, $\vec{j} = -d[\nabla_s \Gamma + \lambda \Gamma \nabla_s \mathcal{K}\Gamma]$, is zero at steady state. Thus $\nabla_s (\ell n \Gamma + \lambda \mathcal{K}\Gamma) = 0$ and hence

$$\ell n \Gamma + \lambda \mathcal{K}\Gamma = H \qquad (20)$$

where H is a constant (essentially the electrochemical potential of Γ) to be determined by a conservation condition as follows. First we choose units so that when uniformally distributed Γ has the value 1. Since Γ is assumed not to be altered by reactions the total amount of the membrane bound molecule, $\int d\omega \Gamma$, is the same regardless of the distribution of Γ and hence

$$\int d\omega \Gamma = \int d\omega = A \qquad (21)$$

where A is the total area of the cell surface. Rewriting (20) in the form $\Gamma = \exp\{H - \lambda \mathcal{K}\Gamma\}$ and using (21) we get $H = \ell n[A/\int d\omega e^{-\lambda \mathcal{K}\Gamma}]$ and hence (20) becomes

$$\ell n \Gamma + \lambda \mathcal{K}\Gamma = \ell n \left[\frac{A}{\int d\omega e^{-\lambda \mathcal{K}\Gamma}} \right], \qquad (22)$$

a convenient closed equation for Γ.

Bifurcation of electrophysiological symmetry breaking patterns occurs in this model when (22) just admits Γ distributions which are a small deviation $\gamma \equiv \Gamma - 1$ from the uniform state $\Gamma = 1$. A convenient parameter to follow is λ (an explicitly given combination of rate, transport and bath medium composition) which directly measures the feedback efficiency at which a disturbance in Γ causes a voltage disturbance that in turn creates a flux of Γ. Indeed at $\lambda = 0$ the only solution of (22) is the uniform state $\Gamma = 1$. To proceed with the bifurcation theoretic calculation of the emerging asymmetric distribution we seek a development of Γ in powers of the deviation of λ from some appropriate critical value λ_c for a given emerging pattern symmetry. It is a standard device in bifurcation theory to introduce a measure ϵ of the amplitude of the emergent pattern. It is not wise to expand directly in $\lambda - \lambda_c$ for it is found here, as in other examples of bifurcation phenomena, that the amplitude of the pattern often emerges as some power other than linear in $\lambda - \lambda_c$. The standard procedure is to introduce expansions as follows:

$$\lambda = \lambda_c + \sum_{n=1}^{\infty} \lambda_n \epsilon^n \qquad (23)$$

$$\gamma = \sum_{n=1}^{\infty} \gamma_n \epsilon^n. \qquad (24)$$

The power of $\lambda - \lambda_c$ at which the amplitude of the pattern emerges depends on the n value of the first nonzero λ_n that the equations allow. A typical case is $\lambda_1 = 0$, $\lambda_2 \neq 0$. Hence for $\lambda \sim \lambda_c$ $\epsilon \propto (\lambda - \lambda_c)^{1/2}$ in this case; [1] $\epsilon \propto (\lambda - \lambda_c)$ is also common.

   To see the structure of the theory let us consider a spherical cell. In that case the kernel K can be written conveniently
in terms of the spherical harmonics

$$K = \sum_\ell \sum_{m=-\ell}^{\ell} k_\ell Y_{\ell m}(\theta,\phi) Y_{\ell m}^*(\theta',\phi'). \tag{25}$$

In this case it is easily seen that the $Y_{\ell m}$ are eigenfunctions of
$\mathcal{K}$,

$$\mathcal{K} Y_{\ell m} = k_\ell Y_{\ell m}, \quad m = -\ell, \; -\ell+1, \ldots, \; 0, \ldots \ell. \tag{26}$$

This property will now be shown to fix the geometries of the
emerging structures.
   The bifurcation theory for a spherical cell proceeds by
putting $(23,24)$ into (22) with (25). To order $\epsilon^0 = 1$, (22) is
satisfied automatically since $\mathcal{K} \cdot 1 = k_o$, independent of θ, ϕ. To
order ϵ we get the linear problem

$$\mathcal{L}(\ell) \gamma_1 = 0, \quad \mathcal{L}(\ell) = 1 + \lambda_c(\ell)[1 - \frac{1}{A} d\omega]\mathcal{K} \tag{27}$$

where the integral over the sphere is applied to the result of
everything to the right. Because of (26) we see that there is one
value of λ_c for each ℓ, denoted $\lambda_c(\ell)$, such that

$$\lambda_c(\ell) = -1/k_\ell. \tag{28}$$

For a given ℓ γ_1 is a (real) linear combination of the $Y_{\ell m}$,

$$\gamma_1 = \sum_{m=-\ell}^{\ell} g_m Y_{\ell m}, \; \ell \geq 1, \tag{29}$$

corresponding to a pattern of "quantum number" ℓ. To this order
in the theory the g_m's are not given.
   To proceed further we collect terms to order ϵ^2 for each
emerging ℓ-pattern. We find

$$\mathcal{L}(\ell) \gamma_2 - 1/2\gamma_1^2 + \lambda_1 k_\ell \gamma_1 = \frac{1}{2A} \int d\omega \gamma_1^2. \tag{30}$$

For the egg of _Fucus_ the pattern most commonly found is the $\ell = 1$
(dipolar) structure. For this case one finds by multiplying by
Y_{1m}^* and integrating $\int d\omega = \int_0^{2\pi} d\phi \int_0^\pi \sin\theta d\theta$ that $\lambda_1 = 0$. One then
may find γ_2 in terms of γ_1. In the next order (ϵ^3) we finally
find that $\lambda_2 \neq 0$ and one obtains a cubic equation for the amplitude factors g_m, $m = 0, \pm 1$. The bifurcation diagram for this
case is shown in Fig. 3a. More details are found in Ref. 19.
   These bifurcation calculations have been within the scope of
the model (18). A bifurcation theory based on the complete
equations of the section on formulation is given in Ref. 7 where
a detailed comparison with experiments on _Fucus_ is presented.

Dynamical Self-Organization. When the parameter λ passes slowly through $\lambda_c(1)$, the bifurcation picture of the previous section accurately describes the system. However, in Fucus, and probably in many other examples, this time scale separation between the characteristic time on which λ varies and the time to obtain the patterned state does not hold. Thus a dynamical theory allowing for the interplay of these two time scales is required to characterize the developmental scenario. A natural formalism to describe this process is that of time dependent Ginzburg-Landau (TDGL) equations used successfully in other contexts of nonequilibrium phase transitions (27).

1. TDGL Formalism. Our object is to obtain a dynamical equation describing the onset of a pattern. The TDGL method has two main features: it (1) identifies a few variables that specify the pattern and (2) develops relatively simple equations for these variables in the limit where the system is not too far from the point of marginal stability. We shall develop these ideas specifically in terms of the Fucus-type theory of the previous section and in particular near conditions wherein the $\ell = 1$ disturbance just becomes unstable.

The formalism is most easily cast in terms of an expansion for $\gamma \equiv \Gamma - 1$ in terms of the spherical harmonics

$$\gamma = \sum_{\ell,m} g_{\ell m}(t) Y_{\ell m}(\theta,\phi). \tag{31}$$

The partial integro-differential equation (18) can be turned into an infinite sequence of equations for the $g_{\ell m}$ by inserting (31) into (18), multiplying by $Y_{\mu\nu}^*$ and integrating over all spherical angles ($\int d\omega$): we find

$$\frac{dg_{\mu\nu}}{dt} = -\mu(\mu+1)(1+\lambda k_\mu) g_{\mu\nu} + \lambda \sum_{\substack{\ell\ell' \\ mm'}} B_{\mu\nu}^{\ell m,\ell'm'} g_{\ell m} g_{\ell'm'} \tag{32}$$

$$B_{\mu\nu}^{\ell m,\ell'm'} = -\ell(\ell+1)k_\ell \int d\omega Y_{\mu\nu}^* Y_{\ell m} Y_{\ell'm'} + k_\ell \int d\omega Y_{\mu\nu}^* \vec{\nabla}_s Y_{\ell m} \cdot \vec{\nabla}_s Y_{\ell'm'} .$$

The key technical and physical assumption is that the system is close to the conditions wherein the $\ell = 1$ modes are just unstable, i.e. λ is near $-1/k$. This implies that if the pattern ($\gamma \neq 0$) is small initially then it will remain so subsequently and will change slowly in time. Thus we introduce a scaling parameter ϵ to measure how close we are to the critical point, i.e.

$$\lambda = -1/k_1 + a\epsilon^2 \tag{33}$$

where a is of the order unity and sweeps through zero as the system passes through criticality for the $\ell = 1$ mode. From the bifurcation theory we expect the $\ell = 1$ pattern amplitude to scale

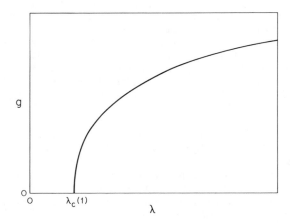

Figure 3a.   Bifurcation plot for Fucus *showing the amplitude of the normal (1 = 1) currents* g *plotted against* λ, *a measure of the time after fertilization.*

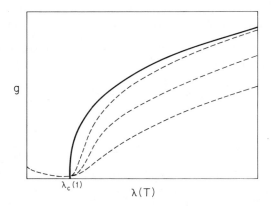

Figure 3b.   Dynamical TDGL-type theory compared to popular bifurcation theory.

The TDGL theory is a dynamical theory that yields the dependence of the mode amplitude g *on time. Such a dynamical theory is needed for many developing biological systems where parameters are changing on the same scale as the growing pattern. The bifurcation theory is limited to the extreme case where the biological parameters in the pattern formation mechanism change very slowly. As the parameter changes more slowly, the TDGL results (– – –) approach the bifurcation theory (———).*

like (i.e. be proportional to) ϵ as $\epsilon \to 0$ whereas the amplitude of the $\ell \neq 1$ modes should come into the next order, i.e. as ϵ^2. Also the lifetime of the critical mode goes like the inverse of the lifetime of small perturbations from the spherical state (obtained by linearizing (32) by simply dropping the quadratic B-terms). Hence the characteristic time for the growth of the pattern is of order $1/\epsilon^2$ and we need an appropriate new time variable τ that characterizes the slow time scale of interest near criticality. Thus we postulate solutions of the form

$$g_{1m} = \epsilon\gamma_{1m}(\tau)$$

$$g_{\ell m} = \epsilon^2\gamma_{\ell m}(\tau), \ \ell \neq 1, \qquad\qquad (34)$$

$$t = \tau/\epsilon^2.$$

As $\epsilon \to 0$ the dynamics of the $\ell \neq 1$ modes is much quicker than that of the slow, $\ell = 1$, modes. Hence putting (34) into (31) and letting $\epsilon \to 0$ we get the "adiabatic following" relation

$$\mu(\mu+1)(k_\mu - k_1)\gamma_{\mu\nu} = \sum_{mm'} B_{\mu\nu}^{1m,1m'}\gamma_{1m}\gamma_{1m'}, \ \mu \neq 1. \ (35)$$

Thus the fast modes follow the slow 1-modes. To obtain the equation for the slow mode amplitudes $\gamma_{1\nu}$, $\nu = 0, \pm1$, we put (34) into (32) for $\nu = 1$, take $\epsilon \to 0$ and insert the adiabatic following relation (35) to obtain

$$\frac{d\gamma_{1\nu}}{d\tau} = -2a\gamma_{1\nu} - \sum_{\substack{mm' \\ m+m'=0}} b_\nu^{mm'}\gamma_{1m}\gamma_{1m'}\gamma_{1\nu} \qquad\qquad (36)$$

where the $b_\nu^{mm'}$ can be related to the $B_{\mu\nu}^{\ell m, \ell'm'}$. This is the sought after TDGL. It gives an equation of motion for the amplitudes $\gamma_{1\nu}$ of the self-organizing electrophysiological pattern.

   2.   Temporal Development of Pattern. The solutions of this TDGL for the amplitude of the pattern are qualitatively as seen in Fig. 3b. Note that this dynamical pattern forming phenomenon is qualitatively different from the bifurcation structure of Fig. 3a when constraint parameters (here λ) change on a time scale comparable to that of the growth of pattern.
   In Fig. 3b we see how a small initial pattern ($\gamma_{1\pm1}$ small, $\gamma_{1\pm1} = 0$ at $t = 0$) first decreases and then begins to grow as λ exceeds $\lambda_c(1) = -1/k$.
   Under typical conditions of development the system has noise, either imposed or inherent molecular fluctuations. To describe this case we must add the effect of noise which may be simulated via a noise source on the RHS of the TDGL. Statistical analysis of TDGL's has been developed in a number of papers (see Ref. 27) and should be of interest in the present situation in evaluating applied electric field experiments on single cell

electrophysiological self-organization to be discussed in the
section on cells in external gradients. Further discussions of
TDGL theory are given in the section on cellular self-organization
mechanisms and in the next subsection in the context of pattern
stability.

Exchange of Stability. The TDGL method provides a procedure
for determining the stability of the patterned states near the
bifurcation point. Let us sketch the main ideas for the $\ell = 1$
steady state patterns under the simplification that the developmental time scale is very long compared to the time to generate
patterns, i.e. we neglect the time dependence of a and b in (36).
With this (36) yields steady state solutions $\bar{\gamma}_{1\nu}$ obeying

$$[-2a + \sum_{\substack{mm' \\ m+m'=0}} b_{\nu}^{mm'} \bar{\gamma}_{1m}\bar{\gamma}_{1m'}]\bar{\gamma}_{1\nu} = 0, \quad \nu = 0, \pm 1. \quad (37)$$

From the symmetry of the problem it is clear that there are
azymuthally symmetric solutions ($\bar{\gamma}_{1\pm} = 0$), implying that the non-
trivial ($\bar{\gamma}_{10} \neq 0$) solution is given by

$$\gamma_{10} = \pm \sqrt{\frac{2a}{b_0^{00}}} \qquad (38)$$

and that all other solutions to (37) are obtained by rotations
of the solution (38).

From the TDGL it is clear that the symmetric state $\bar{\gamma}_{1\nu} = 0$
becomes unstable as a goes from positive to negative. Letting
$\gamma_{10} = \bar{\gamma}_{10} + \delta_{10}$, $\gamma_{1\pm} = 0$, the TDGL for small δ_{10} becomes

$$\frac{d\delta_{10}}{d\tau} = 2a\delta_{10} \qquad (39)$$

and hence the 1,0 pattern is stable where the spherically symmetric state is unstable. Actually this oversimplistic treatment
neglects perturbations of the 1,0 pattern with respect to 1,±
perturbations (not to mention $\ell \neq 1$ perturbations). The main
result of a more complete treatment is that the dipole $\ell = 1$,
pattern is stable except that it is only marginally stable to a
rotation of the axis of the polarity because of the rotational
invarience of the problem.

Other Cellular Self-Organization Mechanisms. Much emphasis
has been placed in this section on the membrane based Ca^{2+} models
involving charged membrane transport mediating species. However,
a host of physically reasonable cellular self-organization phenomena present themselves. In this subsection we shall briefly
discuss some of them.

1. Classic Turing Models. The most well studied models of
spontaneous pattern formation are based on Turing's original idea
that symmetry breaking in biomorphogenesis occurs via an instability in a reaction-diffusion system. In order for this to be
operative the time scales for reaction and diffusion must be
comparable. Since cellular systems are in general quite small
the diffusion term will be very large unless at least one species
involved in the pattern formation has a sufficiently small diffusion coefficient. Thus Ca^{2+} and very large molecules are prime
candidates for relevant pattern forming species. A Turing type
model was used for the study of spherical systems with potential
application to cells but without electrical effects (40, 41).

2. Secondary Bifurcations. A secondary bifurcation occurs
when a pattern that arose from the unpatterned state itself becomes unstable (as a parameter passes beyond a critical value)
and a new pattern of still lower symmetry arises (30). This
phenomenon has interesting biological consequences as pointed out
in Ref. 41 where a spherical model of a biological system (without
electrophysiological processes included) was analyzed. It was
found that, beyond a critical value of a bifurcation parameter λ,
the $\ell = 1$ pattern changed to an $\ell = 2$-like pattern. It would be
very interesting to introduce electrophysiology into this
consideration.
      One particularly interesting application of these ideas is to
the problem of double rhizoid formation in Fucus (19). Indeed do
these arise directly from a $\ell = 2$ bifurcation from the spherically
symmetric state or after the egg passes through the normal $\ell = 1$
pattern? In this context it is useful to combine the TDGL method
and the Keener theory (30) to produce a formalism capable of describing the dynamics of the problem as we discussed in the
section on dynamical self-organization.

3. Membrane Flux Law Feedback. It has been shown that
nonlinearity on the boundary of a system can allow for the existence of waves, static patterns, oscillations or multiple steady
states even when no interesting nonlinear phenomena can occur in
a similar system with no special processes occuring in the bulk
of the medium (55). This idea was applied in Ref. 4 to a model
of spontaneous generation of patterns in which a Ca^{2+} regulated
Ca^{2+} pump played a central role. It was shown that even if the
pump molecule could not move along the membrane, symmetry breaking
could occur. A key feature of Ca^{2+} that made the model work at
physiologically relevant pump and diffusion rates was the small
rate of transport of Ca^{2+} in most cell interiors because of fixed
Ca^{2+} binding sites. The model was fully electric in nature. It
was shown that under cellular conditions the diffusion term can
sometimes dominate the electromigration term in the ion flux so
that positive ions can actually move up a voltage gradient.

4. Autocatalytic Local Incorporation Models. At some
stages of development certain molecules are produced inside a
cell. For example, just after oöcyte fertilization a number of
types of molecules are produced or released from stores. If these
molecules are (1) charged, (2) can be incorporated in the membrane and (3) effect transmembrane fluxes of species (notably
Ca^{2+}) that can build up transcellular gradients (because of low
diffusivity) then a positive feedback loop can be set up that
allows for self-organization. For example, suppose these molecules are positively charged, initially uniformally distributed
(in a burst of release from uniformally distributed stores) and
facilitate the active transport of Ca^{2+} out of the cell. If
there is, for example, a concentration fluctuation of this molecule (denoted M) so as to create a local maximum of M near the
"north pole," then more M will be incorporated in the membrane
there. This would cause a small local increase of Ca^{2+} efflux
and hence a local voltage minimum. But this would tend to attract
more of the positive M ions to the north pole, completing the
positive feedback loop. Note that the slowness of Ca^{2+} diffusion
across the cell is what allows a Ca^{2+} and Ca^{2+} binding site
gradient to build up and hence cause a voltage gradient sufficient
to drive more M ions to the region.

5. Phase Transitions and Freezing in Nonequilibrium
Structures. Turing's theory provides a mechanism for the autonomous generation of biological organization. It has been shown
by Prigogine and Glansdorf and the Brusselles school that a
necessary condition for the existence of these phenomena is that
the system be sufficiently far from equilibrium (29). Thus it
takes a constant flow of free energy to sustain these patterns
and one might wonder if biological systems could, at least in
some cases, invoke some mechanism of freezing in a pattern once
it has been set up to avoid this expenditure (3).
      One possible such mechanism for fixing a pattern is to have
a phase transition. For example, if the pattern is in terms of a
distribution of large molecules on the outer membrane surface, as
in the Fucus-like models discussed here, then a membrane phase
transition from a more liquid-like to a more crystal-like state
of the membrane could essentially immobilize the membrane bound
species and freeze in the pattern. In fact several hours after
fertilization in Fucus the lability (rotatability) of the polar
axis significantly decreases. Indeed this freezing of the Fucus
patterning is not easily explained in terms of a Turing mechanism
since the rotational symmetry of the Fucus egg, as discussed
previously, implies that the electrical polarity is not stable
(or more precisely is marginally stable) to polar axis rotation.
      Other mechanisms for fixing patterns involve laying down
membranes to catch the prepattern (3). For example, if there is
an ($m = 0$, $\ell = 1$)-like composition pattern before cell division
and if division occurs parallel to the equator, then (as in Fucus)

the two progeny are left compositionally different--i.e. certain
molecules that cannot permeate the membrane between the progeny
are forced to be localized in one of the cells.

Cells in External Gradients

Living systems must be able to self-organize in fluctuating
or anisotropic environments and thus, as discussed before, have a
certain degree of autonomy. However, they must also be able to
respond to certain external gradients for survival. Plants, for
example, want to grow with roots down and leaves up. In fact the
direction of polarity of the $\ell = 1$ (see Fig. 2) state of Fucus
can be fixed by unidirectional light, the location of other
neighboring cells or externally imposed electric fields. The response of developing cells to applied fields is the subject on
which we now focus.

Asymptotic Conditions. As a model problem we consider a sin-
gle cell containing the origin of coordinates $\vec{r} = \vec{0}$ and subject to
a uniform external electric field set up by a pair of parallel
planar electrodes at a large distance from the cell. Letting z
denote the direction perpendicular to the electrodes and E be the
electric field set up by the electrodes in the absence of the cell,
we have the asymptotic boundary conditions:

$$V \underset{|\vec{r}| \to \infty}{\sim} -Ez \tag{40}$$

$$\underline{c} \underset{|\vec{r}| \to \infty}{\sim} \underline{c}^{\infty}. \tag{41}$$

Thus all the calculations of the previous section can be extended
by appropriate changes that account for these new boundary conditions at infinity, i.e. we solve (1-7) subject to (40, 41).

Response Phenomena.

1. Hyperpolarizability. In studying cellular electrophysiological self-organization we observed that a cellular system can spontaneously develop a transcellular electrical polarity
and concomitant ionic currents. Thus, as the cell develops, a
condition is approached wherein no external asymmetry is needed to
induce an asymmetry. Close but below this point a very small
applied field of the correct symmetry has a very strong effect,
inducing an anamolously large response.

An example of this phenomenon seems to be the ease with which
the direction of the polar axis of Fucus is fixed by extremely
gentle gradients, most notably the direction of polarization of
polarized light or the coordination of axis direction of neighboring eggs (8). We term this phenomenon "hyperpolarizability." It

is essentially the same phenomenon as the dramatic response of a
system in phase transition (as gas $\rightleftarrows$ liquid) near the critical
point. Perhaps a closer analogy is the response of a ferromagnet
just above the Curie temperature to an applied magnetic field.
The "anamolous" response of reaction-diffusion systems to external influences has been pointed out previously (20).

Hyperpolarizability thus provides a sensitive mechanism
whereby developing biological systems may respond or adapt their
organization to environmental conditions at crucial stages of
development. For example, Fucus would not like to grow with its
roots to the sun. In fact unidirectional light fixes the axis
and sense of the electrical polarity which then, at a later stage,
determines which of the first pair of progeny (after the first
cell division) will be the leaf-stem system and which will be the
presumptive root system.

Hyperpolarizability does not imply that the system is completely at the control of the external gradients. Indeed, the
response is very special--there is a strong tendency for the form
of the response to be essentially that of the modes of the stability analysis which are most weakly stable and, beyond the point
of instability, become the autonomous (imposed gradient free)
pattern.

   2. Lability. The lability of a biological pattern is its
ability to be deformed, rotate or otherwise change in response to
an external influence. For example, the axis of polarity of the
self-sustained voltage patterns of the Fucus egg may be rotated
under the influence of an applied gradient (8, 28).

   As pointed out above in regard to the hyperpolarizability
effect, the lability of a biopattern is closely related to its
stability. Consider, for example, the lability of the Fucus egg
polarity in its early development. In the absence of an applied
gradient, the equations describing the dynamics of the egg are
invarient under a rotation of coordinates about the center of the
egg. This implies that if we have a solution of the form $\Psi(\vec{r}, t)$
then for any rotation operation $\mathcal{R}$ taking a vector $\vec{r}$ to a new
vector $\vec{r}' = \mathcal{R}\vec{r}$, $|\vec{r}'| = |\vec{r}|$, then $\Psi(\vec{r}', t)$ is also a solution
(state) of the Fucus system. This implies that the state $\Psi(\vec{r}, t)$
is only marginally stable as follows. Assume Ψ obeys the
equation

$$\frac{\partial \Psi}{\partial t} = \eta[\Psi]. \qquad (42)$$

This must also hold for a small rotation $\Psi \rightarrow \Psi' = \Psi + \delta\Psi$ where $\delta\Psi$
is small. Since Ψ' also satisfies (42) we have, for small $\delta\Psi$,

$$\frac{\partial \delta\Psi}{\partial t} = \mathcal{L}\delta\Psi \qquad (43)$$

where $\mathcal{L}$ is a linear operator associated with the functional derivative of η evaluated at $\Psi(\vec{r}, t)$. Since the state $\Psi(\vec{r}, t)$ describes

one possible developmental course of the system, $\delta\Psi \equiv \Psi'-\Psi$ must
persist for all times. But (43) is exactly the form of the linear
stability theory for perturbations $\delta\Psi$ from Ψ. Thus there are
infinitely long lived and bounded perturbations from Ψ and hence
Ψ is (at most) marginally stable. The presence of marginal
stability to rotations of the polar axis makes lability quite
plausible. The rigorous mathematical proof of this connection is
somewhat technical and is not given here. Generally invarience of
the dynamics under a continuous transformation group (here rotations) implies marginal stability and lability.

    <u>Imperfect Bifurcation</u>. In the context of spatial self-
organization, the bifurcation diagram of a system is a plot of
the amplitude of a pattern as a function of the various control
parameters. For the cell in a plane parallel applied field of
strength E and with some system parameter λ (as a bath concentration or as in (22)), the pattern amplitude can be described by
the g's in (23-30) and especially (29).
    To briefly give a qualitative idea of how an applied field
effects axis determination consider a <u>Fucus</u>-like spherical cell
about the origin in an imposed field--applied in the z direction
as per (40). Consider now the emergence of an $\ell = 1$ pattern
associated with Y , i.e. $\gamma \sim g\cos\theta$ where γ is the Ca^{2+} pump concentration deviation from uniformity and θ is the angle with respect to the z axis (defined to be the direction of the applied
field as in (40). Then one finds that g satisfies

$$g^3 + a\lambda_2 g + bE_3 = 0 \qquad\qquad (44)$$

where we have assumed the applied field is small $(E = E_3 \epsilon^3)$ as it
certainly is in the highly conductive media in which <u>Fucus</u>
typically grows. Also λ is assumed to be near the critical value
$\lambda_c(\ell = 1)$, i.e. $\lambda-\lambda_c(1) = \lambda_2\epsilon^2$, $\epsilon \ll 1$. The constants a and b
are related to transport coefficients for the cell as explained in
more detail in Refs. <u>7</u>, <u>19</u>. In the nonlinear literature, applied
mathematicians have termed the breaking of the symmetry of a bifurcation diagram, such as that of Fig. 3 for $\ell = 1$ to one like
in Fig. 4b by an imposed "imperfection," an "imperfect bifurcation" (<u>21</u>).
    In the present problem the imperfect bifurcation theory
results in clarifying the close analogy of the development of
polarity in <u>Fucus</u> with a ferromagnetic transition. To demonstrate
this we multiply (44) by ϵ^3 and let $g\epsilon \equiv m$, $a\lambda_2\epsilon^2 \equiv t$ and $bE_3\epsilon^3 \equiv$
h. Then (44) becomes

$$m^3 + tm + h = 0 \qquad\qquad (45)$$

which is recognized as the mean field equation of state for a
ferromagnet for which m is the magnetization, t is the difference
between the temperature and its critical value and h is the
applied magnetic field strength. The equation takes the form of a

cusp in an m, t, h phase diagram as shown and explained further
in Fig. 4. A more complete description wherein all three $\ell = 1$
mode amplitudes are discussed is given in Ref. 7 and 19. The
result of this more complete study is that the only steady state
pattern is that aligned parallel or antiparallel to the applied
field. This may explain why <u>Fucus</u> aligns with an applied
field.

Typically developing systems are in a situation
of dynamical patterning. A bifurcation picture is not relevant
unless there is time scale separation; thus a TDGL formalism is
more appropriate as discussed above in dynamicsl self-organization. We are developing such a theory to study lability in
<u>Fucus</u>-like polarization phenomena.

   <u>Induction of New Phenomena by Imposed Gradients</u>. Studies on
the effects of imposed electric fields on chemical waves (see
below on signal propagation) show that phenomena can be induced
in the system by the imposed gradient that do not exist in the
field free medium. For example, it was found (11) that for a
system wherein only one type of wave existed in the field free
case, two stable types of waves exist in the system subject to
the field. This "induction of multiplicity" implies that beyond
a critical value of the applied field strength new phenomena may
set in that are not simple distortions of field free patterns.
Another strictly imposed field effect is found in the case of a
new two dimensional crescent shaped wave that occurs when a circular wave is subjected to a supracritical field (13).

   Such induction of new phenomena has not been investigated in
the context of bioelectric systems but it would not be unreasonable to expect that such phenomena will be found in the near
future. In fact the induction of the formation of a second head
in certain worms subjected to an external field may be an
example (53).

Bioelectric Patterning in Cell Aggregates

   Strong electric fields and currents have been measured in a
number of multicellular systems ranging from <u>Fucus</u> at the two cell
state, a <u>Cecropia</u> moth oöcyte-nurse cell cyncytum, amphibian and
rodent limbs in regeneration and man (8, 22, 28, 53). Thus it is
imperative to develop a formulation of multicellular phenomena.
A number of complex factors enter in many of these systems. The
simplest situations are those for which the geometry of the
aggregate is fixed so that cells do not change shape or position
as is the case in some stages of <u>Fucus</u> or <u>Cecropia</u> cyncytum
development. However, in most cases of limb development,
innervation (nerve fiber invation) plays a central role. Furthermore, many systems are growing and hence the developing limb, for
example, involves a situation of dynamical geometry. Even more
complex is the phenomenon of cell migration such as that which

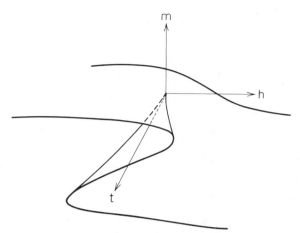

Figure 4a. Imperfect bifurcation showing the breaking of the symmetry of the diagram of Figure 3a due to the imposition of an external electric field of strength proportional to h.

This nonequilibrium phase diagram is in the form of a cusp in (m,t,h) space (see Ref. 45 for definitions). It is a perfect analogue of a ferromagnetic phase transition if we interpret m,t,h as magnetization, temperature (minus its critical value), and applied magnetic field, respectively.

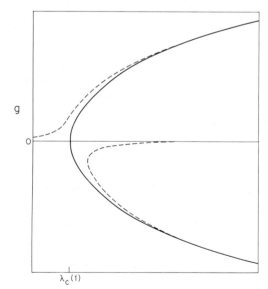

Figure 4b.   Slices through cusp of Figure 4a comparing field-free (E = 0) behavior with that in the presence of an electric field for a Fucus-*like system (where g is proportional to the transcellular electric current).*

The imperfection also may be interpreted as resulting from an inherent cellular asymmetry such as the entry point of the sperm or internal compartmentalization ((——) E = 0; (– – –) E > 0).

often takes place in embryonic development. Here we present a theory for the simplest case of a cell aggregate of fixed overall geometry, fixed cell shape, position and free of mitosis. We first consider a pseudo electro-diffusion theory in the next two subsections and then a more accurate averaging operator formalism in the third subsection. Applications and further developments of these approaches are found in later subsections.

The self-organizational aspect of multicellular systems in the case to be considered here will be in the spirit of the Turing theory except that we shall (1) address the electrophysiology of the problem and (2) consider a more accurate integral operator for the intercellular transport. An important addition to the Turing theory is the idea of size regulation introduced in Ref. 20 in connection with physico-chemical phenomena and in Ref. 44 in the biological context. These considerations are relevant to single cell systems as well and are as follows.

1. Extrinsic Case - Patterns that Scale with System Size
Systems with a conserved quantity, such as the amount of the Γ-species in the single cell models mentioned before, may show a symmetry breaking instability which typically has a first bifurcation that corresponds to a pattern length completely determined by the size of the system and not by any reaction-transport length inherent to the mechanism. These systems develop an overall gradient and the pattern length regulates with system length.   The pattern length is not intrinsic to the mechanism of pattern formation.

2. Intrinsic Case - Patterns that Scale with Kinetic
            Coefficients
This is the classic Turing (1) case wherein, even in an infinite system, the mechanism fixes a pattern length according to the reaction rate and transport coefficients. Thus, roughly speaking, if we double the size of the system, the pattern will be reproduced twice (as long as the system is larger than the inherent pattern length).

Let us now discuss the development of a formalism within which these and other developmental phenomena can be investigated.

Cell to Cell Transport Phenomenology. Consider a mass of cells in an external medium denoted "e" as in Fig. 1. We shall construct a continuum approximation wherein the cells are "smeared out." Such a theory will be accurate when the length scale of interest (i.e., the pattern length) is greater than a cell diameter. An important aspect of the formulation is that the equations derived by taking the continuum limit will relate effective transport rates directly to measurable properties of individual cells or pairs of cells in contact.

Consider an interface between two cells as shown in Fig. 5. The domain III between cells I and II is narrow and hence concentrations are essentially constant across this gap of width Δ and are denoted $\underline{c}^{III}$. For a small contact area A between the cells the column vector of numbers of moles of the various species in this small domain in region III is $A_\Delta \underline{c}^{III}$. Let $\underline{J}^{MI}$ be the transmembrane flux into cell I and similarly for $\underline{J}^{MII}$. Denoting the flux along domain III to be $\vec{\underline{J}}^{III}$ and $\vec{\nabla}_{III}$ to be the gradient along the interface we have the mass balance condition

$$A_\Delta \frac{\partial \underline{c}^{III}}{\partial t} = -A_\Delta \vec{\nabla}_{III} \cdot \vec{\underline{J}}^{III} + A_\Delta \underline{R}^{III} - A[\underline{J}^{MI} + \underline{J}^{MII}] \quad (46)$$

where $\underline{R}^{III}$ are the rates of reaction in domain III, the space between the cells. However, the thickness of the layer between the cells Δ is small. Hence in the limit $\Delta \to 0$ we get

$$\underline{J}^{MI} + \underline{J}^{MII} = \underline{0}. \quad (47)$$

If we assume all cells are the same then we have $\underline{J}^{MI} = \underline{J}^{M}(\underline{c}^{I}, \underline{c}^{III}, v^{I}-v^{III})$, and similarly for $\underline{J}^{MII}$. Thus (47) with the charge neutrality condition in region III,

$$\underline{J}^{M}(\underline{c}^{I}, \underline{c}^{III}, v^{I}-v^{III}) + \underline{J}^{M}(\underline{c}^{II}, \underline{c}^{III}, v^{II}-v^{III}) = \underline{0} \quad (48)$$

$$\underline{z} * \underline{c}^{III} \equiv \sum_j z_j c_j^{III} = 0, \quad (49)$$

yield $\underline{c}^{III}$ and v^{III} as functions of $\underline{c}^{I}, \underline{c}^{II}, v^{I}$ and v^{II}. Substituting $\underline{c}^{III}(\underline{c}^{I}, \underline{c}^{II}, v^{I}, v^{II})$ and $v^{III}(\underline{c}^{I}, \underline{c}^{II}, v^{I}, v^{II})$ into $\underline{J}^{M}(\underline{c}^{I}, \underline{c}^{III}, v^{I}-v^{III})$ we can express the net influx into cell I as a function of the I, II variables only; we denote this function as $\underline{\mathfrak{J}}(\underline{c}^{I}, \underline{c}^{II}, v^{I}, v^{II})$. Hence $\underline{J}^{MI} = -\underline{J}^{MII} = \underline{\mathfrak{J}}$ where, in an obvious notation.

$$\underline{\mathfrak{J}}(I, II) \equiv \underline{J}^{M}(\underline{c}^{I}, \underline{c}^{III}(I, II), v^{I}-v^{III}(I, II)). \quad (50)$$

This function $\underline{\mathfrak{J}}$ shall provide the basis of the link between the "macroscopic" theory and the "microscopic" theory that deals with the properties (such as membrane transport) of a single cell.

A word of caution is in order here in that it may be necessary to account for the fact that the membrane-membrane contact can cause important changes in the individual membranes. Most noteworthy of these is the existence of tight junctions that develop from one cell to another. If such effects are present then we will take them to be included in $\underline{\mathfrak{J}}$.

Small Gradient Theory.

1. General Structure. We expect that the most significant variations in composition occur across a membrane. Thus we neglect variations within a cell and define $\underline{c}(\vec{r}, t)$ to be the concentrations in a cell containing $\vec{r}$. To obtain a weak gradient approximation we calculate the net flux from a cell at $\vec{r} + \hat{n}L$ into one at $\vec{r}$ where $\hat{n}$ is a unit length vector and L is the center-to-center distance between cells. Assuming that the

concentrations and voltage vary on a length scale long compared to L (a "weak gradient approximation") we have

$$\underline{\vec{J}}(\underline{c}(\vec{r},t),\ \underline{c}(\vec{r}+\hat{n}L,t),\ v(\vec{r},t),\ v(\vec{r}+\hat{n}L,t) \approx -\hat{n}\cdot\underline{\vec{J}}_T \quad (51)$$

$$-\underline{\vec{J}}_T = \underline{\underline{\mathcal{D}}}\vec{\nabla}\underline{c} + \underline{\underline{m}}\underline{c}\vec{\nabla}v \quad\quad\quad (52)$$

$$\underline{\underline{\mathcal{D}}} = [(\partial\underline{\vec{J}}/\partial\underline{c}^{II}),\ \underline{\underline{m}}\underline{c} \equiv (\partial\underline{\vec{J}}/\partial v^{II})]\ \text{at}\ \underline{c}^{I} = \underline{c}^{II} = \underline{c},$$

$$v^{I} = v^{II} = v. \quad\quad\quad (53)$$

We have used the fact that $\underline{\vec{J}}(\underline{C}, \underline{C}, V, V) = 0$. The neglect of higher order terms in L may be formalized as follows. Suppose a descriptive variable $\Psi(\vec{r})$ (be it $\underline{C}$ or $\underline{V}$) varies on a length scale L_c. Then we introduce a new variable $\vec{r}' = \vec{r}/L_c$ and write $\Psi(\vec{r}) = \Psi(\vec{r}'L_c) \equiv \Psi'(\vec{r}')$ where Ψ' is a function that varies on a scale of unity. Thus $\Psi'(\frac{\vec{r}+\hat{n}L}{L_c}) = \Psi'(\vec{r}' + \hat{n}\epsilon) \approx \Psi'(\vec{r}') + \epsilon\vec{\nabla}'\Psi'\cdot\hat{n} + \mathcal{O}(\epsilon^2)$.

The weak gradient limit is obtained when $\epsilon \equiv L/L_c \ll 1$.

Using the usual arguments to derive continuity equations in terms of the flux (23) we obtain

$$\frac{\partial\underline{C}}{\partial t} = -\vec{\nabla}\cdot\underline{\vec{J}}_T + \underline{R} \quad\quad\quad (54)$$

where $\underline{R}$ are the reaction rates for processes in the cells. Since a biological ionic strengths are large we have

$$Z*\underline{C} = 0, \quad\quad\quad (55)$$

as in the single cell theory (Z being a row vector of valences).

It is instructive to break $\underline{R}$ into a part due to fast reactions associated with the sticking of mobile species to fixed sites and the rest. For simplicity we assume there is only one type of binding site, Y , that can bind to the s mobile species i = 1, 2,...s to form complexes Y_i. Then letting R denote the remaining reactions we have found that when the chromatographic reactions are fast, the equation of motion (54) for the concentrations $\underline{c}$ of mobile species alone becomes, as for single cells as above,

$$[\underline{I} + \underline{\Delta}(\underline{c})]\partial\underline{c}/\partial t = -\vec{\nabla}\cdot\vec{J} + R \quad\quad\quad (56)$$

$$\underline{z}*[\underline{c} + \underline{y}^{eq}(\underline{c})] + y_0 Y_T = 0 \quad\quad\quad (57)$$

$$(\underline{\underline{\Delta}})_{ij} = \partial Y_i^{eq}/\partial c_j \quad\quad\quad (58)$$

where $Y_i^{eq}(\underline{c})$ is the concentration of the site bound to mobile species i at equilibrium, y is the valence of the empty site, Y_T is the total concentration (empty or bound) of the fixed sites and the sum implied in (57) is over mobile species only. $\vec{J}$ takes the usual form $\vec{J} = -\underline{D}(\underline{c})\vec{\nabla}\underline{c} - \underline{M}(\underline{c})\underline{c}\vec{\nabla}V$ where $\underline{D}$ and $\underline{M}$ are s x s matrices that can easily be related to the $\underline{\underline{\mathcal{D}}}$ and $\underline{\underline{m}}$ and $Y_i^e(\underline{c})$ (see Ref. 5).

2. Relation Between Levels of Description. It is our intention here to make the relation between the macroflus $\underline{J}$ and the individual cell membrane flux law $\underline{J}^M$ more explicit. The diffusion-like coefficients $\underline{\underline{D}}$ of (52) may be written, using (49), as

$$\underline{\underline{D}} = \frac{\partial \underline{J}^{MI}}{\partial \underline{c}^{III}} \frac{\partial \underline{c}^{III}}{\partial \underline{c}^{II}} + \frac{\partial \underline{J}^{MI}}{\partial v^{III}} \frac{\partial v^{III}}{\partial \underline{c}^{II}} \text{ at } \underline{c}^I = \underline{c}^{II} = \underline{c},$$

$$v^I = v^{II} = v. \tag{59}$$

The derivatives $(\partial \underline{J}^{MI}/\partial \underline{c}^{III})$ and $(\partial \underline{J}^{MI}/\partial v^{III})$ can be calculated directly from the cell membrane phenomonology. However, the derivatives of $\underline{c}^{III}$ with respect to $\underline{c}^{II}$ must be determined more indirectly via (48,49). Taking $\partial/\partial \underline{c}^{II}$ of both sides of (48,49) we get

$$\frac{\partial(\underline{J}^{MI}+\underline{J}^{MII})}{\partial \underline{c}^{III}} \frac{\partial \underline{c}^{III}}{\partial \underline{c}^{II}} + \frac{\partial(\underline{J}^{MI}+\underline{J}^{MII})}{\partial v^{III}} \frac{\partial v^{III}}{\partial \underline{c}^{II}} = - \frac{\partial(\underline{J}^{MII})}{\partial \underline{c}^{II}} \tag{60}$$

$$Z_* \frac{\partial \underline{c}^{III}}{\partial \underline{c}^{II}} = 0. \tag{61}$$

In these expressions the derivatives of $\underline{J}^{MI,II}$ are evaluated at the solution of

$$\underline{J}^M(\underline{c}, \underline{c}^{III}, v-v^{III}) = 0 \tag{62}$$

$$Z_* \underline{c}^{III} = 0, \tag{63}$$

since we must evaluate the quantities in (46,47) at $\underline{c}^{I,II} = \underline{c}$, $v^{I,II} = v$. Thus, having solved (62,63) for $\underline{c}^{III}$, v^{III} we can find $\partial \underline{c}^{III}/\partial \underline{c}^{II}$ and $(\partial v^{III}/\partial \underline{c}^{II})$ from the linear equations (60,61). Similar considerations yield expressions for $\mathcal{m}\underline{c}$.

3. Boundary Conditions. The cell mass communicates with the surroundings through its boundaries. Since the flux of nutrients, waste and other agents can profoundly affect development, the conditions at the boundary are quite important. This will manifest itself mathematically in the sensitivity of the system to the boundary conditions on the descriptive variables.

The relevant boundary conditions that are to be imposed depend critically on both the nature of the boundary and the environment. In the latter regard we take the simplest case here wherein the environment is assumed constant in space and time. This is a typical situation because the environment is often quite well stirred and furthermore the diffusion and ionic mobility coefficients in the environment are often much larger than those within the mass. Finally we shall assume that the mass is surrounded by an outer membrane with flux relations $\underline{K}^M$ taken to be positive when directed into the cell mass. Letting ñ be a unit outward normal to the outer membrane (see Figure 1) we have

$$-\hat{n}\cdot\vec{\underline{J}} = \underline{K}^M(\underline{c},v) \text{ at } S(\vec{r}) = 0, \ \hat{n} = \vec{\nabla}S/|\vec{\nabla}S| \qquad (64)$$

where $S(\vec{r}) = 0$ determines the shape of the cell mass, i.e. the location of the boundary membrane. The dependence of $\underline{K}^M$ on the external conditions has been repressed here. The theory is developed further in the section on Patterns generated by the outer membrane and Ref. 43.

A Nonlinear Integral Operator Model of Effective Transport. In many differentiated tissues the cell type changes on a length scale of the order of one cell diamater. Thus, according to the view that cell type is fixed by internal cell composition, the weak gradient approximation of the previous section cannot be applied to these systems. In this section we develop a theory that does not rely on such a small gradient approach by introducing an averaging operator in favor of the usual diffusive flux term of the Turing theory.

1. Interior Cells. To formulate the theory we must consider cells at boundary separately from interior cells that are surrounded by other cells. We take such an interior cell to be crudely described by a sphere of radius R . The concentrations $\underline{C}$ in this cell change due to reaction rates $^O\underline{R}$ and due to flux across its surface. This latter contribution is simply $\underline{J}$ appropriately summed over all neighbor contributions. Thus we get a rate equation for the concentration of each species, $\underline{C}(\vec{r},t)$, in the cell about $\vec{r}$:

$$\frac{\partial \underline{C}(\vec{r},t)}{\partial t} = \underline{\mathfrak{J}}^{(d)} + \underline{R} \qquad (65)$$

$$\underline{\mathfrak{J}}^{(1)} = \sum_{\sigma=\pm 1} \underline{J}(C(r), C(r+\sigma R_o), V(r), V(r+\sigma R_o))$$

$$\underline{\mathfrak{J}}^{(2)} = \frac{1}{\pi R_o} \int_0^{2\pi} d\phi \underline{J}(\underline{C}(\vec{r}), \underline{C}(\vec{r}+\hat{n}R_o), V(\vec{r}), V(\vec{r}+\hat{n}R_o)) \qquad (66)$$

$$\underline{\mathfrak{J}}^{(3)} = \frac{3}{4\pi R_o} \int_0^{2\pi} d\phi \int_0^{\pi} \sin\theta d\theta \ \underline{J}(\underline{C}(\vec{r}), \underline{C}(\vec{r}+\hat{n}R_o), V(\vec{r}),$$

$$V(\vec{r}+\hat{n}R_o)).$$

Here $\underline{J}$ is the cell to cell flux discussed near equation (50) and $\underline{\mathfrak{J}}^{(d)}$ is the flux contribution for d = 1, 2, 3 dimensional systems. A unit vector $\hat{n}$ (depending on an angle ϕ for d $= 2$ and on spherical angles θ, ϕ in the case d $= 3$) is used to average $\mathfrak{J}$ over all neighboring cells in the present continuum model ($\hat{n} = \bar{n}(\phi)$, $\hat{n}(\theta, \phi)$ for d $= 2, 3$ respectively).

Rapid chromatographic reactions may be accounted for as in the case of the small gradient theory. This and charge neutrality lead to

$$[\underline{\underline{I}} + \underline{\underline{\Lambda}}(\underline{c})]\frac{\partial \underline{c}}{\partial t} = \underline{F}[\underline{c}, V] + \underline{R} \tag{67}$$

$$\sum_j z_j[c_j + Y_j^{eq}(\underline{c})] + y_o Y_T = 0. \tag{68}$$

The functional $\underline{F}[\underline{c}, V]$ has the same structure as $\mathfrak{J}$ of (66) except that the zero fluxes for the fixed sites are deleted from $\mathfrak{J}$ and the fixed site concentrations Y_i are held at their equilibrium values $Y_i^{eq}(\underline{c})$; $\underline{\Lambda}$ is given in (58).

   2. Boundary Cells. A cell on the boundary has one wall in contact with the outside world and hence the flux through that wall is $\underline{K}^M$ and not $\underline{J}^M$. Generally we want to replace $\underline{J}^M$ with $\underline{K}^M$ over that fraction of the cell surface in common with the outer boundary. One method for doing so is to replace $\mathfrak{J}$ in (66) by $\underline{K}^M$ in those parts of the d-dimensional sphere surrounding point $\vec{r}$ that stick outside the cell aggregate volume. Thus (67,68) take the same form for the boundary points except that $\underline{F}$ takes on the form, for d $= 3$,

$$4\pi R_o^2 \underline{F}[\underline{c}'] = \int_V d^3r' \underline{J}(\underline{c}(\vec{r}), \underline{c}(\vec{r}'), V(\vec{r}), V(\vec{r}'))\delta(|\vec{r}-\vec{r}'| - R_o) + \int_{\tilde{V}} d^3r' \underline{K}(\underline{c}(\vec{r}), \underline{c}(\vec{r}'), V(\vec{r}), V(\vec{r}'))\delta(|\vec{r}-\vec{r}'| - R_o). \tag{69}$$

Here V and $\tilde{V}$ are the volumes of the aggregate and environment respectively. $\underline{J}$ is $\mathfrak{J}$ with the bound species concentrations replaced by their values $Y_i^{eq}(\underline{c})$ and similarly for the relation between $\underline{K}$ and $\underline{K}^M$. (Both $\underline{K}$ and $\underline{J}$ also have a factor $(4\pi R_o/3)^{-1}$ incorporated in them. Similar expressions can be obtained for one and two dimensions.) Notice that the device of using the Dirac delta functions also allows the use of formula (69) at any point $\vec{r}$ inside the aggregate.

   3. General Remarks. These equations for the dynamics of a cell mass are in the form of a nonlinear partial integro-differential equation. The nonlocal structure and nonlinearity of the transport term allows for short length scale variation on the order of a cell diameter that models the cellular nature of the aggregate. Equations of a similar form arise in the work of

Cowan and coworkers $(\underline{45})$ in the theory of neuronal interactions in the brain. These equations have been shown to yield a great variety of self-organizing phenomena and hence such phenomena are certain to arise in the present theory. Finally we note that in the limit of small R the theory reduces to the small gradient theory. In the section on bioelectric patterning we shall demonstrate some aspects of self-organization in this model.

Patterns Generated by the Outer Membrane. As in the single cell case, the outer membrane itself can generate electrophysiological patterns, even in the absence of reactions in the cell mass, $\underline{R} = \underline{0}$. Such surface induced patterns were first discussed in the context of reaction-diffusion patterns in Ref. $\underline{24}$. Since the environment is taken to be homogeneous the equations $(57,64)$ yield a homogeneous steady state $\underline{c}^h$, V^h if solutions of

$$\underline{K}^M(\underline{c}^h,v^h) = 0 \tag{70}$$

$$y_o Y_T + \sum_j z_j(c_j^h + Y_j^{eq}(\underline{c}^h)) = 0 \tag{71}$$

can be obtained.

Let us investigate the onset of steady bioelectric patterns. For these steady states $\partial c/\partial t = 0$, $\partial V/\partial t = \underline{0}$, and hence we must solve $(56,57)$ with (64) by setting $\partial \underline{c}/\partial t = \underline{0}$ in (57). Bifurcation theory shows that when a critical value of a parameter (such as a bath concentration) attains a critical value, small amplitude patterns arise from the uniform state ($\underline{c}^h$, V^h here) in a pattern dictated usually by the equations linearized about the uniform state. The bifurcation condition for this patterning onset thus occurs when we can find solutions of

$$\nabla^2 \delta \underline{c} = 0, \quad \nabla^2 \delta V = 0 \tag{72}$$

$$\underline{\zeta} * \delta \underline{c} = 0 \tag{73}$$

$$\underline{D}\hat{n} \cdot \vec{\nabla} \delta \underline{c} + \underline{M} c^h \hat{n} \cdot \vec{\nabla} \delta V = \underline{\underline{C}} \delta \underline{c} + \boldsymbol{\mathcal{V}} \delta V \tag{74}$$

$$\zeta_j = z_j + \sum_k z_k \Lambda_{kj} \tag{75}$$

$$(\underline{\underline{C}})_{ij} = (\partial K_i^M/\partial c_j)^h \tag{76}$$

$$\boldsymbol{\mathcal{V}}_i = (\partial K_i^M/\partial v)^h. \tag{77}$$

With this we seek conditions involving the properties $\underline{D}$, $\underline{M}$, $\underline{\underline{C}}$ and $\boldsymbol{\mathcal{V}}$ for which bifurcation to bioelectric patterning can be attained.

The geometry of the cell mass effects the patterns available to the system. First we focus on the simplest case of a

spherical mass. Results on more general ellipsoidal systems
have been obtained in Ref. 46 and below.

    1. The Spherical Cell Mass. For the spherical cell mass
of radius R_M the boundary condition (74) becomes

$$\underline{\underline{D}}\frac{\partial \delta \underline{c}}{\partial r} + \underline{\underline{Mc}}^h \frac{\partial \delta V}{\partial r} = \underline{\underline{C}} \delta \underline{c} + \boldsymbol{\mathcal{V}} \delta V, \quad r = R_M. \tag{78}$$

The dynamics of the problem can then be understood in terms of
the spherical harmonic stability modes: consider solutions of
the form

$$\left. \begin{array}{l} \delta \underline{c} = \underline{\gamma}_{\ell m} Y_{\ell m}(\theta,\phi) r^\ell \\[2mm] \delta V = \nu_{\ell m} Y_{\ell m}(\theta,\phi) r^\ell \end{array} \right\} \quad r < R_M. \tag{79}$$

With this (79) and the charge neutrality condition (73) yield

$$\Omega(\ell,\lambda) \begin{bmatrix} \underline{\gamma}_{\ell m} \\[2mm] \nu_{\ell m} \end{bmatrix} = 0 \tag{80}$$

$$\Omega(\ell,\lambda) = \begin{bmatrix} \dfrac{\ell}{R_M}\underline{\underline{D}} - \underline{\underline{C}} & \dfrac{\ell}{R_M}\underline{\underline{Mc}}^h - \boldsymbol{\mathcal{V}} \\[3mm] \underline{\zeta} & 0 \end{bmatrix} \tag{81}$$

We have identified a particular parameter λ on which to study
the dependence of the system behavior. λ may be a bath concentration, temperature, or transport coefficient or R_M for
example. In order to find nontrivial solutions $(\underline{\gamma}_{\ell m} \neq 0, \nu_{\ell m} \neq 0)$ we have the condition

$$\det \Omega(\ell,\lambda_c(\ell)) = 0 \tag{82}$$

yielding the ℓ-dependent critical value of λ at which patterning
of symmetry ℓ might (but does not necessarily) set in.

    2. Geometric Mode Mixing. The spherical case is mis-
leadingly simple. The most noteworthy feature of the degeneracy
of this case is that the modes that can lead to patterns are
single modes of Laplace's equation $(r^\ell Y_{\ell m}(\theta,\phi))$. In more general
ellipsoidal geometries, for example, this is not the case and
the linear stability analysis involves infinite sums of
ellipsoidal harmonics. It is very interesting that the weight of
mixing depends on chemistry and hence, unlike in the degenerate
case of the sphere, patterns may be determined by kinetics
as well as shape in eccentric cases.
    Perhaps the simplest case displaying geometrical mode mixing

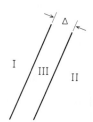

Figure 5. Interface structure between two cells with interiors labeled I and II.

The narrow domain of width Δ between the cells is labeled Region III. This geometry is used to derive equations of multicellular electrophysiology in the section on bioelectric patterning in cell aggregates.

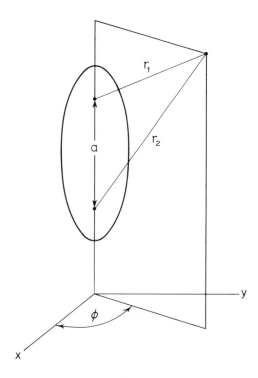

Figure 6. Prolate spheroidal coordinates used to describe an elongated cell mass.

The foci are separated by a distance a along the z axis. See Morse and Feshback (25) for details. Eccentricity of form is found to effect profoundly autonomous current patterns. This geometric mode mixing phenomenon leads to patterns that can be controlled by the chemical kinetics in a manner not found for simple, highly symmetric geometries like the sphere or cube.

is that of the prolate spheroid shown in Fig. 6. It is most convenient to introduce prolate spheroidal coordinates (25) defined as follows:

$$\xi = (r_1 + r_2)/a, \quad 1 \le \xi < \xi_0$$

$$\eta = (r_1 - r_2)/a, \quad -1 \le \eta \le 1 \qquad\qquad (83)$$

$$\phi = \tan^{-1}(y/x), \quad 0 \le \phi \le 2\pi$$

where the prolate ellipsoidal boundary is given by $\xi = \xi_0 =$ constant.

In these coordinates Laplace's equation separates such that functions of the form $P_{\ell m}(\xi)P_{\ell m}(\eta)\binom{\cos}{\sin}m\phi$ satisfy it where the $P_{\ell m}$ are the associated Legendre functions. Thus for this interior problem (i.e. inside the spheroid, not outside it) the general solution of the linear problem is of the form

$$\begin{bmatrix} \delta c \\ \delta V \end{bmatrix} = \sum_{\ell m} \left\{ \begin{bmatrix} a_{\ell m} \\ \alpha_{\ell m} \end{bmatrix} \cos m\phi + \begin{bmatrix} b_{\ell m} \\ \beta_{\ell m} \end{bmatrix} \sin m\phi \right\} P_{\ell m}(\eta)P_{\ell m}(\xi) \qquad (84)$$

where $\alpha_{\ell m}$, $\beta_{\ell m}$, $a_{\ell m}$ and $b_{\ell m}$ are to be determined by the boundary conditions. In our calculations we shall need to determine the normal derivative $\hat{n}\cdot\vec{\nabla}$ at the prolate spheroid and we shall also need to integrate over the surface of the latter. Using Ref. 25 the surface area element $d\omega$ on the spheroid and normal derivative are given by

$$d\omega = h_\eta h_\phi d\eta d\phi \qquad\qquad (85)$$

$$\hat{n}\cdot\vec{\nabla} = \frac{1}{h_\xi}\frac{\partial}{\partial\xi}, \qquad\qquad (86)$$

where the metric h-factors are given by

$$h_\xi = \frac{a}{2}\sqrt{\frac{\xi^2-\eta^2}{\xi^2-1}} \;, \quad h_\eta = \frac{a}{2}\sqrt{\frac{\xi^2-\eta^2}{1-\eta^2}} \;, \quad h_\phi = \frac{a}{2}\sqrt{(\xi^2-1)(1-\eta^2)}. \qquad (87)$$

With (85,87) the boundary conditions (74) and charge neutrality constraint (73) become

$$\frac{1}{h_\xi}\sum_{\ell m}\{\underline{D}(a_{\ell m}\cos m\phi + b_{\ell m}\sin m\phi) + \underline{Mc}^h(\alpha_{\ell m}\cos m\phi + \beta_{\ell m}\sin m\phi)\}$$

$$P'_{\ell m}(\xi_0)P_{\ell m}(\eta) = \sum_{\ell m}\{\underline{C}(a_{\ell m}\cos m\phi + b_{\ell m}\sin m\phi) +$$

$$\mathcal{U}(\alpha_{\ell m}\cos m\phi + \beta_{\ell m}\sin m\phi)\}P_{\ell m}(\xi_0)P_{\ell m}(\eta)\Big|_{\ell m}$$

$$\sum_{\ell m}[\underline{\zeta *a}_{\ell m}\cos m\phi + \underline{\zeta *b}_{\ell m}\sin m\phi]P_{\ell m}(\xi)P_{\ell m}(\eta) = 0. \quad (88)$$

Equations for the $\{\underline{a}_{\ell m}, \underline{b}_{\ell m}, \alpha_{\ell m}, \beta_{\ell m}\}$ can be obtained using the orthogonality relations

$$\int\frac{d\omega}{h_\xi} P_{\ell m}(\eta)P_{\ell' m'}(\eta)\cos m\phi\cos m'\phi = \frac{1}{2}a(\xi^2-1)N_{\ell m}\delta_{\ell\ell'}\delta_{mm'} \quad (89)$$

and similarly for cos → sin. The result for terms like $\cos m\phi$ $\sin m'\phi$ for all m,m' give zero. The normalization $N_{\ell m}$ is a constant. With this

$$[\underline{Da}_{\ell m} + \underline{Mc}^h\alpha_{\ell m}] = \sum_{\ell'} T^m_{\ell\ell'}[\underline{Ca}_{\ell' m} + \mathcal{U}\alpha_{\ell' m}] \quad (90)$$

$$T^m_{\ell\ell'} = \frac{aP_{\ell' m}(\xi_0)}{2P'_{\ell m}(\xi_0)\sqrt{\xi_0^2-1} N_{\ell m}}\int_{-1}^1 d\eta\sqrt{\xi_0^2-\eta^2}P_{\ell m}(\eta)P_{\ell' m}(\eta). \quad (91)$$

A similar equation arises with $a_{\ell m} \to b_{\ell m}$ and $\alpha_{\ell m} \to \beta_{\ell m}$ for the sin terms. Also multiplying the charge neutrality condition in (88) by $P_{\ell' m'}(\eta)\cos m'\phi/h_\xi$ and then $\int d\omega$ we get

$$\underline{\zeta *a}_{\ell m} = \underline{\zeta *b}_{\ell m} = 0. \quad (92)$$

Thus the condition for finding marginally stable modes that correspond to a spatial pattern is that (90,92) have nontrivial solutions. This happens if the determinant of the infinite dimensional matrix Ω formed by writing (92) in the general form $\Omega\Psi = 0$ (where $\Psi = \{a_{\ell m}, \alpha_{\ell m}; \ell = 0, 1, 2,...\}$ has zero determinant.

The most important differences between the prolate spheroid and the sphere is that $T^m_{\ell\ell'}$ is diagonal ($T^m_{\ell\ell'}$ is zero for $\ell \neq \ell'$) for the sphere but not for the spheroid. Points of marginal stability of the system are obtained by finding the eigenvalues of the infinite dimensional matrix Ω and finding which values of system parameters a given eigenvalue passes through zero. The corresponding eigenvector Ψ will yield the form of the marginally stable pattern when inserted into (85). This demonstrates the interesting concept of geometric mode mixing. The bifurcation of patterns in these systems has no trivial relation to the natural harmonics (here the prolate spheroidal harmonics $P_{\ell m}(\xi)P_{\ell m}(\eta)$ {$^{cos}_{sin}$}$m\phi$) for the system. The systems for which mode mixing occurs may be deduced fairly generally. For example, if the system outer boundary can be used to describe a concentric set of surfaces ξ_0 = constant and orthogonal curvilinear coordinates ξ_1, ξ_2, ξ_3 introduced, then mode mixing will not occur if the corresponding metric factor h is independent of the coordinates ξ_2, ξ_3 fixing points on the boundary surface. Examples are found from Morse and Feshback (25); for example, spherical, cubic and cylindrical cell masses will not demonstrate mode mixing whereas more general ellipsoids will.

Bioelectric Patterning in the Integral Operator Formalism.

1. Linear Stability Analysis. Patterns can be studied in the integral operator formalism. Here we demonstrate a stability analysis on an infinite two dimensional tissue. Under homogeneous culture conditions the system has a uniform steady state $\underline{c}^h$, v^h given by

$$\underline{R}(\underline{c}^h, v^h) = 0, \quad y_0 Y_T + \sum_j z_j [c_j^h + Y_j^{eq}(\underline{c}^h)] = 0. \quad (93)$$

We allow $\underline{R}$ to depend on voltage because in a two dimensional medium $\underline{R}$ must contain terms from the exchange of molecules with the culture medium with which the sheet of cells is in contact. Defining the culture medium to have voltage V^∞ then V in $\underline{R}(\underline{c},V)$ is the voltage within a cell minus V^∞, i.e. $V(\vec{r})$ is the voltage drop from the culture medium to the interior of a cell surrounding point $\vec{r}$.

Small deviations $\delta\underline{c}$, δV from the homogeneous state evolve with the linearized equations. It is easy to show that perturbations of the form $\delta\underline{c} = \hat{\underline{c}}e^{zt+i\vec{k}\cdot\vec{r}}$, $\delta V = \hat{V}e^{zt+i\vec{k}\cdot\vec{r}}$ evolve such that

$$\Xi \begin{bmatrix} \hat{\underline{c}} \\ \hat{V} \end{bmatrix} = 0, \quad \det\Xi = 0 \qquad\qquad (94)$$

$$\Xi(z,k) = \begin{bmatrix} \underline{\underline{J}}(1) + f(k^2)\underline{\underline{J}}(2) - z\underline{\underline{I}} & \underline{J}(3) + f(k^2)\underline{J}(4) \\ \zeta^h & 0 \end{bmatrix} \quad (95)$$

$$\underline{\underline{J}}(1) = \frac{\partial\underline{R}}{\partial\underline{c}}, \quad \underline{\underline{J}}(2) = \frac{\partial\underline{J}}{\partial\underline{c}'}, $$

$$\underline{J}(3) = \frac{\partial\underline{R}}{\partial V}, \quad \underline{J}(4) = \frac{\partial\underline{J}}{\partial V'} \qquad\qquad (96)$$

$$f(k^2) = R_0^2 \int_0^{2\pi} d\theta\cos[kR_0\cos\theta]$$

and $J(\underline{c}, \underline{c}', V, V')$ is the modified membrane flux as discussed for the nonlinear integral operator model of effective transport. In this theory only physically interesting perturbations can be studied on the length scale of a cell diameter (R_0) or greater;

hence

$$0 < k < 2\pi/R. \tag{97}$$

Strong deviations from a Turing type reaction-diffusion theory are expected to occur when the pattern length is of order of the cell size, i.e. near the upper limit of (97).

This calculation demonstrates the analysis of the formation of patterns in the integral operator formalism. Indeed bifurcation techniques also follow through fairly straightforwardly.

2. _Traveling Waves_. We now show that constant velocity waves in this model can be studied in terms of time delay equations. Sustained oscillatory or pulse wave propagation seems to control slime mold slug motion and certain aspects of chick embryo development.

A constant velocity and profile wave can be best studied in the frame of reference moving with the wave. Thus if the wave has velocity v the concentration $\underline{c}$ and voltage V must be functions of the single coordinate $\rho = x - vt$ where the plane wave is taken to move along the x direction. With this $(67,68)$ become

$$\underline{J}(\underline{c}(\rho), \underline{c}(\rho+R_o), V(\rho), V(\rho+R_o)) + \underline{J}(\underline{c}(\rho), \underline{c}(\rho-R_o),$$

$$V(\rho), V(\rho-R_o)) + v\frac{d\underline{c}}{d\rho} + \underline{R}(\underline{c}(\rho), V(\rho)) = 0 \tag{98}$$

$$\underline{z}*[\underline{c}(\rho) + \underline{Y}^{eq}(\underline{c}(\rho))] + y_o Y_T = 0. \tag{99}$$

This set of equations is a nonlinear eigenvalue time delay differential equation. Such equations, even for one variable, often have periodic or chaotic solutions and, from the physics of the problem are also certain of having pulse-like solutions in some systems.

It is clear that all the richness of reaction-diffusion systems should persist in the more accurate nonlinear integral operator model. The important difference is, however, that very rapid variations, and posssibly discontinuities in the slope of $\underline{c}$ or V, should be allowed in the integral operator description.

Imposed Field Effects. In this section we have set forth a set of equations to describe pattern formation in a multicellular electrophysiological system. A central goal of the theory is to study the effects of applied electric fields. This is done by imposing appropriate boundary conditions on the equations developed here. For example, assume we subject a one dimensional tissue to fixed ionic currents I_i. Then if the tissue is in the interval $0 \le x \le L_T$ along the x axis, the boundary conditions for the electro-diffusion model of the small gradient theory, i.e. (64), are replaced by $\underline{J} = \underline{I}$ at $x = 0, L_T$. One expects the richness of effects to include hyperpolarizability, induction of new phenomena and imperfect bifurcations to be found in these systems and preliminary results indicate this to be the case (43). Since most theoretical results on the effects of applied fields on non-linear systems have been done on reaction transport physico-chemical systems, we shall now briefly review that subject to more explicitly demonstrate the realm of the possible.

Signal Propagation Under Imposed Electric Fields

The interaction of reaction and transport may lead to the unattenuated propagation of signals in some systems maintained out of equilibrium. These signals usually consist of variations in composition but may also involve variations in temperature, pressure or the physical state of a contractile fiber as in the case of slow waves on smooth muscle. The wave forms that arise range from pulses and periodic trains to fronts; and within each class great variety may occur (see Ref. 26 for a review).

In most cases these chemical waves involve ionic species and hence two interesting possibilities arise: (1) these waves can be affected by applied electric fields and (2) the strong tendency towards charge neutrality and the possible presence of membranes may lead to strong electrical disturbances in association with the propagating compositional disturbance. In this section we review some recent work on the response of reaction-transport waves (10-14) and find strong variations of wave velocity and profile with applied field, induction of new types of waves not found in the field free medium (11), annihilation of waves beyond critical field strengths (11-14) and new two dimensional wave forms with free ends (13).

Experimental Evidence for the Phenomena in Chemical Wave Systems. Although these phenomena were originally predicted theoretically, we first consider the experimental evidence. Using a modification of Winfree's excitable pulse propagating version (31) of the Belousov-Zhabotinskii (BZ) mixture (32), it has been found that electrical effects can be observed (13). The experiments were carried out by subjecting the medium to two parallel electrodes and observing the voltage dependence of the properties of waves induced between them. The modifications of the BZ-Winfree medium were needed to get rid of spectator ions which increased the conductivity so high that joule heating simply boiled the medium when fields sufficiently large to see interesting effects were applied.

Key findings are shown in Figures 7-9. Figure 7 consists of three snapshots taken at regular temporal intervals. At t = 0 a circular wave reached a given radius and the electric field was turned on. In the case shown part of the circular wave going most directly toward the negative electrode was found to disappear! The part of the circle propagating generally toward the positive electrode was found to speed up. In fact the eventual arc or crescent shaped object continues to grow and the

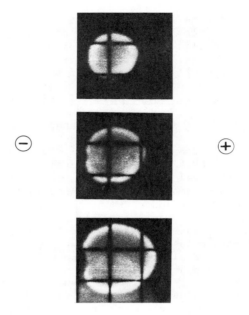

Figure 7.   Evolution of circular wave in BZ medium.

At time zero (top) the circular wave is subject to a plane parallel electric (ohmic) field. The part of the circle propagating towards the negative electrode is annihilated beyond a critical field strength and a crescent wave is observed to propagate (bottom). Note the free ends which are stabilized by the applied field and which become Winfree spirals when the field is turned off. (See Ref. 13 for details.)

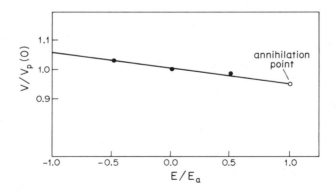

Figure 8.   Velocity response function v(E) yielding the velocity of BZ waves, normalized to the field-free velocity $v_n(O)$, as a function of the applied field E, normalized to the annihilation field E_a beyond which plane waves that would have propagated toward the negative electrode are destroyed. The smooth curve is that predicted by the theory outlined herein, and the dots are experimental values from Ref. 13.

free ends on the negative electrode side are found to be stable.
These crescent waves and their free ends are a purely electrical
phenomenon. It is well known that a free end in the absence of
an applied field will coil into a Winfree spiral (31). But in
the presence of the applied field the end is prevented from
coiling since, if it does so, it gets cut back as it swings into
the annihilating direction--i.e. propagation essentially towards
the negative electrode.

A quantitative measure of the interaction of chemical waves
and steady electric fields is the velocity response curve, i.e.
a plot of the dependence of a plane wave velocity on the
electric field applied along the direction of propagation. Note
that in Figure 8 the curve measured for a modification of the BZ
medium terminates at around 10 volts/cm (for waves propagating
toward the negative electrode) since for larger fields the waves
are annihilated. Further details on these measurements are
found in Ref. 13 where the special chemical wave medium recipes
developed to make the measurements are given.

Theory of Wave-Field Interaction in BZ Medium. A model of
the mechanisms behind the BZ reaction has been set forth by
Field, Körös and Noyes (33) (FKN) and more recently this
mechanism has been modified to incorporate more processes (34).
We have carried out an analysis of the FKN model to determine
the effects of electric fields on BZ chemical wave propagation
(12). Three reductions of the FKN kinetics were studied. The
reductions were based on various assumptions regarding the
existence of wide separations of time scales present in the
system. One reduction, studied by Murray (35), is a two species
model and leads to front propagation only. The evocative
Oregonator three species reduction does not support pulses using
experimentally known rate constants. A more recent reduction,
based on assumptions of the relative time scales of the FKN
kinetics, was termed the "IUator." This model supports pulses
using measured values of rate coefficients and will be focused on
here. Details of the Murray or Oregonator reductions are given
in Ref. 12 and will not be discussed further here.

1. General Considerations. The continuity equations for
a column vector $\underline{c}$ of species taking place in a reaction-
diffusion wave phenomenon take the form

$$\frac{\partial \underline{c}}{\partial t} = \underline{\underline{D}}\vec{\nabla}^2 \underline{c} - \underline{\underline{M}}\vec{E}\cdot\vec{\nabla}\underline{c} + \underline{R}(\underline{c}) \tag{100}$$

where $\underline{\underline{D}}$ and $\underline{\underline{M}}$ are matrices of diffusion and mobility coefficients,
$\vec{E}$ is the applied (assumed constant) electric field and $\underline{R}$ is the
column vector of chemical reaction rates. The simplest wave
phenomenon to study is that for plane waves of constant profile
and velocity. Assuming such a wave to be propagating in the x-
direction with velocity v in the presence of an electric field E
in the x-direction, we have

$$\underline{D}\underline{c}'' + (v + \underline{EM})\underline{c}' + \underline{R}(\underline{c}) = 0 \qquad\qquad (101)$$

where ' denotes an ordinary derivative with respect to a coordinate $\rho = x - vt$ in the Galilean fram fixed to the wave.

The plane wave equation (101) is parametrized by the electric field strength E. Thus the profile $\underline{c}(\rho,E)$ depends on E. Most experimentally accessible is the velocity response function $v(E)$ yielding the dependence of the wave velocity on the electric field as, for example, in Figure 8.

 2. Wave Propagation in Reduced FKN Mechanisms. The full FKN mechanism has many species. However, there are a number of rather fast reactions. Using scalings on concentrations and rate coefficients for concentrations of interest to wave propagation, it has been shown that the FKN mechanism may be reduced to a three variable problem (12). With this procedure it is found that the three reduced concentrations obey the following equations of motion for a wave propagating at constant dimensionless velocity c:

$$x'' + cx' + x(1-x) - xz^2 - (\varkappa xz)^2/4 - xy/\epsilon = 0 \quad (102)$$

$$D_y y'' + (c+\eta)y' + \vee(1+gz-y) - ax^2/6 - axy/\epsilon = 0 \quad (103)$$

$$D_z z'' + (c-e\eta)z' + 2fx(1-z^2-\varkappa^2 xz^2/2) - \delta z = 0. \quad (104)$$

Here x is proportional to [HBrO], $y \propto$ [Br$^-$], z $\propto$ [oxidized form of catalyst, most relevantly Ce^{+4} for the present approximations (36)], $\eta \propto$ applied electric field. All other quantities are given constants except c which is the velocity eigenvalue of the nonlinear system of equations. Matched asymptotic (boundary layer (37)) techniques were used to show (38) that BZ wave propagation could be understood in terms of a Stefan moving boundary problem. (A Stefan problem is one in which the domain on which the equations operate is to be determined as, for example, with a melting ice cube--see citations in Ref. 38 for more details.) The moving boundary turns out to be the interface between domains wherein x and y are alternatively very small. Where y and z are small x obeys the Fisher equation except that the Fisher velocity c = 2 that was believed to be relevant (39) turns out to be too high because the boundary conditions for BZ propagation are not those usually used for the Fisher equation since x is confined to a semi-infinite interval as shown in Figure 9. When z is appreciable the autocatalytic x (Fisher-like) moving boundary wave front dynamics does not operate. Since z (the metal catalyst) is positive it tends to be pushed into the front (as it is being produced by the +2fx term in (104) behind the x front) when a wave is propagating towards the negative electrode. Thus we might expect a slowing down of waves propagating toward the negative electrode as the voltage is increased. The mathematical analysis and the experiments show that the situation is actually more interesting than this little hand waving argument might have us believe. The ionic drift velocity of an ion is the mobility of that ion times the applied field. The theory predicts that when the oxidized metal ion drift velocity increases beyond the field free wave velocity, the wave is annihilated suddenly from a finite amplitude and velocity to no wave at all. This is a strictly nonlinear response phenomenon.

This annihilation phenomenon can be used to explain the crescent wave seen to be developing in Figure 7. The part of the initially circular wave propagating toward the negative electrode with component of electric field normal to the wave front greater than the annihilation field must be destroyed. Results of the theory for the dependence of the velocity on the applied field are shown in Figure 10 where the Oregonator and IUator are compared. In both mechanisms annihilation occurs at the knees of the curve but the velocity responses differ in overall appearance.

3. General Remarks on Wave-Field Interactions. Electric field effects on signal propagation are quite varied. They stem from the fact that since different ions have different mobilities and charge they can be driven quite differently, potentially significantly disturbing the balance of composition attained in the field free reaction-diffusion profile. This leads to the possibility of creating new wave phenomena significantly different from field free wave propagation. Thus direction reversal, annihilation, creation of new types of waves and enhancement of propagation are all possible.

It is not known yet whether these effects are important in any examples of biological signal propagation although the potential richness of phenomena here makes investigation of such a possibility a tempting future area of investigation. A key factor in making these phenomena be accessible is to insure that the background ionic conductivity is sufficiently small so that large enough fields can be attained without boiling the system due to ohmic heating. As found in the experiments on BZ mixtures ($\underline{13}$) such modifications of the wave medium are sometimes attainable.

Electrified Periodic Precipitation. In the banded precipitation of PbI_2 from KI and $Pb(NO_3)_2$ in a Liesegang experiment ($\underline{47}$) diffusion drives the I^- ion into the Pb^{2+} gel as seen in Figure 11. It is observed that the incursion of the banded region into the gel slows down and the band spacing gradually increases as one proceeds down the tube from the KI solution end. However, if one puts a negative electrode into the KI solution and a positive electrode in the $Pb(NO_3)_2$ end of the gel tube, the ionic drift term will, in the absence of precipitation, cause the

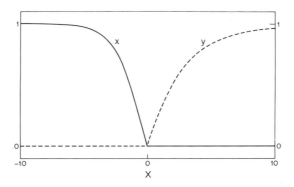

Figure 9.   Approximate $x(\propto [BrO_2])$, $y(\propto [Br^-])$ *wave profiles for BZ leading wave front as described by a Stefan moving boundary scheme discussed in Refs. 12 and 38, and the section on signal propagation under imposed electric fields.*

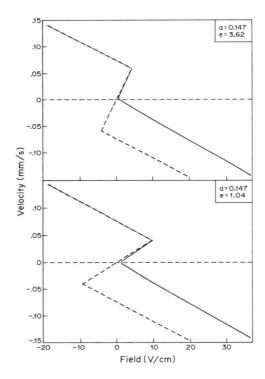

Figure 10.   Comparison of velocity response of Oregonator and IUator models for two cases: (1) catalyst is Mn^{2+}/Mn^{3+} *(top curves); (2) catalyst is* $Fe(phen)_3^{2+}/Fe\text{-}(phen)_3^{3+}$ *(bottom curve). (———) IUator predictions; (———) the FKN-consistent Oregonator solution (see Ref. 12 for details).*

coprecipitates (I^-, Pb^{2+}) to move toward each other at constant
(but different) velocities. This makes it plausible that the
resulting precipitation bands will become periodic--i.e. with
equal spacing--under certain ranges of applied potential.

In Figure 12 the result of the above electro-precipitation
banding experiment is shown. Note that for the many bands
observed, the spacing is constant, unlike the zero voltage
experiment shown schematically in Figure 11.

The theory of field free precipitation banding is in somewhat of a state of controversy. The traditional Ostwald-Prager
theory is based on an interplay of nucleation and diffusion and
relies on the cross diffusion geometry of the coprecipitates (48).
However in recent experiments (49, 50) it was shown that
spontaneous patterns evolve from a homogeneous sol as shown in
Figure 13. To account for this phenomenon a new theory was
developed based on the competition between precipitate particles
of different sizes (42, 50). This competition arises because
larger particles, due to surface tension, have an equilibrium
salt concentration which is lower than that of smaller
particles. Thus a patch of the system with slightly larger
average particle size will lead to an influx of salt and hence
growth at the expense of the particles in the neighborhood. This
leads to an instability in the state of the homogeneous sol
and consequent development of spatial pattern. The theory also
allows for sequential banding in the Liesegang configuration.

Currently, we are attempting to provide a unified theory
that incorporates both nucleation and competitive particle growth.
We shall then examine the electrical effects. This should not
only provide a basis of explanation of the electro-banding
phenomenon, but perhaps more importantly, provide a means of
discriminating between the two mechanisms of band formation--i.e.
how they interplay and which dominates. Indeed the competitive
particle theory could explain the phenomenon of secondary banding
as follows. Secondary banding is the development of bands from
an initially uniform single band of the Liesegang experiment.
But a single Liesegang band can be conceived of as a region of
uniform sol. A uniform sol is, according to the competitive
particle theory, unstable to pattern formation. In this picture
the regularity of the secondary bands is a consequence of the
existence of a small gradient in particle size across the initial
band. Such a small gradient in the competitive particle theory
leads to regularity of banding--i.e. not random as the patterns
of Figure 13.

Since phase transitions take place in biological systems, as
for example in membranes, it may be quite fruitful to investigate
precipitation bands and their electrical manifestations in biological systems, especially the ability of electrical fields,
possibly generated by the organism itself, to regularize a
precipitation pattern.

Figure 11. Schematic Liesegang experiment to show that the normal trend is for band spacing to increase down the tube. The main difference between Figures 11 and 12 is that in the regularizing conditions, the electromigration dominates diffusion.

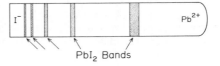

Figure 12. Schematic Liesegang experiment to show that the normal trend is for band spacing to increase down the tube. The main difference between Figures 11 and 12 is that in the regularizing conditions, the electromigration dominates diffusion.

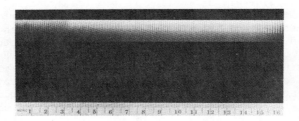

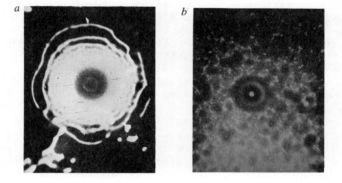

Figure 13.   Swirl (a) and halo (b) patterns obtained in a supercooled PbI₂ experiment.   Width of photographs represents 7.5 mm.

Growth, Inherent Asymmetry and Other Effects

Perhaps the key issue in the study of electrical effects in development is to determine to what degree the observed electric fields are an inherent part of a developmental process or merely a consequence of it. To conclude our discussions we now address some facets of this question.

Inherent Asymmetry as an Imperfection. Much is made in the developmental literature and in particular in critiques of the invocation of Turing mechanisms, that, for example, eggs are inherently asymmetric. It is stressed in these discussions that this inherent asymmetry or pattern is what fixes the later developmental axis, for example. In this regard the location of the point of entry of the sperm is believed key. However, recent experiments involving the manipulation of developing eggs seems to put some doubt into the universal applicability of this dogma (56). The question we wish to address here is to what extent these inherent asymmetries are causes or simply perturbations of more fundamental organizational phenomena.

The concepts of hyperpolarizability and of imperfect bifurcations come to bear most heavily on this issue. Near a point of instability of a system to pattern formation it is very sensitive to small perturbations. Thus any inherent asymmetry will in some sense be greatly amplified. Qualitatively speaking, the hyperpolarizability concept would say that the response of the system to the inherent asymmetry will not only be large, but will be in a particular form--typically of the inherent symmetry of the patterning modes of the stability analyses which are most long lived. Thus, for example, if there is some granule or perhaps localization due to centrifugation in Fucus that is found to fix the axis of polarization, then is this not just an imperfection that selects among the inherent degenerate patterning modes and not the determining factor in deciding pattern symmetry? To study this it is useful to consider the case of a weak asymmetry as an imperfection and use the machinery of imperfect bifurcation theory. The analysis of cells in external gradients or imposed electric fields discussed earlier carries over quite straightforwardly here (51). Consider a single spherical cell with a small asymmetry due to the internal distribution of sites of reaction or barriers to transport. Let this asymmetry be analyzed in terms of the complete set of solutions $r^\ell Y_{\ell m}$ of Laplace's equation. Then if the $\ell = 1$ patterns would arise in the imperfection free system the cubic equations for the mode amplitudes found in (36) $(d\gamma_\nu/dt = 0)$ will become

$$-2a\gamma_{1\nu} - \sum_{m+m'=\nu} b_\nu^{mm'} \gamma_{1m}\gamma_{1m'}\gamma_{1\nu} + I_\nu = 0 \qquad (105)$$

where I_ν is a measure of the degree to which the imperfection is of symmetry $\ell = 1,\nu$. For example, if the imperfection is the point of entry of the sperm, taken to be the "north pole," then $I_{\pm 1} = 0$ and the bifurcation diagram looks exactly as in Figure 4 where h is to be interpreted as I_o, the axis being fixed along the north/south pole.

Thus for a weak imperfection in a system near criticality we see than an imperfection in the presence of a pattern formation mechanism effects the pattern only in regards to its orientation but not its inherent configuration. Indeed the amplitude of the mode is somewhat altered but we notice that the mode itself (in the weak imperfection case) is unchanged. (It is the stability mode that, for example, fixed the ratios of the individual ion currents in the Fucus problems (7).)

In order to resolve the issue of whether the observed pattern is due to an inherent asymmetry or a Turing type self-organization mechanism, one must make a calculation to see if the former can, in fact, explain the amplitude and ratios of ionic currents and other details of the pattern.

Growth in Developmental Bioelectrics. Growth and changes of geometry are very important features of many developmental processes. The fact that geometry profoundly affects the electric field of a system and that the growth dynamics is strongly affected by the distribution of molecules, many of which are ions, suggests a potential mechanism for the presence of morphological instability driven by a feedback loop involving the electric field in a nontrivial way. This is, in fact, well known in electroplating where the tendency for the smooth plating state to become unstable to the growth of bumps is an industrial nuisance.

The mechanisms for coupling morphology changes to electric fields in biological systems can be quite complex. For example, the invasion of nerves into a growing limb is known to promote growth; nerves in culture are found to grow along electric fields (8, 53). This and other mechanisms of morphological instability coupling bioelectrics and evolving geometry are presently under investigation (52). Indeed since small bumps can profoundly affect the current density into the bump, it appears that this mechanism is a strong driving and controlling force for the ability of systems to grow limbs, sprout roots or other essential features (8, 22, 28, 53).

The Future. True advances in this field can only come if detailed model making and experimentation are closely coordinated. Since so many effects are usually going on at the same time, responsible bookkeeping in the form of detailed mathematical descriptions are needed to keep track of and organize the data if issues of mechanism of development or organization are to be resolved. A promising case in this regard is the formulation of a detailed model of Fucus (5-7) capable of explaining the

published <u>Fucus</u> data. What is now needed for the <u>Fucus</u> problem
is more experiments directed at probing the predictions of the
model so as to proceed in an orderly way towards refining the
present picture and, indeed, checking its validity. We are quite
enthusiastic that this can be done successfully becasue of the
physico-chemical orientation of some investigators in this area.

A very challenging and important field of theoretical research is in regards to the effects of high frequency electric
fields as reviewed in Refs. <u>53</u>, <u>54</u>. The pioneering experimental
work of Pilla (<u>54</u>) seems to connect these effects to cell surface processes. It has also been shown that these effects are
strictly nonlinear in nature opening up the interesting theoretical area of nonlinear response of membrane systems.

Enthusiasm in science should always be tempered with humil-
ity. The 1947 study by Lund (<u>28</u>) and the work of many investigators over the last century points out that the role of electric forces in development has long been appreciated. It is our
hope that recent advances in the theory of nonlinear equations,
and the contributions of Turing, will enable theoreticians, in
collaboration with experimentalists, to make a real contribution
here in order to complement the evergrowing body of very interesting experimental data. The potential medical applications of
the field to the control of regeneration and wound healing (as it
is already being used in bone healing (<u>53</u>)) makes interest in
this field of great relevance.

Literature Cited

1. Turing, A. M.   Phil. Trans. Roy. Soc., London, 1952, Ser. B
    <u>237</u>, 37.
2. Hodgkin, A. L.   Physiol., 1976, <u>263</u>, 1.
3. Ortoleva, P.; Ross, J.   Develop. Biol., 1973, <u>34</u>, F19; ibid.
    Biophys. Chem., 1973, <u>1</u>, 87.
4. Larter, R.; Ortoleva, P.   J. Theoret. Biol., "A Theoretical
    Basis for Self-Electrophoresis," (to appear).
5. Larter, R.; Ortoleva, P.   J. Theoret. Biol., "A Study of
    Instability to Electrical Symmetry Breaking in Unicellular
    Systems" (submitted for publication).
6. Larter, R.; Strickholm, A.; Ortoleva, P.   Cell, "A Detailed
    Model of the Electrical Symmetry-Breaking Transition in
    Early <u>Fucus</u> Egg Development" (submitted for publication).
7. Larter, R.; Ortoleva, P.   J. Theoret. Biol., "Bifurcation of
    Autonomous and Induced Polarity in <u>Fucus</u> Eggs" (submitted
    for publication).
8. Jaffe, L. F. in <u>Membrane Transduction Mechanisms</u>, Cone, R. A.
    and Dowling, J. E., Eds.; Raven Press, New York, 1979; p.
    199.
9. Zhabotinskii, A.   Proc. Aacken Symposium of the Bunsengesell-
    eschaft, 1979, p. 657.

10. Schmidt, S.; Ortoleva, J. J. Chem. Phys., 1977, 67, 3771.
11. Schmidt, S.; Ortoleva, J. J. Chem. Phys., 1979, 71, 1010.
12. Schmidt, S.; Ortoleva, J. J. Chem. Phys., 1980, "Electrical Field Effects on the FKN Chemical Waves" (to appear).
13. Feeney, R.; Schmidt, S.; Ortoleva, P. Physica D, "Experimental Evidence of Electrical Field-Chemical Wave Interaction: Annihilation and Comet Waves" (to appear).
14. Larter, R.; Schmidt, S.; Ortoleva, P. in Synergetics Conference Proceedings, Haken, H., Ed.; Springer-Verlag, Schloss, Elmau, West Germany, 1979.
15. Poo, M-m.; Robinson, K. R. Nature, 1977, 265, 602.
16. Poo, M-m.; Poo, W-J. H.; Lam, J. W. J. of Cell Biol., 1978, 76, 483.
17. Scarpa, A.; Carafoli, E., Eds. "Annals of the New York Academy of Sciences"; 1978.
18. Sattinger, D. "Topics in Stability and Bifurcation Theory," Springer Advanced Mathematics Series, 309; Springer, New York, 1973.
19. Smiley, M.; Ortoleva, P. "Bifurcation of Current Patterns in Developing Cells" (in preparation).
20. Ortoleva, P.; Ross, J. J. Chem. Phys., 1972, 56, 293; ibid. 1972, 56, 287; Nitzan, A.; Ortoleva, P.; Deutsch, J.; Ross, J. J. Chem. Phys., 1974, 61, 1056.
21. Gurel, O.; Rossler, O., Eds. "Proceedings of the Conference on Bifurcation Theory and Its Applications"; Ann. N. Y. Acad. Sci. 316.
22. Smith, S. D. Ann. N. Y. Acad. Sci., 1974, 238, 500; Becker, R. D. Sci. News, 1971, 100, 322; Illingworth, C. M. J. Pediatr. Surg., 1974, 9, 853; Douglas, B. S. Austr. Pediatr. J., 1972, 8, 86.
23. deGroot, S. R.; Mazur, P. Nonequilibrium Thermodynamics; North Holland, Amsterdam, 1962.
24. Ortoleva, P.; Ross, J. J. Chem. Phys., 1972, 56, 4397; Bimpong Bota, K.; Ortoleva, P.; Ross, J. J. Chem. Phys., 1974, 60, 3124.
25. Morse, P. M.; Feshback, H. Methods of Theoretical Physics; McGraw Hill Book Co.; New York, 1953.
26. Hanusse, P.; Ortoleva, P.; Ross, J. Adv. Chem. Phys., 1978; Ortoleva, P. "Selected Topics from the Theory of Nonlinear Physico-Chemical Phenomena"; Theoretical Chemistry, Eyring, H. and Henderson, P., Eds.; Academic Press; New York, 1978).
27. Nitzan, A.; Ortoleva, P. Phys. Rev. A, 1980, 21, 1735 and many references cited therein.
28. Lund, E. J. Bioelectric Fields and Growth; U. of Texas Press; Austin, Texas, 1947.
29. Nicolis, G.; Prigogine, I. Self-Organization in Nonequilibrium Systems; Wiley; New York, 1977.
30. Keener, J. P. Studies in Applied Math., 1976, 55, 187.

31. Winfree, A. T. in <u>Theoretical Chemistry</u>, Eyring, H. and Henderson, P., Eds., 1978; p. 1.

32. See $\underline{9}$ and $\underline{31}$ and references cited.

33. Field, R.; Koros, E.; Noyes, R. <u>J. Am. Chem. Soc.</u>, 1972, $\underline{94}$, 8649.

34. Edelson, D.; Field, R.; Noyes, R. <u>Int. J. Chem. Kinet.</u>, 1977, $\underline{88}$, 814; Zhabotinskii, A., Ref. $\underline{9}$ above.

35. Murray, J. <u>J. Theoret. Biol.</u> 1976, $\underline{56}$, 329.

36. The kinetics of BZ medium with $Fe(phen)^{3+}$ replacing Ce^{4+} appears to be somewhat different and other approximations to the dynamics may be needed--see Noyes, R. M. (preprint).

37. Nayfey, A. <u>Perturbation Methods</u>; Wiley; New York, 1973.

38. Schmidt, S.; Ortoleva, P. <u>J. Chem. Phys.</u>, 1980, $\underline{72}$, 2733.

39. Tyson, J. <u>The Zhabotinskii Reaction: Lecture Notes in Biomathematics</u>; Springer; New York, 1976.

40. Billing, G.; Hunding, A. <u>J. Chem. Phys.</u>, 1978, $\underline{69}$, 3603.

41. Hunding, A.; Billing, G. <u>J. Chem. Phys.</u>, 1980, $\underline{45}$, 359.

42. Lovett, R.; Ortoleva, P.; Ross, J. <u>J. Chem. Phys.</u>, 1978, $\underline{69}$, 947.

43. Feinn, D.; Ortoleva, P. "Electrophysiological Instabilities in Multicellular Systems" (in preparation).

44. Larter, R.; El-Badewi, M.; Merino, E.; Ortoleva, P. "Developmental Bioelectricity and Geochemistry"; <u>Proceedings of a Workshop on Instabilities, Bifurcations, and Fluctuations</u>; Austin, Texas, 1980.

45. Ermentrout, G. B.; Cowan, J. D. <u>Biol. Cybernetics</u>, 1979, $\underline{34}$, 137.

46. Huntington, C.; Feinn, D.; Auchmuty, G.; Ortoleva, P. "Mixed Mode Electrophysiological Self-Organizing Patterns in Ellipsoidal Systems" (in preparation).

47. Liesegang, R. T. <u>Phot. Archiv.</u>, 1896, $\underline{21}$, 221.

48. Ostwald, W. <u>Kolloid-Z</u>, 1925, $\underline{36}$, 380.

49. Flicker, M.; Ross, J. <u>J. Chem. Phys.</u>, 1974, $\underline{60}$, 3458.

50. Feinn, D.; Ortoleva, P.; Scalf, W.; Schmidt, S.; Wolff, M. <u>J. Chem. Phys.</u>, 1978, $\underline{69}$, 27.

51. Ortoleva, P. "Inherent Asymmetry and Imperfect Bifurcation in the Developmental Scenario" (in preparation).

52. Chadam, J.; Ortoleva, P. "Electrophysiological Aspects of Shape Changes in Biological Systems" (in preparation).

53. Brighton, C. T.; Black, J.; Pollack, S. R., Eds. "Electrical Properties of Bone and Cartilage: Experimental Effects and Clinical Applications"; Grune and Stratton; New York, 1979.

54. Pilla, A. A. "Electrochemical Information Transfer at Cell Surfaces and Functions: Applications to the Study and Manipulation of Cell Regulation" (preprint).

55. Ortoleva, P.; Bimpong-Bota, K.; Ross, J. <u>J. Chem. Phys.</u>, 1974, $\underline{60}$, 3124; Ortoleva, P.; Bimpong-Bota, E.; Nitzan, A.; Ross, J. <u>J. Chem. Phys.</u>, 1977, $\underline{66}$, 3650.

56. Chung, H.; Malacinski, G. <u>Develop. Biol.</u>, 1980, $\underline{80}$, 120.

RECEIVED January 28, 1981.

Coherent Processes in Biological Systems

H. FRÖHLICH

Department of Physics, Oliver Lodge Laboratory, The University of Liverpool, Oxford Street, Liverpool, L69 3BX, U.K.

The success of molecular biology is based on the derivation of the detailed molecular structure of biologically important molecules such as enzymes, DNA. Frequently the opinion has been expressed that the activity of biological systems can be understood in terms of standard chemical reactions, based on a knowledge of structure, in conjunction with diffusion of molecules. It must be pointed out, therefore, that biological systems exhibit sensitivities, at times, that equal those of the best available modern instrumentation.

As an example we mention the sensitivity at low light intensities of the human visual system which according to a careful analysis by Rose (1) is close to the theoretical limit. The system thus can be considered as an image converter of the highest possible sensitivity, though it uses materials of quite a different nature from those used by technologists.

In a more general sense, biological systems receive energy through metabolism (or light), and use a part of this energy to develop and maintain a complex organization. In simple physical systems, in general, supply of random energy leads to an increase in temperature. Exceptions arise in the case of machines which require complex arrangements. More simple, in principle, is the case of laser where the supply of energy yields the well-known coherent laser states.

Long range coherence, moreover, is a very general concept which may arise subject to a few material properties, and it has been proposed, therefore, that biological systems make considerable use of this possibility (2,3,4). Do biological materials, from the point of view of physics, possess some common material properties? They do in their extraordinary dielectric properties (5). Most remarkable, here, are the strong electric fields, of order 10^7 volt/m, that are maintained in all biological membranes, although the only use that classical biology has made of this is restricted to nerve membranes. Such fields, clearly, lead to a strong electric polarisation of all materials in a membrane; oscillation of these materials then lead to electric polarisation waves.

0097-6156/81/0157-0213$05.00/0

Coherent Electric Polarisation Waves

Electric polarisation waves can be classified in terms of their normal modes. In general, these normal modes form bands, though in some cases isolated modes may also exist. The lowest frequency of all these modes is different from zero. A band of normal modes covering a frequency range between ω_1 and ω_2,

$$0 < \omega_1 \leqslant \omega \leqslant \omega_2, \tag{1}$$

is assumed to be in very strong interaction with the rest of the system which is treated as a heat bath wtih temperature T. It is essential that not only first but also second order terms in this interaction are of importance, whereas terms leading to an interaction between the modes of polarisation wave are considered negligible. These are the main requirements which the material must exhibit in order to be capable of showing excitation of a single mode under the influence of random supply of energy arising from metabolic processes. For let n_k be the number of quanta in the mode with frequency ω_k, let s_k be the rate of supply of energy to this mode, and let ϕ_k and $\chi_{k\ell} = \chi_{\ell k}$ be appropriate transition probabilities, then the rate $\dot{n}_k$ of change of n_k satisfies the kinetic equation (2,4)

$$\dot{n}_k = s_k - \phi_k[n_k e^{\beta\omega_k} - (1+n_k)] -$$
$$- \sum_\ell \chi_{k\ell}[n_k(1+n_\ell)e^{\beta\omega_k} - n_\ell(1+n_k)e^{\beta\omega_\ell}] \tag{2}$$

where

$$\beta = h/KT \tag{3}$$

A formal stationary solution of (2) can be easily presented (6) though we shall give here only the solution for the simplified case in which all ϕ_k are equal to ϕ, and all $\chi_{k\ell}$ equal to χ,

$$n_k = [1 + \frac{s_k}{s} \frac{\phi}{\chi}(1-e^{-\beta\mu})][e^{\beta(\omega_k-\mu)} -1]^{-1} \tag{4}$$

where

$$s = \sum_k s_k \tag{5}$$

and

$$e^{-\beta\mu} = \frac{\phi + \chi \sum_\ell (1+n_\ell)}{\phi + \chi \sum_\ell n_\ell e^{\beta\omega_\ell}} \tag{6}$$

Thus $\mu = 0$ in thermal equilibrium (s=0), when (4) becomes a Planck distribution, and

$$0 = \mu < \omega_1 \tag{7}$$

Now from (2) it can be shown that for sufficiently large s, the total number of quanta $N = \Sigma n_k$ increases proportionally to the total rate of supply s. Equation (4) then shows that a critical rate of supply s_0, exists, such that for $s > s_0$ something analogous to Einstein condensation of a Bose gas must occur. This implies that μ, which acts as chemical potential, must approach ω_1 very closely such that the occupation, n_1, of ω_1 becomes very large. Since ω_1 represents a normal mode, it follows that this excitation is coherent.

The above observation has been confirmed with the use of a number of more specific models, some using field theory, others using a finite number of modes (7-14).

Consequences

The possibility of coherent excitation, discussed in the previous section, rests on the introduction of the non-linear χ-terms. For if χ=0, then (6) yields $\mu = 0$ and the possibility of coherent excitation disappears. When the excitation is achieved, on the other hand, then the system is capable of collective behaviour and can exhibit properties that at first sight do not appear to be inherent in the unexcited system. Most important is a frequency-selective long-range interaction of such excited systems (15,4) which may lead, it has been suggested, to control of cell division in an organ, to long-range attraction (e.g. of enzyme and substrate) and to other consequences. Once such attraction has been achieved, of course, the usual short-range chemical interactions will take over. These, together with the spatial rearrangements due to long-range interaction, will, in general, lead to new frequencies which, if excited, will lead to the attraction of different groups, so that a unidirectional development of the system may be anticipated.

Amongst possible frequencies, 10^{10}–10^{11} Hz has been estimated for polar membrane vibrations, higher frequencies, up to 10^{13}–10^{14} Hz, for proteins, lower frequencies (16), of order 10^9 Hz, for RNA. These frequency regions include those corresponding to millimeter and centimeter electromagnetic waves, and it may be expected then that biological processes that make use of electric vibrations in these frequency regions may be influenced by externally applied electromagnetic waves. This should particularly arise when the relevant size of the material is small compared with the vacuum wavelength. Otherwise, however, external radiation will interact with optically-active modes only, and it is unlikely that those modes are relevant for biological purposes. In such cases, interaction is restricted to surface effects and effects of irregularities.

Consider now a complex biological process that is initiated by the consequences of strong excitation of a certain mode, leading to selective long-range interaction. Let t_1 be the time required for this process, and let t_2 be the time of the subsequent chains of biological processes. The total rate R thus is

$$R = \frac{1}{t_1 + t_2} \tag{8}$$

Now the first process requires coherent excitation, which in turn requires the rate of energy supply s to be larger than the critical s_0. Thus $t_1 \to \infty$, i.e., $R \to 0$, if $s < s_0$. When $s > s_0$ then we shall assume

$$t_1 = \frac{a}{(s - s_0)^n} \tag{9}$$

where $n = 1$, and $\underline{a}$ is a constant. Together with (8) it follows that

$$R = \frac{1}{t_2} \frac{(s - s_0)^n}{(a/t_2) + (s - s_0)^n}, \quad s \geqslant s_0 \tag{10}$$

i.e., R is a step-like function whose value becomes $1/t_2$, independent of s when s is very large.

Consider now that the system is preparing for the particular process by supplying energy at a rate $s_B < s_0$, say $s_B = s_0 - \Delta$. Then, if the relevant frequency region is in the microwave or millimeter-wave region, and if electromagnetic energy is supplied at a rate $s_m > \Delta$, then the process will take place, i.e., it will be triggered by the externally supplied energy. The dependence in this intensity will again be step-like, with the step starting at the rate $s_m = \Delta$, which might be very low. A slight modification of the s_m-independent region will arise when the absorption of the external wave in the system is relevant. This case has been treated in (6). As a whole, however, these processes are characterized by their step-like dependence on intensity, and by their restriction to certain frequency regions. Furthermore, as first discussed in (12), equation (2) implies that a certain non-negligible time of irradiation will be required to approach the stationary state.

Experiments

Electromagnetic waves may, under certain circumstances, trigger biological events with the use of relatively low intensities, as discussed above. To test this possibility experimentally, it is required to investigate the triggered biological event in its dependence on the intensity, frequency, and duration of the applied radiation. A great number of experiments at a single fre-

quency (usually 2450 MHz) do exist; they are not suitable to test
the theory, though some of them do exhibit effects at very low
intensities so that thermal action is unlikely.

In a report of the USSR Academy of Science (January 1973)
(17) the required set of experiments have been carried out on a
number of biological materials with the use of coherent millimeter
waves, vacuum wave length 6-7 mm, a large range of intensities
and of duration of irradiation, as required to test the theory.
They confirm, quite in general, the theoretical results and can
thus be considered as confirmation of the theory (18).   Subsequently experiments on the influence of the growth of yeast cultures have exhibited the existence of narrow frequency resonances
(19), and recently, Grundler (20), working with very high resolution, has been able to demonstrate conclusively the existence of
very narrow resonances.

Reproducibility of results is sometimes difficult to achieve,
and this may be due to a number of reasons.   Thus Grundler finds
a narrow positive maximum adjunct to two negative minima.   As a
consequence, working with lower resolution will average over these
and yield no noticeable effect.   Other parameters, however, of
both physical and biological nature are likely to be relevant;
investigations to determine these are in progress.

At higher frequencies, the laser-Raman effect affords, in
principle, the possibility of detecting non-thermal excitation
of vibrations.   These would be found from a higher than thermal
ratio of anti-Stokes to Stokes lines.   The Raman effect in biological systems has recently been reviewed by Webb (21).   Unfortunately only two relevant measurements have been carried out,
so far, but both demonstrate non-thermal excitation.   A difficulty
affecting reproducibility arises here from the effect of a laser
beam on a biological system as discussed in (21), in the case of
individual cells.   The best way to avoid this appears to be the
use of a flow instrumentation so that each cell is subjected to
the laser beam for a very short period only (22).

Finally, one may question whether the activated polar vibrations in individual cells can be expected to have exactly the same
frequency for all cells.   For assume that, through a fluctuation,
a water molecule or a hydrogen ion is attached to the vibrating
region in one cell but not another.   The non-homogenuous part of
the arising field will then alter the relevant frequency by an
amount which is small compated with this frequency but may well
be of order of the frequency distance between resonances reported in (19) and (20).

NOTE ADDED IN PROOF
Meanwhile literature has been found (e.g., B.L. Epel in
Photophysiology 8, 209, 1973) according to which visible light
inhibits various biological processes in E coli.   Also experimentation with flow instrumentation has begun and appears to yield
interesting results which will be published in due course by
F. Drissler.

ABSTRACT
    The model leading to the excitation of coherent electric
vibrations in biological systems is reviewed and the experimental
evidence for it is briefly discussed.

LITERATURE CITED
1. Rose, A. Image Technol. 1970, 12, 13.
2. Fröhlich, H. Int. J. Quantum Chem. 1968, 2, 641.
3. Fröhlich, H. Riv. Nuovo Cimato 1973, 3, 490.
4. Fröhlich, H. IEEE Trans. Microwave Theory Tech. 1978, 26, 613.
5. Fröhlich, H. Proc. Natl. Acad. Sci. U.S.A. 1975, 72, 4211.
6. Fröhlich, H. "Advances in Electronics and Electron Physics"
    Vol. 53, Academic Press, New York, 1980, 85.
7. Bhaumik, D.; Bhaumik, K.; Dutta-Roy, B. Phys. Lett. 1976, 59A,
    77.
8. Bhaumik, D.; Dutta-Roy, B.; Lahiri, A. Phys. Lett. 1978, 68A,
    131.
9. Wu, T.M.; Austin, S. Phys. Lett. 1977, 64A, 151.
10. Wu, T.M.; Austin, S. J.Theor. Biol. 1978, 71, 209.
11. Wu, T.M.; Austin, S. Phys. Lett. 1978, 65A, 74.
12. Wu, T.M.; Austin, S. Phys. Lett. 1979, 73A, 266.
13. Mills, R.E. Phys. Lett. 1972, 39A, 153.
14. Moskalenko, S.A.; Miglei, M.F.; Khadshi, P.I.; Pokatilov, E.P.;
    Kiselyova, E.S. Phys. Lett. 1980, 76A, 197.
15. Fröhlich, H. Phys. Lett. 1972, 39A, 153.
16. Prohofsky, E.W.; Eyster, J.M. Phys. Lett. 1974, 50A, 329.
17. Devyatkov, N.D. Soviet Physics US PEKHI(Translation) 1974,
    16, 568.
18. Fröhlich, H. Phys. Lett. 1975, 51A, 21.
19. Grundler, W.; Keilmann, F.; Fröhlich, H. Phys. Lett. 1977,
    62A, 463.
20. Grundler, W. Personal communication
21. Webb, S.J. Physics Reports 1980, 60, 202.
22. Drissler, F.; MacFarlane, R.M. Phys. Lett. 1978, 69A, 65.

RECEIVED October 31, 1980.

Coherent Modes in Biological Systems

Perturbation by External Fields

FRIEDEMANN KAISER

Institute of Theoretical Physics, University of Stuttgart, Pfaffenwaldring 57, 7000 Stuttgart – 80, West Germany

In recent years considerable attention has been given to understanding both the stability of biological systems and their interactions with nonionizing electromagnetic waves. Toward this aim a special effort has been made by many authors using either refined experimental techniques or a modelling approach. The problem has gained increasing interest both, through rather exciting experimental results and through theoretical considerations (1).

Well documented biological effects exist, arising from irradiations at very low intensities where thermal effects certainly are to be excluded (vid. Refs. 2, 3 for details). The reported nonthermal effects occur in certain frequency regions only. They usually exhibit saturation at rather low intensities. In addition, these effects might be masked by thermal ones. In these cases the energy transfer from the radiation to the system varies slowly with frequency and is largely determined by dielectric losses.

A detailed and very successful investigation of the complex structure has shown that there exists no spatial order in these systems (vid. Ref. 3, chapter 2 for details). However, it is well-known in modern physics that, besides spatial order, other types of order do exist, e.g. order of motion. In many cases this type of order can be described by long range coherence.

As early as 1967 Fröhlich (4) emphasized that biological systems exhibit a relative stability for some modes of behaviour. In their active state (in vivo) these modes remain very far from thermal equilibrium. One manifestation of the stable behaviour is a coherent excitation, which means that a single mode is strongly excited. Fröhlich has suggested that coherent oscillations (as a special realization of long range coherence) ought to be of great importance in biological systems (4, 5).

To give an interpretation of the specific behaviour and stability of biological systems, one should primarily look for basic physical ideas, which may serve as working models to establish physical theories for a description of order and function. The idea of making models is suggested by the enormous complexity, which characterizes biological systems. With the aid of models it is

0097-6156/81/0157-0219$05.75/0

possible to pass over the complexity of the system by restricting
to the relevant mechanisms which might be responsible for both,
the internal function and the interaction with an external stimulus.

From our point of view, the following basis seems appropriate
for theoretical considerations:
1. the functional complexity of biological systems necessitates
    the application of macroscopic theories, e.g. the concepts of
    Synergetics (6) and Dissipative Structures (7),
2. the existence of some modes of behaviour very far from ther-
    mal equilibrium requires nonlinear interactions between the
    relevant subunits,
3. the specific modes, which are thermally decoupled from the
    remaining part of the system, must be stabilized by a sui-
    table energy and/ or matter input,
4. the interaction with external fields can lead to additional
    transport instabilities (i.e. nonequilibrium phase transiti-
    ons), which can lead to new stable or unstable states of
    function within the system.

It should be stressed that Fröhlich's concept of coherent
oscillations agrees with these four rather general requirements.
However, it should be emphasized that theoretical physics can only
provide us with the relevant concepts, which can point to a number
of possibilities, but it cannot predict in which way the system
has evolved. The actual state of function can only be found in
close collaboration with experiments.

General Concept and Theoretical Basis

Nonlinear Systems. Nonlinearities play a dominant role in
physics and many other disciplines. For example, all material laws
have a nonlinear characteristic. In many cases, the usually applied
linearization procedures are suitable and well established methods,
which might lead to satisfying results. However, nonlinear systems
can exhibit a behaviour, which is completely absent in the regime
of linear dynamics. Both, the development and the maintenance of
such a behaviour seem to be provided by a general mechanism: nonlinear dissipation.

Dissipation as an organizing factor can only occur under certain conditions, necessary prerequisites are: energy input (open
system), nonlinear dynamics and stabilization far away from thermal equilibrium i.e. beyond the regime of linear irreversible thermodynamics (vid. the requirements of Chapter I).

Oscillating phenomena and hysteresis behaviour (bi-, multi-
stability) are the most important phenomena in systems far from
thermal equilibrium, excluding spatial structures (patterns,
travelling waves). Examples of both types of temporal structures
can be found in all disciplines where nonlinear dynamics play a
significant role. In biophysics it appears that dissipation provides a general mechanism and may also account for the functional

stability and specific sensitivity of cooperative systems to environmental influences.

Nonlinear Oscillations (Limit Cycles). We want to restrict ourselves to nonlinear oscillations of limit cycle type (LC), which means that we are only dealing with selfsustained oscillations. This type of nonlinear oscillations can only occur in nonconservative systems, it is a periodic process, which is produced at the expense of a nonperiodic source of energy within the system.

It should be stressed that oscillatory phenomena are wellknown in biology. They span a wide range of periods, reaching from fractions of seconds (neuronal and EEG activities) and minutes (biochemical oscillators) to hours and days (circadian rhythm...). Besides these cooperative oscillations on an intra-, inter- and supercellular level, the usual oscillations on a microscopic basis (e.g. electronic transitions, intra- and intermolecular vibrations, rotational relaxation,...) must be taken into account.

Externally driven limit cycles can exhibit a great variety of behaviour. Quite generally, one gets a nonlinear superposition of an internal nonlinear oscillation with an external oscillatory perturbation. Details of the resulting behaviour (including sub- and superharmonic oscillations, entrainment, quenching...) depend on both, the frequency and intensity of the applied fields and on the internal nonlinear kinetics of the considered system.

To extend the special concept of coherent electric oscillations to further phenomena, we assume two rather general postulates:

1.   observable biological oscillations must be stable limit cycles or coupled sets of nonlinear modes of this type,
2.   stable limit cycles are a proper description for coherent oscillations in active systems.

To include the description of externally driven oscillating systems, a third postulate is suggested:

3.   externally driven limit cycles are a suitable basis for a description of the effects of external fields on biological and related systems.

The limit cycle concept reveals a possible explanation of the specific sensitivity of biological systems to a weak external stimulus through the following mechanism: the internal LC represents a storage of (metabolic) energy, which can be used to build up a signal, whereas the externally supplied field energy (with appropriate frequency and intensity) only causes the LC to collapse. This trigger effect of the external signal makes plausible the existence of nonthermal effects in irradiated biological systems, though the external energy supply is too weak to create a response of the system.

The LC concept has been applied to describe collective chemical and physicochemical reactions with an oscillatory kinetics, circadian and cardiac rhythm, brain function and rhythm etc. Details of this concept may be found in a recent article (8), where

a large number of both, theoretical model oscillators and experimentally found oscillatory phenomena have been presented.

Models

To give an illustration of our concept, we want to present
some rather simple model systems. These models are examples of a
typical nonlinear behaviour and they might perhaps serve as an
explanation of some specific effects found in experiments (vid.
Refs. 1, 2, 3). It should be emphasized that the models are rather
speculative. However, they are based on both, the physical properties and the relevant physical laws, which determine the dynamics
of the system under consideration.

Model 1: Generalized Van der Pol Oscillator

The Van der Pol oscillator is a well-known and best studied
example of a limit cycle oscillation. It has its origin in nonlinear electric circuits. We take a generalized version of it,
which in its normalized form reads:

$$\ddot{X} - \mu(1 - X^2 + \alpha X^4 - \beta X^6)\ \dot{X} + X = F(t) \qquad (1)$$

($\dot{} = \dfrac{d}{dt}$, X = amplitude of oscillation, e.g. a measure for time dependent polarization in membranes, bonding state of ions etc.;
$\alpha, \beta = 0$ is the usually applied Van der Pol limit).

The r.h.s. of the equation represents the external drive; for
simplicity we restrict to a harmonic one, $F(t) = F_o \cos \lambda t$.

Without the external field, two stable oscillations with fre-
quencies ω_1 and ω_2 and amplitudes x_1 and x_2 exist; an unstable LC
is situated between the two LCs. The stable oscillations are shown
in Figure 1. By external means and by parameter variations the system can be driven from one stable oscillation to the other one,
exhibiting a threshold and excitability. Furthermore, the external
field can lead to a complete collapse of the small amplitude oscillation. The closer the external frequency λ is to the internal
one, ω_1, the smaller is the critical field strength F_{oc}, which is
necessary for the breakdown of the small oscillation and the subsequent transition to the other one. For $F_o > F_{oc}$, the system can
only exist in the large amplitude state. This state is stable with
respect to F, but there exists a region, where partial quenching
of the oscillation can occur.

In the resonance region the system oscillates with the external frequency λ and with an increased amplitude (entrainment region). Far away from resonance, the internal free oscillations are
present. This behaviour is completely absent in systems, where no
self-sustained oscillations can exist. A typical example of such a
system is a nonlinear conservative system. The resonance diagram
has been drawn in Figure 2 for both, the small and the large amplitude oscillation.

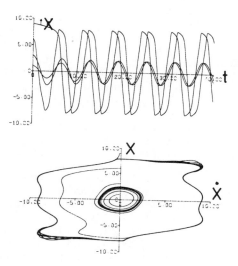

Figure 1. X(t) — t *(amplitude as a function of time) and* X(t) — X(t) *(phase-plane) computer diagram of the generalized Van der Pol oscillator with* $F_o = 0 = \lambda$ *for 4 different values of initial conditions. Both the small and large amplitude oscillations are shown.*

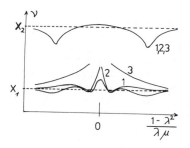

Figure 2. Resonance diagram (steady-state amplitude v as a function of the detuning parameter $(1 - \lambda^2)/(\lambda\mu)$*) for 3 different values* F_o *(*$F_{o1} < F_{o2} < F_{o3}$*). Note the instability region of the small limit cycle.*

The resulting frequency and the steady state amplitude for both oscillations are given in Figure 3 as a function of the external field amplitude for a certain frequency λ. The transition from one LC to the other one occurs below that point, where the latter LC gets entrained ($F_{oc} < \tilde{F}_{oc}$).

The important result is that, whereas the small oscillation can be influenced by very weak external fields, leading to a total collapse of the LC, the large amplitude cycle is rather stable against perturbations. This means that the system can be driven from a perturbable state to a nearly unperturbable one. Typical examples of entrained or perturbed oscillations are given in Figure 4.

A multiple LC model has been suggested by the author (9) to explain some rather interesting experimental results with respect to Ca^{2+} - efflux measurements in the ELF- and microwave irradiated brain. On the basis of the generalized Van der Pol oscillator, two stable and oscillating calcium states would exist. With regard to the frequency and intensity specific behaviour of this model, both, the frequency and intensity windows (which are the dominant features of the experiments) receive a possible explanation. However, a physical basis for our mathematical model is still lacking. Work towards this direction is going on.

Furthermore, the concept of externally driven limit cycles can yield an explanation of the extremely narrow frequency ranges of these effects. One can easily show that the nonlinear damping term vanishes, if one averages over one period of oscillation. This means that the energy supply per cycle is consumed during one period, i.e. the internal damping gets compensated by internal energy sources. A stable internal oscillation with fixed frequency results.

Model 2: Coherent Oscillations in Membranes

Fröhlich's suggestion that long range coherence might be important in biological systems, has found a profound demonstration and verification in two model calculations. In the coherent oscillation model he has shown that a Bose condensation-like excitation results, if a set of nonlinearly coupled oscillators is pumped by external energy supply above a certain threshold (5). In the high-polarization model he has been able to show that metastable highly-polarized oscillating states can exist in dielectric materials of suitable properties. Both, a few rather exciting experimental results and some model calculations on a strongly physical basis seem to support these ideas (vid. Ref. 1 for details).

Recently Fröhlich has extended his ideas to give a possible explanation of the extraordinary high sensitivity of certain biological systems to very weak external electric and magnetic signals (2). The model is a combination of both, a nonlinear chemical reaction, which is based on long range interactions, and a ferroelectric term, which represent the specific dielectric properties of membranes. The model equations read:

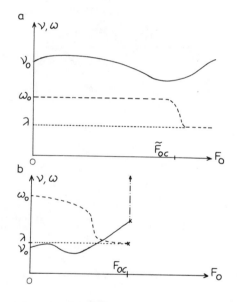

Figure 3.   Steady-state amplitude ν and steady-state frequency ω of both limit cycles as a function of the external field strength F_o for a fixed and arbitrary external frequency λ. For $F_o = F_{oc}$, the small limit cycle becomes unstable; for $F_o = F_{oc}$, a complete entrainment results. (———) ν; (– – –) ω; (a) $ν_o = X_2$, $ω_o = ω_2$; (b) $ν_1 = X_1$, $ω_o = ω_1$).

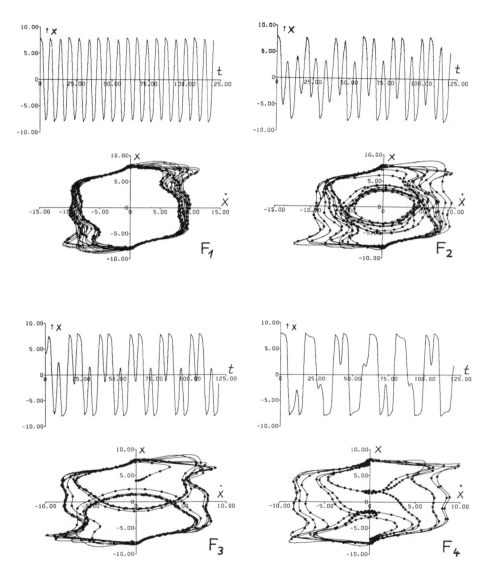

Figure 4.   Oscillation and phase-plane diagrams (see Figure 1) of the externally driven limit cycles for 4 different values of the external field strength F_o and for a fixed external frequency λ with $\lambda < \omega_1, \omega_2$ ($F_1 < F_2 < F_3 < F_4$).

$$\dot{\nu} = \gamma \, \sigma + \alpha \, A \, \sigma \, \nu + (c^2 e^{-\Gamma^2 \nu^2} - d^2) \, \nu + F(t) \qquad (2)$$

$$\dot{\sigma} = - \beta \, \nu - \alpha \, A \, \sigma \, \nu$$

with $\nu = N - \gamma | \alpha A$, $\sigma = S - \beta | \alpha A$, $\alpha, \beta, \gamma > 0$.

N, A are the concentrations of excited and unexcited enzyme molecules, ν, σ are the corresponding excess concentrations i.e. the
deviations from chemical equilibrium. S is the number of substrate
molecules per unit volume. $\gamma\sigma$ results from the long range interaction, $\beta\nu$ and $\alpha A \sigma \nu$ originate from the nonlinear enzyme-substrate
reactions. Aside from "chemical" terms we have an additional "dielectric" term which consists of two parts: a term describing the
system's tendency to become ferroelectric, i.e.

$$c^2 e^{-\Gamma^2 \nu^2} \nu \qquad (2a)$$

and frictional losses (electric resistences), i.e. $- d^2\nu$. F results
from the interaction of the system with its surrounding. Equs. (2)
have been investigated in great detail (11, 12, 13). The most important result is the existence of a LC, representing a chemical
lowfrequency oscillation to which corresponds an electric vibration
due to the highly polar states of certain enzymes. It should be
stressed that the high frequency coherent dipole oscillation is
contained in the parameters of the equations. In addition, the model fits well to our requirements and postulates of the LC concept.
    We only want to present some results for the externally driven
system. We confine ourselves to a harmonic electric field, $F(t)$
$= F_o \cos \lambda t$. Again one has to investigate the competition between
an internal nonlinear oscillation and an external oscillatory
field.
    Figure 5 shows the unperturbed LC with a fixed frequency ω_o
and a steady state amplitude ν_o, respectively. The complete behaviour of the perturbed system is given in the resonance diagram
Figure 6. One gets a slightly asymmetric diagram. Remarkable is the
extreme increase of the amplitude in the resonance region (entrainment regime), a quenching behaviour close to the high frequency
side of the resonance peak (i.e. partial suppression of the oscillation) and free oscillations with the internal frequency outside
these regions. This behaviour is well-known for self-sustained
oscillations. However, contrary to the results of our model 1, the
system can be driven into a completely unstable situation, which
leads to the collapse of the oscillatory state. Summing up, one
finds a series of transitions, which for a fixed frequency λ and
an increasing field F yields the scheme:
    unperturbed free LC → multifrequency and multiamplitude oscil-
    lations (quasiperiodic state) → transition to a new LC with fre-
    quency λ (entrainment) → collapse of the LC (instability) and
    onset of travelling waves (nonlinear response signal).

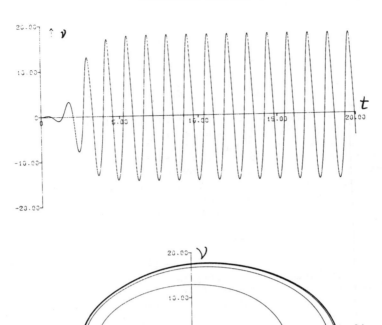

Figure 5. $v(t) - t$ *(amplitude as a function of time) and* $v(t) - \delta(t)$ *(phase-plane) diagrams of the coherent oscillation model (Model 2) with* $F_o = 0 = \lambda$. *The computer plot shows a typical limit cycle oscillation.*

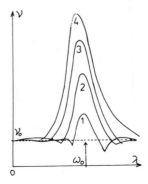

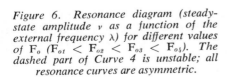

Figure 6. Resonance diagram (steady-state amplitude v *as a function of the external frequency* λ*) for different values of* F_o $(F_{o1} < F_{o2} < F_{o3} < F_{o4})$. *The dashed part of Curve 4 is unstable; all resonance curves are asymmetric.*

A similar scheme can be given for a varying external frequency. Typical examples of perturbed oscillations are shown in Figure 7. Figure 7e demonstrates that after some oscillations with increasing amplitude (transients) the system gets unstable. The different regions of behaviour have been drawn in Figure 8.

The critical strength F_{oc}, which is necessary for the LC to collapse and to create a response signal, is given by the external as well as by the internal parameters. Predominant are the dielectric ones (c^2, d^2), since these parameters determine the frequency and amplitude of the internal oscillation. We have been able to show that pulsed and modulated external fields can only shift the instability point towards smaller or higher values of the critical field strength per cycle. Qualitative changes in the overall behaviour of the driven LC system are impossible.

The relevance of the model is a matter of controversal discussions. Though the chemical reaction is a rather speculative one, one should realize that the special type of nonlinear reaction can be replaced by an other one. The important step is the combined existence of both, a special chemical kinetics and a related electric behaviour. Both terms can be modified, but they must be based on physical laws and the extraordinary dielectric properties of the material.

Model 3: Extended High-Polarization Model

The possible existence of highly polarized metastable states in biological model membranes has led us to a preliminary model for specific interactions in membranes (14). We have assumed that biomolecules are capable of nonlinear polarization oscillations, when they are sufficiently excited by metabolic energy or by external means, e.g. electric fields. Restricting to the case of two interacting molecules for simplicity, the dynamics of the system is given by a set of nonlinear differential equations for the polarization P_i of the molecule i:

$$\ddot{P}_i + \mu_i \dot{P}_i + \omega_i^2 P_i - \alpha_i P_i^3 + \beta_i P_i^5 + \gamma_{ij}(R)\, P_j = F_{o,i} \cos \lambda t \quad (3)$$

$$(i=1,2;\ j=2,1;\ \mu_i,\ \alpha_i,\ \beta_i > 0).$$

$\mu_i \dot{P}_i$ has been introduced as a phenomenological damping term to prevent the system from becoming unstable, when only a very small amount of energy is supplied and to account for always present loss processes. $\gamma_i(R)\, P_i$ results from the dipole-dipole interaction, i. e. $\gamma_{ij}(R)\, P_i P_j$; higher coupling terms have been neglected. We have restricted to the first three odd powers in P_i, these terms correspond to a symmetric nonlinear potential.

The two molecule model may be viewed as a starting point to discuss the dynamics of highly polarizable biomolecules in mema

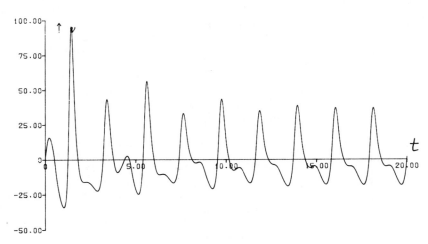

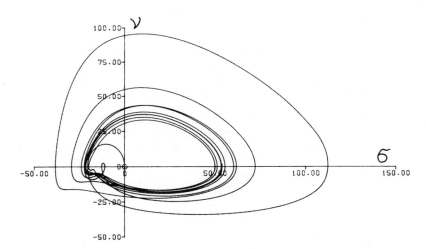

Figure 7.   Oscillation and phase-plane diagrams of the externally driven limit cycle of the coherent oscillation model.

(a) $\lambda_1 < \omega_0$, $F_o < F_{oc}$; (b) $\lambda_2 = \omega_0$, $F_o < F_{oc}$; (c) $\lambda_2 = \omega_0$, $F_o \rightarrow F_{oc}$; (d) $\lambda_3 > \omega_0$, $F_o < F_{oc}$; (e) $\lambda_3 > \omega_0$, $F_o = F_{oc}$: collapse of oscillation ($\omega_0 = $ frequency of unperturbed limit cycle; Figures (a)–(d) belong to Region III, Figure (e) to Region IV of Figure 8).

b

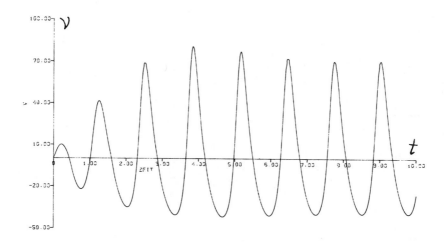

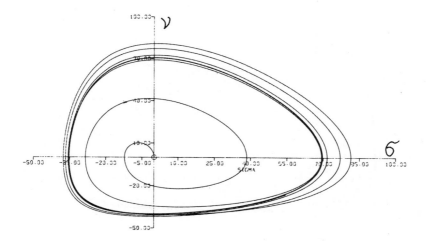

Figure 7.   Continued

c

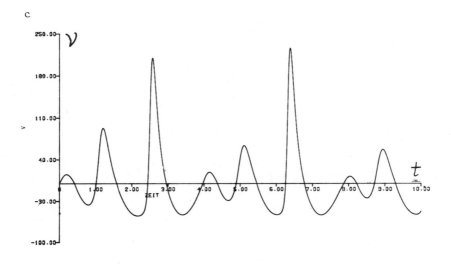

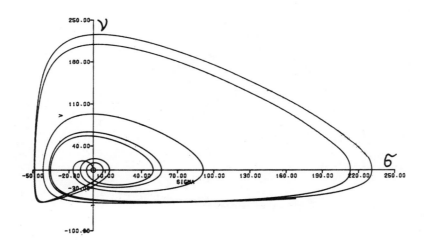

Figure 7.   Continued

d

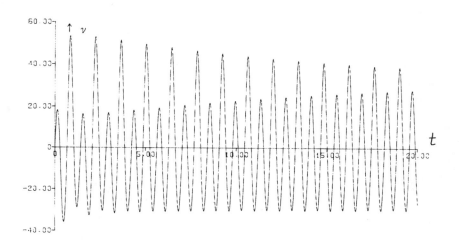

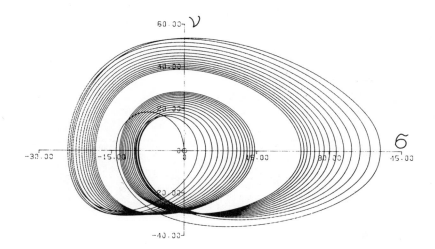

Figure 7. Continued

e

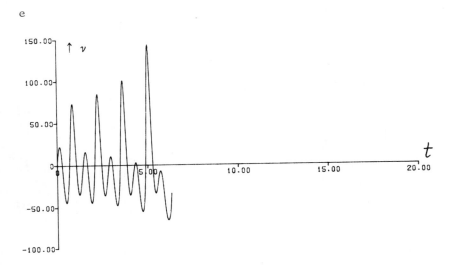

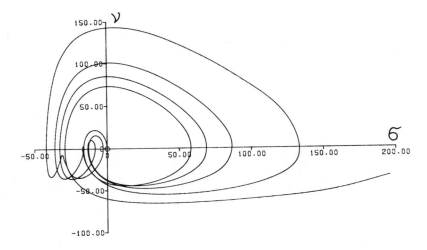

Figure 7.   Continued

branes. Depending on both, the initial condition (total energy) and
the externally supplied energy (given by the frequency and intensity of the external electric field), the oscillators can be stabilized in a highly polar oscillating state. For each molecule
three types of stable states ($P_{i,0} = 0$, $\pm P_{i,1} \neq 0$) are possible,
if there is no coupling between the molecules. Consequently three
types of stable oscillations can exist:

a.   oscillations around $P_{i,0}$ with small amplitudes (the usually
     found linear behaviour)

b.   oscillations around $P_{i,0}$ with large amplitudes (giant dipole
     oscillations with zero mean value)

c.   nonlinear oscillations around $\pm P_{i,1}$ (with nonzero mean value).
The three types of oscillatory behaviour are shown in Figure 9,
with $P_{i,0}$ and $P_{i,1}$ written as P_0 and P_i, respectively. $P_{i,1}$ must
not necessarily be a stable state, a metastable state is conceiv-
able and perhaps more probable. Details depend on the parameters
α_i and β_i.

Energy can be exchanged from one oscillator to the other one,
a typical situation is given in Figure 10. This behaviour can explain functional changes of irradiated systems: the highly polarized molecule A absorbes additional energy, which is transferred
partially to molecule B. After some transient periods, B is highly
excited and it can exhibit a new function. A direct excitation of
molecule B may be forbidden, whereas A is already stabilized in the
highly polar state by internal means.

Furthermore, a typical nonlinear resonance behaviour of non-
self-sustained oscillators results, it includes hysteresis effects
(bistability) and transitions to a new state (upper curve in Figure 11). This new state can either be a small or a large amplitude oscillation; in both cases a stable state of non-zero polarization ($P_{i,1}$) is included. Provided that the system is prepared in
a certain state, small external influences can drive it into a
state with a completely different vibration. A possible realization
is given in Figure 11, the system can jump from one resonance curve
to the other one. However, since we are dealing with a linearly
damped, but otherwise conservative system, the response of the system is predominantly governed by the initial conditions. No competition between internal and external oscillations is possible, the
resulting oscillating state is completely determined by the external constraints.

Model 4: Local Excitation Model

The possible existence of strong excitations of some modes of
behaviour might allow for energy storage mechanism in certain biological subunits. Some years ago we discussed the possibility of
exciting some or at least one additional degree of freedom by a
flux of energy through the system. For a simple model system (a
linear chain of molecules to which a singular degree of freedom is
coupled), we have found that the single mode gets strongly excited,

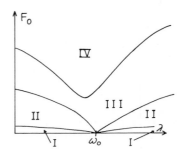

Figure 8. Regions of different behavior of the externally driven limit cycle of Model 2 (see Figures 5–7): (I) free oscillation (limit cycle with ω_0); (II) quasi-periodic oscillation; (III) entrainment (limit cycle with λ); (IV) unstable region → onset of traveling waves.

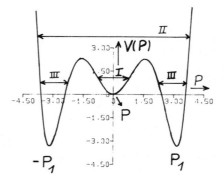

Figure 9. Schematic of possible types of oscillations for Model 3 (potential $V(P)$ as a function of polarization P); (I) harmonic oscillations (linear regime); (II) nonlinear oscillations with a large amplitude, $< P >_T = 0$; (III) nonlinear oscillations around the stable states $\pm P_1$, with $< P >_T \neq 0$.

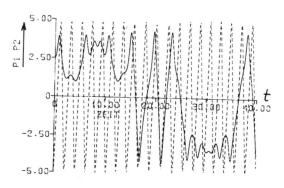

Figure 10. $P_i(t)$ — t *diagram (computer plot of the polarization as a function of time) ((——) $P_1(t)$; (– – –) $P_2(t)$)*

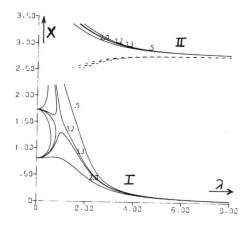

Figure 11.   Resonance diagram (computer plot of the steady state amplitude of one oscillator as a function of the external frequency λ) for 4 different values of the damping term μ *(μ = 0.5; 1.2; 1.3; 2.0) ((I) oscillations around P_o; (II) oscillations around P_1)*

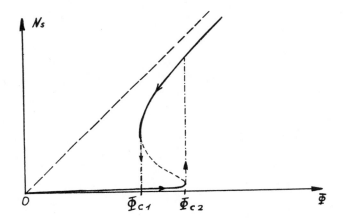

Figure 12.   Excitation of the singular mode N_s as a function of the external pump parameter (phonon flux Φ) of the local excitation model (Model 4). Both the steady-state excitation (hysteresis) and the possible oscillations on the hysteresis are shown.

when the flux exceeds a critical value. In addition, there is a
hysteresis in the dependence of the number of excitations N on the
pump power or flux Φ (15).

The steady state results are shown in Figure 12. For Φ_{c2}, the
single mode gets strongly excited, i.e. the energy is preferentially channeled into this mode (Bose condensation-like excitation).
If, by internal means, the system is near Φ_{c2}, only a small amount
of energy is necessary to drive the system into the highly excited
state. Furthermore, we have been able to show that oscillations on
the hysteresis are possible for $\Phi_{c1} \leq \Phi \leq \Phi_{c2}$. A detailed inspection of the transport equations (generalized nonlinear Peierls-
Boltzmann equations for phonons) shows that nonlinear kinetics,
dissipation and energy supply via transport are indispensable for
such a behaviour to occur.

A description of the rather complicated transport formalism is
beyond the scope of this article and will be omitted. For our purposes the important result is the excitation and stabilization of
a single mode. Contrary to the results of the other models with a
Bose condensation-like excitation, the coherently excited mode is
the mode with the highest and not with the lowest frequency.

Conclusions

Interaction with External Fields. The models considered exhibit cooperative behaviour through nonlinear internal oscillations
(models 1, 2, 4) or through nonlinear resonances (model 3). This
makes plausible the existence of effects, when the system is driven
by weak external fields of appropriate frequency.

On the basis of Fröhlich's suggestions and the properties of
biological systems (vid. models 2, 3) one may take into account the
following possible interactions of an electromagnetic field with
biological systems (16, 17):
1. the membrane intrinsic electric field (10^5 V/cm), which is
    responsible for the metastable highly polarized state,
2. the coherent electric oscillations ($10^{10} - 10^{12}$ Hz), leading
    to collective biochemical reactions through long range inter-
    actions,
3. the resulting ELF branch (10 - 100 Hz region), which may des-
    cribe EEG activities.
It should be stressed that the different regions are not independent from each other, interactions are not restricted to the above
frequency regions and to membranes.

General

Our models may be viewed as a rather speculative and very simplified version of any actual situation, nevertheless they may
serve as a starting point to get more insight into the function of
biological systems and their interactions with external fields. As
a result of these models, the limit cycle concept seems to be a
relevant basis for theoretical investigations.

We would like to comment particularly on four remarkable aspects of this concept:

1. nonlinear oscillations are the result of cooperativity in complex systems; they are intimately linked with nonequilibrium constraints and irreversibility,

2. limit cycles exhibit a pronounced behaviour with respect to the frequency and intensity of an external stimulus; they are capable of explaining extreme sensitivities by a mere trigger action of the external signal,

3. nonlinear systems (in an oscillating or bistable state) can be driven to a new state of order or function; in certain cases, extremely small changes of the external constraints are sufficient for the transitions, i.e. very weak perturbations can create drastic changes, if one applies the appropriate frequencies,

4. both, the general limit cycle concept and the more specific concept of coherent oscillations require the supply of energy (metabolic energy, biological pump) to create and stabilize the active state.

It should be emphasized that the relevance of the concept can only be checked by very accurate experimental investigations. To establish a clear picture, it is absolutely necessary to measure both, the frequency and the intensity dependence of the effects. In addition, the measurements should include the duration of irradiation and both, an increase and decrease in the applied field intensity to detect possible hysteresis effects.

From a theoretical point of view, one has to solve the problem of the onset of a propagating pulse after the LC collapse. This necessitates the introduction of space dependent variables and of appropriate boundary conditions. This problem has already been discussed for model 2 (13).

Literature Cited

1. Kaiser, F., Z. Naturforsch., 1979, 34a, 134
2. Adey, W.R., Bawin, S.M., Neurosci. Res. Progr. Bull., 1977, 15, 67
3. Fröhlich, H., "The Biological Effects of Microwaves and Related Questions"; Advances in Electronics and Electron Physics. Vol. 53, 85-152, 1980
4. Fröhlich, H., in "Theoretical Physics and Biology", Versailles 1967, Marois, M., Ed., North-Holland: Amsterdam, 1969
5. Fröhlich, H., Int. J. Quant. Chem., 1968, 2, 641
6. Haken, H., "Synergetics, an Introduction", Springer: Berlin, 1978
7. Nicolis, G., Prigogine, I., "Self-Organization in Nonequilibrium-Systems", J. Wiley: New York, 1977
8. Kaiser, F., Nonlinear Oscillations (Limit Cycles) in Physical and Biological Systems p. 343-389, in "Nonlinear Electro-

magnetics", Uslenghi, P.L.E., Ed.,Academic Press: New York, 1980

9. Kaiser, F., Workshop on the "Mechanism of Microwave Biological Effects", University of Maryland, May, 1979
10. Adey, W.R., Bio Systems, 1977, 8, 163
11. Kaiser, F., Biol. Cybernetics, 1977, 27, 55
12. Kaiser, F., Z. Naturforsch., 1978, 33a, 294
13. Kaiser, F., Z. Naturforsch., 1978, 33a, 414
14. Kaiser. F., Szabo, Z., (to be published)
    Szabo, Z., diploma thesis, University of Stuttgart, 1980
15. Kaiser, F., Z. Naturforsch., 1977, 32a, 697
16. Illinger, K., Workshop on the "Physical Basis of Electromagnetic Interactions with Biological Systems", University of Maryland, June, 1977
17. Kaiser, F., Symposium on the "Biological Effects of Electromagnetic Waves", Helsinki, Finland, 1978
    Radio Science (in print 1980)

RECEIVED December 9, 1980.

The Response of Biochemical Reaction Systems to Oscillating Stimuli

L. K. KACZMAREK

Division of Biology, California Institute of Technology, Pasadena, CA 91125

In this paper I shall discuss, in a general way, some basic dynamical properties of biochemical reaction schemes that are subjected to an external perturbation that oscillates in time. The first part of this paper will deal with the ways in which a weak external oscillating stimulus is able to alter the concentrations of metabolites in a biochemical system. This part will, in particular, consider what happens when the reaction system already oscillates in a limit cycle mode due to non-linearities in its reaction kinetics. It will be shown that such an autonomous biochemical oscillator may exhibit an enhanced sensitivity to a narrow range of externally applied frequencies.

The second part of this paper will examine the behavior of "labeled" metabolites in a system that is forced to oscillate. A labeled metabolite is defined as one that closely resembles the natural metabolite and is, therefore, subject to the same catabolic reactions as the natural metabolite. The addition or formation of the labeled form is, however, considered to be an unique event and there is no resynthesis of the labeled form through anabolic reactions. Examples of the labeling of metabolites include a) the addition of a trace amount of radioactively labeled metabolite, b) the impairment of the function of macromolecules through external radiation, or c) chemical modifications of enzymes or membrane receptors by their binding to exogenous agonists, antagonists or toxins. It will be shown that the flux of labeled metabolites through a pathway whose rate is forced to oscillate may be markedly enhanced relative to the same system at a stationary steady state, even though the mean concentrations of metabolites in the oscillating and stationary states may be the same.

The Perturbation of Non-linear Reaction Schemes By Oscillating Stimuli

If an external perturbation is able to influence the rate of any step in a biochemical reaction, changes in the concentration of

0097-6156/81/0157-0243$05.00/0

reactants will take place. For linear reaction schemes, the magnitude of the change in concentration is a simple function of the strength and duration of the perturbation. If the external perturbation oscillates in time, the concentrations of the metabolites will be forced to oscillate.

For nonlinear reaction schemes, maintained far from chemical equilibrium, a variety of more interesting interactions are possible ($\underline{1}$). These include threshold phenomena in which a small transitory external perturbation may induce a permanent change in the steady state concentrations of metabolites. In such a case the magnitude of the change may be independent of that of the stimulus beyond a certain threshold value. Nonlinear reactions may also display a form of resonance when the perturbation oscillates in time. This can be inferred by examining the stability properties of linearized forms of nonlinear reaction schemes ($\underline{2}$, $\underline{3}$). A complete description of this form of interaction, however, usually requires numerical computations ($\underline{4}$). I shall now describe the results of some computations in which a nonlinear reaction scheme that is capable of autonomous oscillations was perturbed by an oscillating stimulus applied over a range of frequencies ($\underline{5}$).

The model used for this analysis comprises three reaction steps interconnecting four reactants, A, X, Y, and B.

$$A \underset{k_{-1}}{\overset{k_1}{\rightleftharpoons}} X \qquad\qquad (1)$$

$$X \underset{Qe^{\eta Y}}{\overset{Pe^{\eta Y}}{\rightleftharpoons}} Y$$

$$Y \underset{k_{-3}}{\overset{k_3}{\rightleftharpoons}} B$$

The rate constants k_1, k_{-1}, k_3 and k_{-3} may be considered to incorporate the effects of enzymes that catalyze these steps and whose concentrations remain constant and in excess of the concentrations of A, X, Y and B. The three reaction steps may therefore represent biological interactions such as ionic binding, protein-lipid interactions, membrane transport of metabolites or ions, or changes in the conformations of proteins. The ringed arrow on the second step denotes that molecules of the species Y interact in such a way as to enhance the catalysis of X to Y. This positive cooperativity is represented by making the rate constants for the second step exponentially dependent on the concentration of Y. The strength of the cooperative interaction is given by the constant η. For the analysis of the frequency sensitivity of this reaction scheme, I shall consider the back reaction rates for the second and third steps, i.e., Q and k_{-3} to be vanishingly small. Then, assuming that the reaction system is an open one such that the concentrations of A and B are maintained constant, the kinetic equation for the time evolution of the concentrations X and Y within a fixed volume are

$$\frac{dX}{dt} = k_1 A - k_{-1} X - Pe^{\eta Y} X \qquad (2)$$

$$\frac{dY}{dt} = Pe^{\eta Y} X - k_3 Y \qquad (3)$$

This pair of equations can generate a variety of interesting dynamical behaviors including multiple stationary states, limit cycle oscillations, and co-existing stationary and oscillating states for a single set of parameters (5). When these parameters are themselves forced to oscillate, the resultant X,Y trajectories may become highly complex. How to quantitate the sensitivity of such a reaction scheme to external perturbations at differing frequencies may therefore become a problem. The solution adopted here is to examine the properties of the system at a set of parameters at which multiple steady states exist, one of these being a stable limit cycle oscillation and another being a stationary stable steady state. Beyond a finite threshold value, a perturbation to one state induces a transition to the other state. The efficacy of differing frequencies of external perturbation to induce a transition from the oscillating limit cycle state to the other stationary state can then be examined.

Figure 1 shows Y_0, the steady state value of Y, as a function of P with other parameters held constant. Over a range of values of P, three steady states co-exist. The stability of these states has been examined by normal mode analysis (5) and unstable states are depicted by the broken line. Over the range of values of P associated with the asterisks, the "upper" steady state has the characteristics of an unstable focus and computer integration of equations (2) and (3) demonstrates the existence of a stable limit cycle around this state. This region can therefore provide the required co-existence of a stable limit cycle and a stationary state.

The phase plane plot of Figure 2 illustrates the behavior of the concentrations of X and Y within this region. Initial concentrations of X and Y corresponding to a point above the broken line will evolve in time to the limit cycle. The broken line represents the separatrix of the middle unstable steady state which has the stability characteristics of a saddle point. Initial values for X and Y corresponding to a point below the separatrix will evolve to the stable state to the right of the diagram.

An external oscillating perturbation may be introduced into this reaction scheme by allowing one of the rate constants to be a function of time, for example,

$$k_1 = k_1' [1 + g \sin (\omega t + \emptyset)] \qquad (4)$$

or

$$P = P' [1 + g \sin (\omega t + \emptyset)] \qquad (5)$$

with

$$g < 1$$

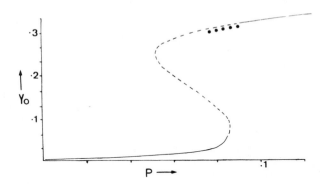

Biophysical Chemistry

Figure 1.   Steady-state value of Y *in Equations 2 and 3 as a function of* P *for the parameters* $k_1A = 1.0$, $k_{-1} = 1.0$, $k_3 = 3.0$, *and* $\eta = 16.0$ *(5). ((– – –) Unstable states; (*) the region for which numerical integration revealed a stable limit cycle.)*

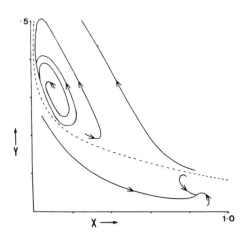

Biophysical Chemistry

Figure 2.   Representation of the behavior of X *and* Y *in the phase plane for Equations 2 and 3 with parameters* $k_1A = 1.0$, $k_{-1} = 1.0$, $k_3 = 3.0$, $\eta = 16.0$, *and* P = 0.077 *(5).*

In the context of the present symposium, this perturbation could be considered to result from the interaction of an external oscillating electric field with a reaction step involving a charged species.

Numerical integration of equations (2) and (3) with initial values for X,Y on the limit cycle and with one of the rate constants oscillating as in equation (4) or (5) may result in a transition of the X,Y trajectory across the separatrix towards the stationary state. The occurrence of a transition is dependent on the parameters g, ω and $\emptyset$. For extremely small amplitude perturbations (g $\rightarrow$ 0), the trajectory continues to oscillate close to the limit cycle. As g is increased, however, transitions may occur. The time taken for a transition is then primarily a function of the frequency of the perturbation. The time from the onset of the oscillating perturbation to the time at which the trajectory attains the lower steady state (Δt) is plotted in Figure 3 as a function of ω with all other parameters held constant. The arrow marks the minimum value for Δt which occurs when the frequency of the external perturbation exactly equals that of the unperturbed limit cycle itself. The second minimum occurs at the first harmonic of the limit cycle. Qualitatively similar results are obtained when numerical integration is carried out with differing values for g and $\emptyset$.

Using the ability to displace the trajectory of a limit cycle across a fixed boundary (the separatrix) as a measure of sensitivity to an external perturbation, it can therefore be seen that nonlinear oscillating reaction systems are able to respond most sensitively to a range of externally applied frequencies close to their endogenous frequency.

The Flux of Labeled Metabolites Through Oscillating Reactions

I shall now turn to the behavior of labeled metabolites in reaction systems where rates are forced to oscillate. The previous section dealt with the interaction of external perturbations with a nonlinear reaction system. An enhanced flux of labeled compounds through a reaction pathway may, however, occur even when a linear reaction system is made to oscillate and when the imposed oscillation produces no change in the mean concentrations of the metabolites (6).

Consider first the formation and catabolism of a metabolite according to the following kinetic equation for the time evolution of its concentration X with a fixed volume.

$$\frac{dX}{dt} = \alpha(t) - \beta(t)X \qquad (6)$$

All anabolic reactions are represented here by the term α whereas βX represents all catabolic reactions. In the most general case, α and β could each be functions of other metabolites and of X itself and are always positive. Initially, however, I shall

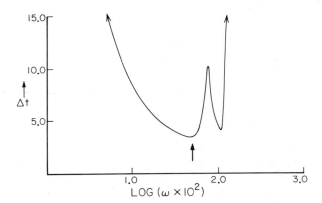

Biophysical Chemistry

Figure 3.   Frequency sensitivity of Equations 2 and 3 with the parameters $A = 1.0$, $k_{-1} = 1.0$, $k_3 = 3.0$, $\eta = 16.0$, $P = 0.077$, *and with* k_1 *given by Equation 4* ($k_1' = 1.0$, $g = 0.015$, $\phi = 0$) (5).

The abscissa is the logarithm of the stimulating frequency ω. *Initial values for* X *and* Y *are points on the unperturbed limit cycle (see Figure 2) and the ordinate* Δt *is the time computed for the trajectory to approach the lower stationary state.*

consider them to be independent of X. If we disregard the case of random changes in α or β, there are two general types of steady state solutions for equation (6) as $t \to \infty$. If α and β are represented as time-independent constants, the concentration X will reach an unique stationary steady state value as $t \to \infty$. On the other hand, if the parameters α and/or β oscillate regularly in time a steady state oscillation will be forced in X.

For the oscillating system, the mean chemical flux $\bar{\alpha}$ is given by

$$\bar{\alpha} = \frac{1}{T} \int_0^T \alpha(t)dt = \frac{1}{T} \int_0^T \beta(t)X(t)dt \tag{7}$$

where T is the period of oscillation. Similarly, for the mean value, $\bar{X}$, of the concentration X

$$\bar{X} = \frac{1}{T} \int_0^T X(t)dt \tag{8}$$

Now consider that at time $t = 0$ some proportion R(0) of the concentration X is present as its labeled form. Assuming that the rates of catabolism and anabolism are unaffected by labeling, the disappearance of labeled X is given by

$$\frac{dR}{dt} = -\beta(t)R \tag{9}$$

with the solution

$$R(T) = R(0)\exp \left\{- \int_0^T \beta(t)dt\right\} \tag{10}$$

In the case that the system is free of perturbations or oscillations at its steady state

$$\beta = \frac{\bar{\alpha}}{\bar{X}} \tag{11}$$

and equation (10) becomes

$$R(T) = R(0) \exp \left\{ \frac{-\bar{\alpha}T}{\bar{X}} \right\} \tag{12}$$

This exponential decay rate for R in a stationary system will now be compared with that for a system in which X oscillates due to oscillations in α or β. First, if the oscillations are driven solely by the anabolic term α and the rate of catabolism β remains time-independent, inspection of equations (6-10) shows that, for the steady state oscillation, relations (11) and (12) hold true. That is, the rate of removal of labeled compounds remains independent of the oscillations in α and X. On the other hand, if the rate of reaction through which the flux of R is occurring is made to oscillate, i.e., if $\beta(t)$ oscillates, $\frac{dR}{dt}$ will be a function of this oscillation. If

$$X(t) = \bar{X} + x(t)$$

where $x(t)$ is a periodic function whose integral vanishes over the period T and $x(t) << \bar{X}$ it can be shown (6) that

$$R(T) \gtrsim R(0) \exp \left\{ -\frac{\bar{\alpha}T}{\bar{X}} - \frac{\bar{\alpha}}{\bar{X}^3} \int_0^T x^2(t)dt \right\} \qquad (13)$$

Because $x^2(t)$ must always be positive, a comparison of equations (12) and (13) indicates that the rate of removal of R will be enhanced by these small amplitude oscillations of undefined waveform. Similarly, for the case of sinusoidal oscillations in X

$$X(t) = \bar{X} + x_1 \sin \left(\frac{2\pi t}{T} \right); \qquad |x_1| < \bar{X}$$

it may be shown (6) that

$$R(T) = R(0) \exp \left\{ -\frac{\bar{\alpha}T}{\sqrt{\bar{X}^2 - x_1^2}} \right\} \qquad (14)$$

Again the argument of the exponent here must always be more negative than that of equation (12) for the stationary state indicating an enhanced removal of labeled metabolites due to the oscillations. For the case of very large oscillations in $X(t)$ such that $x_1 \to \bar{X}$, equation (14) shows that complete removal of R occurs with one period of oscillation. This can also be shown to be true for large oscillations of undefined waveform (6).

Although these arguments have been presented for reaction systems whose rates are forced by an external oscillator, they remain true for autonomous biochemical oscillations where α and β are nonlinear functions of metabolite concentrations. That is, the rate of removal of a labeled compound through a reaction step whose rate is oscillating due to nonlinear kinetics will be enhanced over an equivalent system that maintains the same mean chemical flux and mean concentrations of metabolites but does not oscillate. This has been demonstrated numerically (6) on the reaction system (1) from the previous section using the full kinetic equations

$$\frac{dX}{dt} = k_1 A - k_{-1} X - Pe^{\eta Y} X + \frac{Pe^{\eta Y} Y}{K} \qquad (15)$$

$$\frac{dY}{dt} = Pe^{\eta Y} X - \frac{Pe^{\eta Y} Y}{K} - k_3 Y + k_{-3} B \qquad (16)$$

where
$$K = \frac{P}{Q} \qquad (17)$$

The removal of labeled X and Y from the system is given by the equations

$$\frac{dR_X}{dt} = -k_{-1} R_X - Pe^{\eta Y} R_X + \frac{Pe^{\eta Y} R_Y}{K} \qquad (18)$$

$$\frac{dR_Y}{dt} = Pe^{\eta Y}R_X - \frac{Pe^{\eta Y}R_Y}{K} - k_3 R_Y \tag{19}$$

where R_X, R_Y represent the proportions of labeled X and labeled Y, respectively. This system is compared with an analogous linear system in which the second reaction step which converts X to Y exhibits no cooperativity, i.e., $\eta = 0$. Denoting the concentrations of X and Y and the proportions of labeled compounds in such a linear system by lower case letters provides a set of equations

$$\frac{dx}{dt} = k_1 A - k_{-1}x - px + \frac{py}{K} \tag{20}$$

$$\frac{dy}{dt} = px - \frac{py}{K} - k_3 y + k_{-3}B \tag{21}$$

$$\frac{dr_x}{dt} = -k_{-1}r_x - pr_x + \frac{pr_y}{K} \tag{22}$$

$$\frac{dr_y}{dt} = pr_x - \frac{pr_y}{K} - k_3 r_y \tag{23}$$

When

$$p = \frac{(k_{-1}\bar{X} - k_1 A)k_3 K}{k_1 A - k_{-1}\bar{X} + k_{-3}B - k_3 K\bar{X}} \tag{24}$$

this set of equations (20-24) describes a non-oscillating system that, at steady state, maintains the same mean chemical flux as the nonlinear system of equations (15-19) and whose steady state value for x is equal to $\bar{X}$, the mean value of X in the nonlinear system.

Figure 4A shows X_0 the stationary state value of X for the nonlinear system as a function of P. With this set of parameters no multiple steady states exist but the steady states marked by the broken line are unstable and evolve to stable limit cycles. The amplitude of the limit cycles is shown in Figure 4B.

With initial conditions $R_x(0) = 1$, $R_y(0) = 0$, $r_x(0) = 1$, $r_y(0) = 0$ it is now possible to compare the rate of removal of R_x and r_x in the nonlinear and linear systems. When the nonlinear system oscillates (Figure 5A), it can be seen that at the end of one oscillation and at all times thereafter $R_x < r_x$ (Figure 5B). The ratio of R_x to r_x at the end of one period of the oscillating system is given in Figure 4C for the same range of values of P as in Figures 4A and 4B. When the nonlinear system does not oscillate the removal of R_x and r_x from the two systems proceeds at the same rate. When the nonlinear system evolves to a limit cycle, however, $R_X(T)$ is very much less than $r_x(T)$ indicating a profound enhancement of the removal of labeled X in the nonlinear system even though both systems maintain the same mean chemical flux and mean metabolite concentration $\bar{X}$.

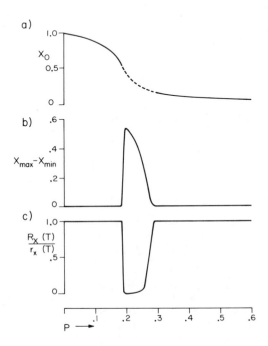

American Journal of Physiology

Figure 4. (6).

(A) Steady-state value of X in Equations 15 and 16 as a function of P. Unstable states are indicated by the broken line. (B) Magnitude of the stable limit cycle oscillations associated with the unstable stationary states in A. The magnitude of the oscillation is expressed as the difference between the maximum and minimum values for X. (C) Ratio of label $R_X(T)$ remaining in this oscillating system (Equations 15–19) to $r_x(T)$, the label remaining in a corresponding nonoscillating system that maintains the same chemical flux and mean metabolite concentration (Equations 20–24). Abscissa for all three graphs is at the bottom and in all cases the other parameters are $k_1A = 1.0$, $k_{-1} = 1.0$, $k_3 = 3.0$, $k_{-3}B = 10^{-6}$, $\eta = 10.0$, $K = 10^6$, $R_X(0) = 1$, $R_Y(0) = 0$, $r_x(0) = 1$, and $r_y(0) = 0$.

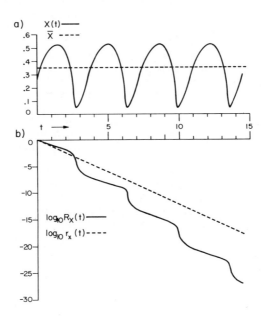

American Journal of Physiology

Figure 5. (6).

(A) Stable limit cycle in X(t) *is the numerically determined solution to Equations 15 and 16 for the parameters* $k_1A = 1.0$, $k_{-1} \equiv 1.0$, $k_3 = 3.0$, $k_{-3}B = 10^{-6}$, $\eta = 10.0$, $K = 10^6$, *and* $P = 0.22$. *The broken line gives* $\overline{X}$ *for this oscillation (Equation 8). (B) Logarithm of* R_X *is shown as a function of time for the system of Equations 15–19 with the same parameters as in A and with* $R_X(0) = 1$, $R_Y(0) = 0$. *The dotted line gives the logarithm of* r_x *as a function of time with the same parameters for Equations 20–24, and with* $r_x(0) = 1$, $r_y(0) = 0$.

Discussion

All biological cells have evolved to respond to their external environment in a specific way. Sensory cells respond to stimuli of a particular sensory modality while nonsensory cells respond in a specific manner to stimuli that are chemical or electrical changes in their extracellular environment often produced by other cells of the same organism. The first part of this paper showed that it would be possible for a cell to be "tuned" by means of a cellular oscillator of biochemical origin, to respond to only a discrete range of frequencies of stimuli. The period of a biochemical oscillator may range from fractions of a second to many hours. A stimulus impinging on the oscillator may markedly alter the concentration of reactants when its frequency matches that of the oscillator but produce little or no change at other frequencies.

The second part of the paper showed that either external oscillations or the occurrence of autonomous oscillations in a biochemical pathway can enhance the flux of labeled compounds in that pathway. This feature can prove to be useful to the experimentalist. Suppose that a biochemical system is exposed to a weak external oscillating stimulus. If the frequency of oscillation is high, it may not be possible to determine if the concentrations of metabolites are being forced to oscillate at the same frequency. If, however, the metabolites can be labeled, e.g., by the addition of trace amounts of radiolabeled compounds, the flux of these labeled compounds may be markedly enhanced relative to the unperturbed system, indicating that forcing of the metabolite concentrations is taking place. For example, using radiolabeled calcium ions, it has been possible to show an enhancement of calcium fluxes in avian forebrain in response to weak amplitude-modulated VHF fields. This effect is most sensitive to a range of imposed frequencies close to 16 Hz, suggesting that the field interacts with an endogenous oscillation at this frequency (7).

Acknowledgement

This work was supported by National Institutes of Health grant NS-07071.

Literature Cited

1. Nicolis, G; Prigogine, I.   "Self Organization in Non-Equilibrium Systems"; Wiley-Interscience: New York, 1977.
2. Ortoleva, P. J.; Ross, J. J. Chem. Phys., 1972, 56, 293-294.
3. Hyver, C. Bull. Math. Biol., 1975, 37, 1-9.
4. Boiteux, A.; Goldbeter, A.; Hess, B. Proc. Nat. Acad. Sci. (USA), 1975, 72, 3820.
5. Kaczmarek, L. K. Biophys. Chem., 1976, 4, 249-251.
6. Kaczmarek, L. K. Amer. J. Physiol., 1979, 237, R350-R354.
7. Bawin, S. M.; Kaczmarek, L. K.; Adey, W. R. Ann. N.Y. Acad. Sci., 1975, 247, 74-81.

RECEIVED December 9, 1980.

Nonlinear Impedance and Low-Frequency Dispersion Effects of a Polyelectrolyte Under High Sinusoidal Fields

CHIA-LUN J. HU and FRANK S. BARNES

Department of Electrical Engineering, University of Colorado, Boulder, CO 80309

In understanding the electrical characteristics of biological materials such as tissue which is a complex, inhomogeneous, aniso-tropic, and nonlinear material, we feel it is necessary to first understand the electrical properties of the simpler biological fluids. Additionally since the fields in the vicinity of mem-branes may be quite large ($\approx 2 \times 10^4$ volts/cm) it is important to understand the high field behavior as well as the more commonly measured small signal characteristics.

Most biological solutions are polyelectrolytes consisting of polymer ions (enzyme or protein ions) and small counter ions (Na^+, K^+, Ca^{++}, etc.). These polyelectrolytes are generally good con-ducting mediums. Therefore, it is usually very hard to apply high sinusoidal voltages to these mediums if one wishes to see their behavior under high fields because the ohmic heating will raise the temperature and damage the medium before any other phenomena can be observed. To avoid the ohmic heat damage, the usual tech-nique is to use short pulses. The nonlinear conductance and other behavior of many electrolytes under high pulsed fields are gener-ally classified as *Wien effects*. However, there exists a problem that the results under *pulse excitation* cannot generally be used to derive the results under high *sinusoidal fields* because the superposition principle is not applicable when the medium behaves nonlinearly. With the technique to be described, both the magni-tude and the phase of the medium impedance under high *sinusoidal fields* are measured as functions of frequency, voltage, and con-centration of the medium.

Since the two major results we obtained in our experiments are a nonlinear impedance and a low frequency dispersion effect of polyelectrolytes under *high fields*, it is logical for us to provide the readers with some background review in the field of nonlinear effects and high-field dispersion effects of electro-lytic solutions. Most of the studies in these fields were devoted to Wien effects and DFW dispersion theory which are briefly dis-cussed here. A detailed discussion of these two groups of studies with their recent developments is reported in a separate review chapter in Nonlinear Electromagnetics.

0097-6156/81/0157-0255$05.00/0

There are two effects discovered by Wien and others in a
period from 1927 to 1931. They found that under high pulsed
fields, there is a significant increase of conductivities in many
strong electrolytes (first Wien effect) and even *stronger* increase
of conductivities in some electrolytes with much *weaker* ionic
strengths (second Wien effect). This nonlinear conductance effect
is explained by the decrease of ionic-cloud dragging on the heavy
ions drifted under high fields. Since their discovery, many investigations were subsequently carried out using different experimental schemes. On the other hand, around the same time, Debye,
Falkenhagen and Williams reported some experimental and theoretical
studies of certain electrolytes that show a ramp increase of conductivity under constant high pulses when frequency is scanned
across a certain region. This was explained by the ionic cloud
relaxation effect. Both of these groups of high voltage experiments were carried out by using pulse excitations to avoid ohmic
heat damage to the medium.

Thin-Film I-V Sampling Technique

In contrast to the pulse technique reported in the literature
for observing nonlinear and other effects under high fields, we
designed a thin-film structure as shown in Figure 1 for applying a
moderate sinusoidal field (about 500 V/cm, peak to peak) to the
medium. We cover a standard microscope slide with two pieces of
aluminum foil (about 0.5 mil or 1.3×10^{-3} cm thick) with 2 mm
spacing between them. Then we cover the whole slide with scotch
tape, except for a small exposed area near the center as shown in
Figure 1 (1 mm x 4 mm of foil is exposed on each side. No tape is
used in the 2 mm x 4 mm gap). A small drop of polyelectrolyte
(sodium polystyrene sulfonate or NaPSS) or saline (0.9% salt in
distilled water) is then placed onto the exposed area and it is
spread around to form a "thin-film" impedance by putting a piece
of cover glass on top of it. The cover glass and the slide are
then clamped in place by two special clips. Now, if we apply a
d.c. or an a.c. voltage across the two pieces of aluminum foil as
shown, the impedance of this thin-film electrolytic "cell" can be
measured as shown later and it ranges from 4 KΩ (a.c.) to 200 KΩ
(d.c.), depending on the frequency of the excitation voltage and
the liquid medium used. The high impedance shown here is the result of the thin-film structure or the thin cross-section of the
sample. Also the large surface to volume ratio used here reduces
the temperature rise significantly because of thermal conduction
across the large surface. The small amount of heat generated is
conducted away efficiently through the aluminum foil and the cover
glass which are placed in direct contact with the solution.

To measure the impedance of the thin-film electrolyte we used
a current and voltage sampling (i-v sampling) method as shown in
Figure 1. Because the impedance across the electrolyte slide
(about 200 KΩ d.c.) is much higher than the current sampling

resistor ($r = 10\Omega$ to 50Ω) which is connected in series in the circuit, the presence of this small sampling resistor in the circuit
will not significantly affect the i and v across the solution.
Therefore, the current i through the electrolyte can be monitored
by monitoring $v_r \equiv ri$ across the sampling resistor. Similarly,
the voltage drop across the sample slide can be monitored by monitoring (through a 10x attenuation probe) the voltage drop across
the generator because these two voltage drops are approximately
equal. The monitoring device we use is a dual-trace oscilloscope
(Tektronix 561). By calculating the amplitudes and phases of the
i-v curves shown on this oscilloscope, we can determine the complex impedance $\hat{z}$ of the electrolyte sample. (Note: For the
case of nonlinear impedance, as shown by the non-sinusoidal i
under the sinusoidal v in the first picture of Figure 2, etc., we
take the impedance to be defined by the ratio of the amplitudes of
the maximum points in the i-v curves monitored (with proper cali-
bration factor inserted, of course) and the phase difference
between these two maximum points. This is realized as being tech-
nically different than that obtained from a Fourier analysis of
the waveform. However, the v:i ratio still provides useful insight into the physics of the liquid.) Figures 2, 3 and 4 are the
i-v curves monitored by the oscilloscope at various frequencies,
various applied voltages, and various relative concentrations of
the NaPSS solutions. Figures 5 and 6 are the dispersion and the
nonlinear characteristics calculated from Figures 2-4. For example, in the third picture on the top row of Figure 2, the
admittance $\hat{Y}$ is calculated as

$$(2.7\,\text{div.} \times 10\ \text{ma/div.})/(2\ \text{div.} \times 50\ \text{v/div.}) \cdot \exp j(0.2\ \text{div.}/1.8\ \text{div.})$$

$$\times\ 360° = 2.7\ e^{j40°}/Z_o$$

where $Z_o \equiv 10\ K\Omega$. This is indicated by the 10.0 KC points of
the $\rho = 1.0$, $v = 100$ v or $E = 500$ v/cm, y, θ curves shown in
Figure 5. In general, it is seen from Figures 5 and 6 that admittance tends to increase as any of the following parameters
increases: frequency, voltage, and concentration of the solution.
       The reproducibility of these data is checked by repeating the
experiments with the same applied voltages, same frequencies, but
fresh polymer samples. By averaging the measured data under the
same conditions, we see that the fluctuation of the amplitude
measurements is less than 10% of the average amplitude, and that
of the phase measurements is less than 30% of the average value.
The main reason for these fluctuations occurring is found to be
due to the variation of the thickness of the thin film. That is,
although the thin-film samples prepared here are *clamped* between
the covering glass and the microscope slide as mentioned earlier,
it is found that when the clamping position or the clamping pressure is changed, the i-v curves on the oscilloscope will change.

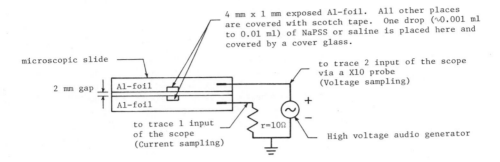

4 mm x 1 mm exposed Al-foil. All other places
are covered with scotch tape. One drop (~0.001 ml
to 0.01 ml) of NaPSS or saline is placed here and
covered by a cover glass.

microscopic slide

2 mm gap

Al-foil

Al-foil

to trace 2 input of the scope
via a X10 probe
(Voltage sampling)

to trace 1 input
of the scope
(Current sampling)

r=10Ω

+

−

High voltage audio generator

Figure 1. Experimental setup

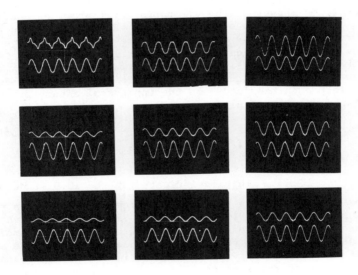

*Figure 2. The i–v curves for NaPSS under 100 V, 50 V, 20 V; ρ = 1.0. Left
column: 0.1 KC; middle column: 1.0 KC; right column: 10.0 KC. Vertical scale
(upper trace is for i; lower trace is for v): top row: i in 10 ma/div., v in 50 V/div.;
middle row: i in 4 ma/div., v in 20 V/div.; bottom row: i in 2 ma/div., v in 10
V/div.*

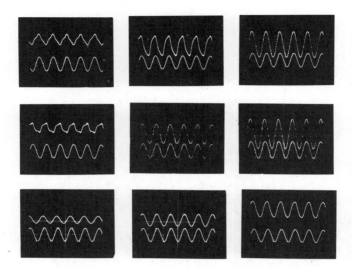

Figure 3.   The i–v curves for NaPSS under 100 V, 50 V, 20 V; ρ = 0.5. Frequency and voltage scales are the same as in Figure 2; i scales are 2.5 ma/div., 1 ma/div., 0.5 ma/div., from top to bottom.

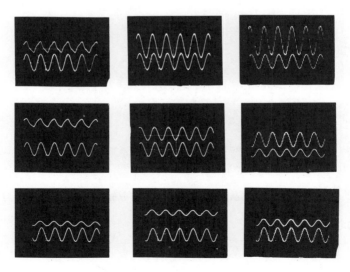

Figure 4.   The i–v curves for NaPSS under 100 V, 50 V, 20 V; ρ = 0.1. Frequency and voltage scales are the same as in Figure 2; i scales are 5/3 ma/div., 2/3 ma/div., 1/3 ma/div., from top to bottom. For 10 KC displays (last column) chopper mode is used because alternation mode is not stable.

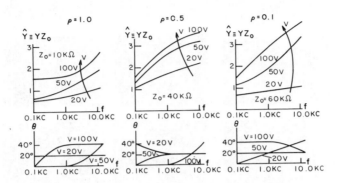

Figure 5.   Dispersion characteristics (Nomenclature: (v) applied voltage (peak to peak); (ρ) relative concentration of NaPSS; (Y) admittance of the sample in mho; (Ŷ) normalized admittance of the sample; (Zₒ) normalization factor in ohm; (θ) angle of Y).

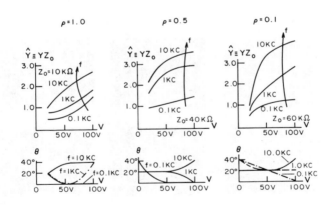

Figure 6.   Nonlinear characteristics (nomenclature as in Figure 5)

This indicates that a change of the thin-film thickness will affect significantly the i-v relations of the thin-film sample. This is of course to be expected theoretically, because the current is parallel to the thin-film surface and the resistance of the sample is inversely proportional to the cross-section of the thin-film. Therefore, a change of say 10% of the thickness, which may not be detected by naked eyes at all, will change the admittance of the sample by also 10%. Following this line of thought, we designed a special device as shown in Figure 7 for hoping to get better control on the liquid film thickness. The base of this device is made of an aluminum plate. A is the slide guide milled out of the plate for sitting the microscope slide. B and C are two clamps fixed on the base plate. The ends of these clamps are screwed onto the base plate. The central screw on each clamp is a plastic screw for holding the slide tightly in place. D and E are two micrometer-type screws for pressing the covering glass on the slide. The traveling distance of D or E screw can be read out accurately by the dial reading on the head of this screw as shown in the enlarged part of Figure 7. By adjusting the micrometer screws to the same dial readings every time we have a fresh sample we can then obtain much better control on the liquid film thickness. Indeed, using this device, we have obtained $\bar{z}$ data with amplitude variation less than 6% and phase variation less than 3° around the average values shown in Figures 5 and 6.

Results

There is a build-up phenomenon observed after the turn-on of the voltage. That is, at high fields of 500 v/cm, the i or current curve is sinusoidal at the beginning. But it starts to deform to the non-sinusoidal curves shown in Figures 2-4 in a time less than five minutes, depending on the voltage, the frequency, and the sample used. At steady state, if the frequency or the voltage is swept, the non-sinusoidal i curve is usually symmetrical with respect to the peak of the v curve when frequency is lower than 50 Hz. But when frequency is increased at fixed field strengths, the leading and the trailing parts of the i curve start to rise at different rates. The leading part always rises faster than the trailing part. Eventually, at high frequencies, the i curve becomes sinusoidal but with its peak shifted forward in time. See, for example, the top row of Figure 2. The shift of this peak and the change of the i curve depend also on the applied voltage as well as on the concentration of the solution as can be seen by comparing pictures row to row in Figures 2-4. On the other hand, when the frequency is kept fixed and the voltage increased, the current waveform changes from a pure sinusoidal waveform at low voltage to a non-sinusoidal waveform with considerable harmonic content at high voltages.

Figure 8 is the i-v curves of a 0.9% saline sample under 500 v/cm. The slide and the electrodes used are the same as those used in the polyelectrolyte measurements. It is seen that the

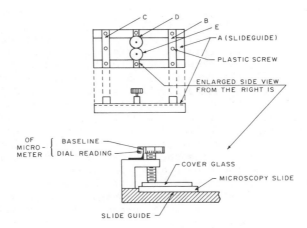

Figure 7. Clamping setup for controlling the thin-film thickness of the sample

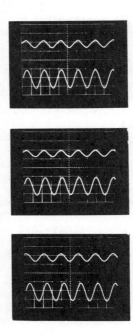

Figure 8. The i–v curves for saline under 100 V of various frequencies. Vertical scale of upper trace: i in 1/3 ma/div.; vertical scale of lower trace: v in 50 V/ div. Frequency = 0.1 KC, 1.0 KC, 10.0 KC from top to bottom.

nonlinearity and the dispersion are *not* significant as compared to
those in the polyelectrolyte.

To check the temperature rise in the liquid sample under high
fields, we have tried two preliminary approaches. First, we used
a radiometer designed in our Instrument Development Laboratory.
A special IR bandpass filter is used in the radiometer which
allows us to calibrate the reading of the meter by facing the
meter input window against an icy water surface. The angular input aperture of this instrument is very sharp which thus allows a
temperature measurement on a selected small area. In spite of
some noise and stability problems of the instrument, the increment
temperature of the solution under a medium applied voltage (40 V
peak to peak) is seen to be around 8°C. The second method we
used to measure the solution temperature is to insert a fine-wire,
E-type thermocouple into the solution. This thermocouple is made
by Omega Company in Connecticut. Its wire diameter is only 0.0005
inches or half a mil. The thermally-induced voltage at the far
end of this thermocouple is measured by an HP d.c. micro-volt-
meter. This measurement is done when the applied voltage is
temporarily switched off such that the thermo-electric output is
not affected by the large applied voltage. The reference junction
of this thermocouple is exposed to room temperature environment,
hence the voltmeter reading can be taken directly as proportional
to the temperature increment of the sample if the slight nonlinearity of the thermocouple response is neglected. The measured
temperature increments of our samples ($\rho = 1.0$) under high applied
fields are shown in Table I.

It is seen from these measurements that the highest steady
state temperature rise is about 27°C when 100 volt sinusoidal
voltage is applied across the 2 mm gap where the liquid sample is
deposited. The time required for the steady state temperature to
decay to 1/3 of its initial value after the applied voltage is
turned off is seen to be 20 seconds to 1 minute.

We have also carried out some preliminary measurements, by
using Kerr effect, on time constants for the alignment of the
macromolecules in the NaPSS solution under high fields. We use a
pair of crossed polarizers placed around the sampling slide and
pass a He-Ne laser beam through the sample as shown in Figure 9.
When a high a.c. voltage is applied to the aluminum electrodes on
the slide, the output He-Ne intensity increases slowly but significantly as detected by an RCA 1P22 photomultiplier tube. This
increase eventually approaches a limit level and the time constant
for reaching this level is about the same as that for the current
wave form to reach the a.c. steady state. This seems to indicate
that the build-up phenomenon mentioned earlier is probably due to
the molecular alignment and not due to the thermal equilibrium
effect.

Summarizing the experimental data, we have the following results on the polyelectrolyte NaPSS. In the range of
0.1 KHz $\leq$ f $\leq$ 10.0 KHz and 100 v/cm $\leq$ E $\leq$ 500 v/cm (peak to peak):

TABLE I

Applied voltage V	20 V peak to peak		
Frequency f	10 KHz	1 KHz	0.1 KHz
Steady state thermo-couple output v_{th}	0.1 mv	0.2 mv	0.4 mv
ΔT at steady state	1.7°C	3.3°C	6.7°C
Applied voltage V	40 V peak to peak		
Frequency f	10 KHz	1 KHz	0.1 KHz
Steady state thermo-couple output v_{th}	0.2 mv	0.6 mv	1.3 mv
ΔT at steady state	3.3°C	10°C	21.7°C
Applied voltage V	100 V peak to peak		
Frequency f	10 KHz	1 KHz	0.1 KHz
Steady state thermo-couple output v_{th}	0.6 mv	1.0 mv	1.4 ~ 1.6 mv (not stable)
ΔT at steady state	10°C	16.7°C	23.4° ~ 26.6°C

1. admittance Y increases as frequency increases;

2. Y increases as applied voltage increases;

3. Y increases as concentration increases;

4. i always leads v by an angle less than 40°;

5. there is a definite build-up format for the current wave-form which takes one to five minutes to reach the steady-state after the voltage is turned on;

6. the time constants in this build-up seem to be correlated to the time constants for aligning the macromolecules under high fields as detected by our Kerr effect experiments;

7. higher harmonics in i-curve are most prominent at low frequencies and high voltages;

8. there is no such significant nonlinear and dispersion effects when saline is used as samples;

9. the steady-state temperature rise ΔT in the sample under 500 v/cm is around 27°C. For lower applied fields, ΔT's are much lower than this.

In addition to these results, we have observed also another interesting phenomenon, i.e., resonance of polymer impedance under high intensity but low frequency fields (1 KHz to 10 KHz). At the present time, we are checking the reproducibility of this phenomenon. We hope to publish this in a subsequent article.

Discussion

Because the nonlinear and the dispersion data of our experiments are obtained at CW sinusoidal fields of less than 500 v/cm, while the Wien effects and the high voltage dispersion effects reported in the literature were investigated under pulse excitations of 10 to 200 KV/cm strengths, we feel that the theories discussed in Wien effects and high voltage dispersion effects may not be completely suitable for explaining all the phenomena we observed. The following are some other possible mechanisms which we can think of that may relate to the experimental results we obtained.

Non-Newtonian Fluid. Many viscous mediums, for example, most lubricants used in automobiles are non-Newtonian fluids. That is, their viscosities depend on the shearing velocity and many of them decrease as velocity increases (up to a certain limit). (Note: This is why most automobiles are most efficient

at 20 to 55 miles/hour, because the viscosity of the lubricant is
minimum in a certain range of shearing velocity corresponding to
these speeds (1).). At low voltages, the velocity of current
carrying ions in an electrolyte is very low and viscosity variation is small. Therefore, the resistance of the medium is a constant independent of the applied voltage. But when the voltage is
high, the velocities of ions are higher. For Wien's experiments
using 100 KV/cm pulses, the velocities of certain ions are calculated by Debye and Falkenhagen, as around 1 meter/sec (2). The
nonlinearity of viscosity may thus play an important role in the
nonlinear impedance and other related phenomena under high fields.
Both Wien's experiments and our experiments show that when voltage
increases, in general, resistance of the medium decreases, which
is compatible to the nonlinear nature of the viscosities exhibited
in many lubricants. Of course, more quantitative studies (for
example, measuring the viscosities of biological solutions at
various shearing speeds) must be made before we can claim that the
nonlinear viscosity indeed contributes to the nonlinear impedance
phenomenon we observed.

     Space Charge Effect. Space charge effect of electrical
properties of liquids have been studied in at least two aspects.
One is the "concentration effect" in electrochemistry and the
other, the "SCLC effect," or, the space-charge-limited-current
effect in liquid crystals. We would like to discuss these two
effects separately in the following.

(1) Concentration Effect in Electrochemistry. In a bulk electrolytic cell, the resistance of the liquid layers near any of the
electrodes is generally nonlinear and current-dependent, because
the ionic concentrations near the electrodes are generally inhomogeneous due to electrolysis and contact potentials. This space
charge, or concentration effect, as usually called in electrochemistry (3,4), will contribute a modification or an over-voltage
to the total voltage between the electrodes in the cells. That
is, the voltage between the electrodes is deviated from that of
the (linear) Ohm's law by an over-voltage which, in part, is contributed by the space charge near the electrodes. This modification in a bulk electrolytic cell is generally very small because
the bulk part of the liquid in the cell is still homogeneous. But
when the two electrodes are placed very close to each other as
those shown in Figure 1 here, the liquid between the electrodes
may be inhomogeneous everywhere. Therefore, the space-charge induced nonlinearity may be very prominent because of this inhomo-
genity of the ion distribution.

(2) SCLC in Liquid Crystals. The conductivity of a liquid crystal medium is generally much smaller than that of an electrolyte,
because its physical properties are closer to those of an insulator or a semiconductor. The conductivities of many liquid

crystals were measured by several people in the last decade (5-8) and they generally show significant nonlinear and temperature dependent behaviors. Shaw and Kuffman reported a one-dimensional space charge theory, similar to the one used in insulator break-down effects, for explaining the nonlinear resistance behavior of liquid crystals. The agreement between the theory and the experi-ments are quite good for several liquid crystals. But, Yoshino, etc., found experimentally several other cases which are quite apart from Shaw's theory. Shaw's theory lies in the fact that mobility of electrons or ions in an insulator-like medium is generally small, hence *space charge* may build up easily if charge is "injected" into the medium by high applied fields. The result of this is a nonlinear resistance effect in the bulk medium. Although polyelectrolyte is a good *conductor* in contrast to the *insulator-like* liquid crystal, yet the space charge calculation used to explain the *d.c.* nonlinear effects in liquid crystals may still be adopted to the explanation of the *a.c.* nonlinear impe-dance effects reported in this article because the qualitative behaviors of the two are quite similar.

Thermal-Chemical Effect. Although the heating problem in our experiments is much reduced as compared to that in the bulk sys-tems, there is still a temperature rise in the medium. But this temperature rise reaches a steady-state due to the balance between heat generation and heat conduction. This steady-state tempera-ture is lower than the irreversible damage threshold of the medium such that the medium is not permanently damaged. Because of this temperature rise more giant molecules will be decomposed into polyions which will result in an increase of conductivity of the medium. This increase of conductivity will in turn generate more ohmic heat and produce more decomposition -- consequently, a nonlinear conduction mechanism exists. (Note: some years ago, the authors published a paper on the thermal-chemical effects in bio-mediums under laser heating (9). The mechanism described there can be adopted to the thermal-chemical decomposition effect here with only slight modification.) We have done some indepen-dent experiments on bulk samples of beef flank to check this thermal-chemical effect on the medium conductivity. The method we used is the same i-v sampling technique as described above. In spite of the rather poor reproducibility, we found that the im-pedance does decrease as the temperature rises. The temperature rise can be felt by touching the meat sample and it can reach to a very high level such that the meat can be seen to have been permanently damaged. The result of this experiment on one typical meat sample is shown in Figure 10. The polyelectrolyte experi-ments reported above may be partly contributed to by the same mechanism described here.

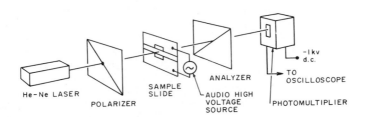

Figure 9.   Kerr effect experiment setup for checking the molecule alignment time under high fields

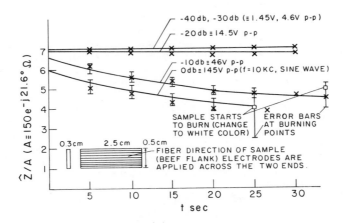

Figure 10.   Impedance of a beef flank sample with fiber along current direction

Conclusion

In summarizing our results, we have shown

(1) A new thin-film technique for reducing the effects of ohmic heating on measurements of the i-v (or current-voltage) characteristics of conductive liquids at sinusoidal fields up to 500 v/cm.

(2) The i-v sampling technique used here provides a real-time oscilloscope display of the i-v characteristics. This allows us to measure both amplitude and phase of the medium impedance at a.c. steady state. It also allows us to monitor the build-up phenomenon as well as the continuous variation of the i waveform when f or V is swept.

(3) For polyelectrolyte NaPSS samples, significant nonlinear effects and significant dispersion effects in audio frequency range were recorded quantitatively. Figures 5 and 6 summarize these results. Qualitative behaviors of these phenomena are also summarized at the end of the Results section. These phenomena were not observed significantly in saline solutions as shown in Figure 8.

Abstract

A simple thin film technique has been developed to measure the electrical properties of polyelectrolyte solutions under sinusoidal electric fields of 100-500 v/cm at frequencies of .10-10 KHz. Ohmic heating is largely avoided by the rapid transfer of heat to the electrodes and by the high surface to volume ratios. The resulting temperature is not sufficient to damage the medium. Current and voltage wave forms are monitored directly so that dispersion and nonlinear phenomena of the medium can be viewed directly as functions of frequency, voltage, and concentration of the solution. Possible mechanisms for the observed phenomena are discussed.

Literature Cited

1. Langlois, W.L.; "Slow Viscous Flow"; Macmillan and Co., Inc.: New York, N.Y., 1964.
2. Falkenhagen, H.; Williams, J.W.; J. Phys. Chem. 1929, 33, 1121.
3. Kortüm, G.; "Treatise on Electrochemistry"; Elsevier Publ. Co.: 1965. Chapter 12.
4. Glasstone, S.; "Introduction to Electrochemistry"; D. Van Nostrand and Co., Inc., 1942. Chapter 13.
5. Shaw, D.G.; Kauffman, J.W.; Phys. Stat. Sol. (a), 1971, 4, 467-477.

6.   Shaw, D.G.; Kauffman, J.W.; J. Chem. Physics, March 1971,
     54, 2424-2429.

7.   Yoshino, Y.; Yamashiro, K.; Tabudii, Y.; Inuishi, Y.; IEE
     Conference Publications #129, 1975, 295-298.

8.   Yoshino, Y.; Yamashiro, K.; Tabudii, Y.; Inuishi, Y.; Jap.
     J. Appl. Phys. 1974, 13, 1471-1472.

9.   Hu, C.; Barnes, F.; IEEE Transactions on Biomedical Engi-
     neering July 1970, BME-17, 220-229.

RECEIVED October 31, 1980.

Ionic Nonequilibrium Phenomena in Tissue Interactions with Electromagnetic Fields

W. R. ADEY

Jerry L. Pettis Memorial Veterans Hospital, Loma Linda, CA 92357 and
Departments of Physiology and Surgery, Loma Linda University
School of Medicine, Loma Linda, CA 92350

With few exceptions, plant and animal cells maintain internal concentrations of cations that differ sharply from levels in the surrounding fluid. Typically, this partitioning involves the selective intracellular accumulation of K^+ and the extrusion of Na^+. The lipid bilayer or plasma membrane forms the essential skeleton of the cell against free ionic movement in either direction. Transmembrane movement of ions is said to occur through pores or channels which are highly hydrophobic and behave selectively towards different ionic species. Removal of Na^+ from the interior of the living cell involves active transport by "pumps" that require metabolic energy. To a first approximation, these ionic relationships in the "resting" condition of the cell have been effectively modeled on the basis of ionic equilibrium states, as expressed in the Goldman and Nernst equations ([1]). These equations offer an adequate basis for the development of the negative membrane potential of 70 to 90 mV. Excitation as a process characterizing nerve and muscle cells is associated with a transient reduction or abolition of this membrane potential, and in some cases with a temporary "overshoot" or reversal of its polarity. Just as for the membrane potential, these major but transient perturbations in the production of action potentials have been adequately modeled in dynamics of ionic equilibria by Hodgkin and Huxley ([2]).

The Hodgkin-Huxley model elegantly describes major ionic phenomena in excitation of the squid giant axon. Its subsequent application to motor nerve cells of the mammalian spinal cord ([3]) was based on some of the first microelectrode records from within nerve cells, which disclosed with striking clarity the hyperpolarizing and depolarizing shifts in membrane potential associated with activation of inhibitory and excitatory synaptic nerve fiber endings on the surface of the cell. Interest and excitement occasioned by these findings were universal, but scarcely justified the giant intellectual leap in the inference that the neurobiologist held within his grasp "the neurophysiolgical basis of mind." In the interim, it has become clear that we should

approach an understanding of structural and functional substrates
of brain as the organ of mind in more subtle ways, placing renewed
emphasis on neglected or discarded aspects of its tissue organization. Even so, we may remain baffled and confused by apparent
causality that we would attribute to brain maps and models of
particular regions or systems, since for example, any one brain
region may be depicted in terms of molecular biology of its
synaptic transmitter substances, or of the immunological identity
of its membrane surface glycoproteins, or of the extent of dendritic branching of its neurons, or of the "local circuitry" of
its intrinsic neuronal networks, or by the major afferent and
efferent paths connecting it with other cerebral nuclei. We
have come to recognize the importance of hierarchical organization
in these superimposable schemata that depict a particular brain
region.

Nevertheless, it is not clear that any of these models has
considered the possibility that one cell may influence another
in brain tissue through modulation of their shared electrochemical
environment; whether this be by altered cationic concentrations
in the extracellular medium, or by changing the binding of opioids
and other peptides at receptor sites on cell surface glycopro
teins, or by possible susceptibility of an individual cerebral
neuron to the weak oscillating electrochemical field that surrounds it as the electroencephalogram (EEG). This oscillating
pericellular field appears to arise principally by "leakage"
from the multitude of fine dendritic branches that spread from
the small cell body of typical cerebral neurons. Though weaker
by about six orders of magnitude than the electric gradient of
10^5 V/cm across the lipid bilayer of the cell membrane, evidence
from a wealth of experiments that have mimicked these oscillations
in brain, bone and pancreatic tissue unequivocally confirm their
capacity to modify interrelated cell surface receptor mechanisms
that include ion binding characteristics, hormonal binding ability
and immunological capacities. This growing body of evidence from
quite disparate tissues suggests that cell-to-cell communication
through weak electrochemical perturbations in the pericellular
environment may be a quite general biological property. The
effectiveness of such weak stimuli in triggering a cascade of
intracellular processes at far higher energy levels implies a
series of amplification mechanisms before or during the transmembrane coupling of the initial stimulus. At least a partial
answer to this amplification and extension of the weak triggering
event at the membrane surface may lie in cooperative processes
within and around those glycoprotein molecules that form a
specific receptor site. In seeking an understanding of aspects
of these elemental processes of intercellular communication,
there is a modest prospect that they may ultimately be equated
with the processes by which storage of experience and its recall
occur in brain tissue.

Imposition of weak electromagnetic fields oscillating or modulated at low frequencies is a valuable tool in studies of transductive coupling of pericellular electrochemical stimuli to cellular mechanisms. Observed sensitivities involve responses to stimuli far weaker than those initiating massive ionic perturbations characterizing excitation according to the Hodgkin-Huxley model. Some of these responses also show sharply lowered thresholds in certain narrow ranges of frequency and amplitude. Jointly, these data indicate that these sensitivities are based on nonequilibrium reactions. Further supporting evidence comes from studies of membrane phase transitions that show sharp thermal dependence.

Nonlinear Transitions in Cell Membrane States

As discussed below, new knowledge about cell membrane ultrastructure emphasizes the importance of a layer of stranded glycoprotein material external to the lipid bilayer in a wide range of functions. These functions range from modulation of transmembrane ion fluxes through membrane ion channels to formation of receptor sites for antibody molecules. These capabilities depend in great measure on the polyanionic terminal structure of these stranded protrusions. Clearly, the two examples cited present extremes in the complexities of membrane organization. Nevertheless, both types of process exhibit similar sharp transitions as a function of temperature that are consistent with cooperative processes.

The accumulation of potassium in smooth muscle shows a critical thermal transition that can be described in terms of a cooperative accumulation process ($\underline{4}$). Steady-state levels of potassium and sodium of taeniae coli of guinea-pig are critically affected by varying temperature in the narrow range 12° to $17^{\circ}C$. Electrolyte distribution within these muscle cells undergoes abrupt readjustment around a critical temperature. For both cations, the critical temperature, T_c, is $13.8^{\circ}C$ in the presence of 5 mM external potassium. T_c decreases to $10.0^{\circ}C$ with an external potassium concentration of 10 mM (Figure 1). These findings are in good agreement with the following predictive model of a cooperative mechanism.

Using a cooperative adsorption isotherm developed by Ling ($\underline{5}$) to derive a cooperative absorption isotherm that explicitly relates intracellular potassium content to external potassium concentration, Reisin and Gulati ($\underline{4}$) have expressed the cooperative isotherm for the intracellular potassium as a function of K_{ex}/Na_{ex}. This isotherm K_{ad} is defined

$$K_{ad} = F_{T}/_2 \left\{ \frac{\xi - 1}{[(\xi - 1)^2 + 4\xi n^{-2}]^{\frac{1}{2}}} \right\} \tag{1}$$

where F_T represents the amount of fixed negative charge sites on the membrane surface (in $\mu M/g$) which can interact cooperatively

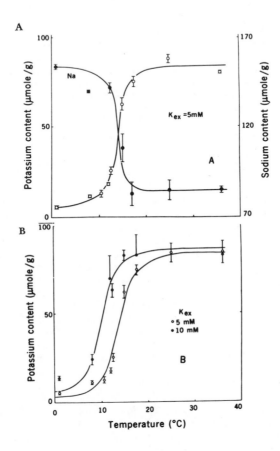

Figure 1.   (A) Effect of temperature on the steady-state potassium (○) and sodium (●) contents of taenia coli smooth muscle fibers. The high sodium content above 17°C is mainly attributable to the large extracellular space in smooth muscles. (B) Effect of K_{ex} on T_c for the thermal transition, developed from theoretical curves derived from Equations 1 and 3 (see text). For these curves, the potassium levels in the sorbitol space (2.15 μmol/g at 5mM K_{ex}, and 4.3 μmol/g at 10mM K_{ex}) were added to the theoretically calculated values. (4)

with cations; ξ is defined as $K^{oo}_{Na \to K}(K_{ex}/Na_{ex}$, where $K^{oo}_{Na \to K}$ is the intrinsic equilibrium constant (selectivity ratio of potassium over sodium); K_{ex} and Na_{ex} are the external potassium and sodium concentrations; and $\underline{n}$ is a function of the energy of nearest neighbor interactions, and gives a measure of cooperation among sites. When the potassium concentration approaches $\frac{1}{2}$ F_T, Eq. 1 can be rearranged

$$\ln \left(\frac{K_{ad}}{F_T - K_{ad}} \right) = \underline{n} \ln \frac{K_{ex}}{Na_{ex}} + \underline{n} \ln K^{oo}_{Na \to K} \qquad (2)$$

If F_T and $\underline{n}$ are not significantly affected by temperature, Eq. 2 can be differentiated with respect to the reciprocal of absolute temperature

$$\frac{\partial \ln[K_{ad}/F_T - K_{ad}]}{\partial(1/T)} = \underline{n} \frac{\partial \ln K^{oo}_{Na \to K}}{\partial(1/T)}$$

$$= \underline{n} \frac{\Delta H^{oo}_{Na \to K}}{R} \qquad (3)$$

where

$$-RT \cdot \ln K^{oo}_{Na \to K} = F^{oo} = \Delta H^{oo} - T\Delta S^{oo} \qquad (4)$$

and ΔF^{oo}, ΔH^{oo} and S^{oo} are changes in the intrinsic free energy, intrinsic enthalpy, and intrinsic entropy, respectively, for the exchange of potassium by sodium on adsorptive sites. The relationship in Eq. 3 emphasizes that for an adsorptive process there must be a critical thermal transition. In non-cooperative mechanisms (when $\underline{n} = 1$), thermal transitions also occur, but for a fixed value of ΔH^{oo} the cooperative transition is steeper by a factor of $\underline{n}$. Reisen and Gulati conclude that this model correctly predicts the behavior of smooth muscle around the transition temperature with respect to cell electrolyte levels as a function of temperature, and in predicting a lower transition temperature when K_{ex} is raised. For sodium-rich frog muscles, the reaccumulation of potassium to a steady state condition is related to K_{ex} by a sigmoidal cooperative curve for experiments performed at 0°, 10° and $25^o C$ (6).

Accumulation of potassium within the cell by a cooperative process is a transmembrane event. However, there is also good evidence that movement of potassium ions through membrane channels is modulated by the binding of calcium ions at channel sites -- the "plug in the bath" model (7). Membrane surface glycoproteins with polyanionic terminal strands offer a broad and powerful substrate for these cationic interactions. Competition between hydrogen and calcium ions at these sites has been modeled as the initial transductive step in excitation (8).

These same surface glycoproteins have been modeled as receptors for antibody molecules and in the binding of lectin molecules, such as concanavalin A. On the lymphocyte membrane,

cross linking between sites in these processes recodes the surface in length and in area by "patching" and "capping." Patching
and capping are inhibited by prior treatment of the cell surface
with lectin molecules, a process described as anchorage modulation (9, 10, 11). Patching and capping occur at a more complex
level of structural organization than in simple cation binding to
a polyanionic substrate. By comparison, the dimensions of Y-
shaped antibody molecules or of tetravalent concanavalin A
molecules, and the size of resulting patches and caps, all bespeak
processes on a galactic scale. Yet these, too, are calcium
dependent and exhibit sharp thermal transitions in the range
20-25°C, consistent with cooperative processes. They are
dependent on metabolic energy supplied from within the cell,
and this requirement for nonequilibrium conditions also supports
a cooperative model.

Tissue Sensitivities and Membrane Models of Transductive Coupling to Weak EM Fields

For the squid axon, the transmembrane current density to produce a nerve impulse has a threshold around 1.0 mA/cm^2. Many
nerve cells, including the motor nerve cells of the mammalian
spinal cord, require a similar current density through the
membrane of the cell body to induce firing. The neuronal
membrane offers a resistance of 2000-5000 Ω/cm^2. By contrast,
tissue fluid surrounding nerve cells in brain and other nervous
ganglia has a much lower specific resistance in the range
5-25 Ω.cm^{-1}. Thus, in the context of either intrinsic tissue
fields generated by the leakage of bioelectric activity from
cells to the fluid that surrounds them, or in effects attributable
to tissue components of environmental EM fields, transmembrane
paths do not form a preferred pathway for tissue current flow,
and only a small fraction of the total tissue current actually
penetrates cell membranes. Based on differential conductance
characteristics cited above, these transmembrane components would
be about three orders of magnitude less than those in the extracellular space. Thus, if we assume a transmembrane current
density of 1.0 mA/cm^2 at threshold for nervous excitation, a
current density of 1.0 A/cm^2 in extracellular fluid would be
necessary to achieve this transmembrane level.

We may extrapolate from these basic considerations in two
ways. We may evaluate the extracellular electric gradients
associated with intrinsic or imposed tissue fields against the
magnitude of the gradients in the membrane potential, both in
resting conditions and in association with modification of the
membrane potential during synaptic excitation. In this way, we
may appraise the probability of direct effects of extracellular
tissue fields in excitation of nerve cells. A second approach
will consider the observed biological sensitivities to these
fields. This will lead to the crux of our current dilemma. A

rapidly widening series of observations in cells of bone (12, 13, 14) and blood (15), as well as in nervous tissue (16, 17, 18) have confirmed sensitivities to electrochemical gradients in fluid around these cells as much as six orders of magnitude less than the electrical gradient across the cell membrane (the membrane potential). What are the mechanisms by which these weak oscillating electrochemical gradients are coupled to the vast tides of cations known to move across the cell membrane in the ensuing stages of excitatory depolarization and inhibitory hyperpolarization? Hitherto, the latter processes have held pride of place in all models of excitation, despite the very large triggering energies necessary for their initiation. The clear evidence for effectiveness of stimuli much weaker than those producing cell membrane depolarization through massive direct perturbation of ionic equilibria raises a second question. What is the significance of these newly disclosed sensitivities for internal communication in normal and abnormal tissue? How are they utilized in cell-to-cell communication in defining aspects of homeostasis, or in modulating sensitivity to the myriad extrinsic electrochemical and neurohumoral stimuli that constantly pervade a tissue? Recent studies provide partial answers to some of these questions, and also point the way to needed future research.

    Bioelectric Organization of Nervous Tissue. The membrane potential of 70 mV is developed across the lipid bilayer of the cell membrane. This layer is approximately 40 Å thick, so that the transmembrane electric gradient is of the order of 10^5 V/cm. This extraordinary dielectric strength is not easily replicated in artificial materials. It is noteworthy that the resting membrane potential maintains this dielectric bilayer within a factor of two of electrical breakdown (19). Release of neural transmitter substances from synaptic terminals on the nerve cell surface transiently snifts the membrane potential at the site of release by a few millivolts. In terms of an altered transmembrane gradient, this shift is of the order of 1.0 kV/cm.
    Cerebral cortex has an intrinsic oscillating field in the extracellular fluid, the EEG. It appears to originate principally in the enormously branched dendrites that characterize cerebral neurons. Measured over cellular dimensions, the EEG has a typical gradient of 50 mV/cm (20, 21), and a frequency spectrum from 1 to 100 Hz, with most energy in the band from 1 to 20 Hz. Records from intracellular microelectrodes in many but not all cerebral neurons display large slow oscillations up to 15 mV in amplitude that resemble the EEG from the same cortical region in spectral analyses. However, with an amplitude of 20–50 μV, the EEG is less than 1.0 percent of the amplitude of the intracellular neuronal waves from which it is derived, due to its attenuation in the neuronal membrane.

Until recently, extracellular gradients as weak as the EEG in cerebral tissue have not been considered physiologically signifi- cant in information transfer, nor in the modulation of tissue functional states. As discussed below, there is now good evidence that impressed gradients that mimic the EEG, either simply as low frequency fields or as RF or microwave fields amplitude modulated at low frequencies in the EEG range, can elicit altered efflux of calcium ions and of transmitter substances (22-26). Moreover, these weak imposed extracellular fields are capable of either modifying or entraining the EEG at the rate of low frequency field components (27, 28), implying that these fields with gradients of 50 mV/cm are capable of influencing the much larger membrane potential of 10^5 V/cm. Clearly, this requires a form of transductive coupling with considerable "amplification" of the weak triggering oscillation. Possible models of these inter- actions will be discussed.

Bioelectric Sensitivities of Organisms to Environmental EM Fields. As background to current research on biophysical mechanisms that might underlie these sensitivities at the molecu- lar level, we may enumerate some of the interactions reported in whole organisms (for reviews, see Adey, 29, 30).

Behavioral effects have been reported with tissue components of environmental extremely low frequency (ELF) fields between 10^{-7} and 10^{-8} V/cm in the spectrum below 10 Hz. They include navigation and prey detection by sharks and rays (31, 32), bird navigation (33, 34), altered daily biological rhythms in man and birds (35, 36), and subjective time estimates in monkeys (37, 38). Rats exposed to 60 Hz 1 kV/m fields show reduced nocturnal motor activity in the first 2 or 3 days of exposure and increased alerting behavior during and following 30 days of exposure to these fields (39). Rays could be trained to seek a food reward in a circular tank in which the earth's magnetic field became an essential cue (40). Calculated tissue electric gradients based on the rate of the animal's movement through the natural magnetic field were 0.5 μV/cm. These responses faded out with magnetic fields weaker than the natural level, and were not observed with fields two orders of magnitude greater, suggesting an intensity "window." These low frequency perturbations are sensed by tubular receptors opening on the skin of the head. Their extremely high wall resistance (6 $M\Omega/cm^2$) contributes to a low-pass frequency characteristic with an effective upper frequency limit of about 10 Hz, thus establishing a frequency "window." No such special- ized electroreceptors are known to exist in the mammalian periph- eral or central nervous systems. However, intracellular ferro- magnetic bodies have been described in bacteria that orient to the earth's magnetic field (41), in the thoracic banding of bees (42), and in the skull or muscles of pigeons (see 43). The possible role of these inclusions in tissues of bees and pigeons in orienting to environmental magnetic fields is not yet known.

These behavioral responses to ELF fields suggest "windowed" sensitivities to nervous tissue gradients around 10^{-7} V/cm, with an effective upper frequency limit between 10 and 100 Hz. This tissue component is produced by fields in air of 10-100 V/m. It is approximately six orders of magnitude weaker than the EEG gradient of 10-100 mV/cm over cellular dimensions. Induction of EEG level gradients by environmental low frequency electric fields is not practical, by reason of weak coupling of such a field in air to the aqueous conducting medium of tissue (29). It would require an environmental field of 500 kV/m. However, EEG level fields are easily induced in tissues by weak radio and microwave fields at frequencies of 100-1000 MHz with incident energies around 1.0 mW/cm^2, and electric gradients in air of 60-100 V/m. When sinusoidally modulated at ELF frequencies, particularly below 20 Hz, they alter cation binding in cerebral tissue. These are also "windowed" reactions, as discussed below, and relate to the low frequency modulation of the imposed field.

Only a few behavioral studies have so far been reported with these modulated RF fields. Chicks exposed to 450 MHz, 1 or 5 mW/cm^2 fields sinusoidally modulated at 3 or 16 Hz during performance of a fixed-time 30 sec schedule of water reinforcement showed trends towards longer latency of response (44). In Soviet studies, rabbits and rats chronically exposed for 120 days to extremely low levels of 50 or 2500 MHz continuous fields or 10 GHz fields pulsed at 1000 or 20 Hz showed statistically significant alterations in conditioned reflexes with field intensities between 1.9 and 2.0 μW/cm^2. A 2450 MHz, 1 mW/cm^2 microwave field pulsed at 1000/sec had a synergic effect on the action of Valium (chlordiazepoxide) on fixed-interval behavior in rats (46).

Cell Membrane Models of Transductive Coupling of Weak EM Fields. The arrangement of stranded glycoprotein molecules outside the lipid bilayer (plasma membrane) of the cell membrane was noted above. Their organization and functional role have been addressed in a series of membrane models which have developed the concepts of "the greater membrane" (47) and the "fluid mosaic" model (48). The fluid mosaic model embraces most of the recent data on membrane molecular biology. The phosophlipid bilayer of the plasma membrane behaves as a fluid whose viscosity is modified by the presence of intramembranous particles (IMPs) within it (49). The IMPs range in molecular weight from about 300 for the prostaglandins and related "molecular switching" molecules to about 50,000 for β-microglobulins associated with antibody receptor sites (9). Many of these molecules have both external and internal termini. The internal protrusions may connect with microtubules and thus with the nucleus of the cell. Many of the external protrusions are glycoproteins with terminal amino-sugars (sialic acids) that have numerous fixed-charge anionic binding sites. The cell surface thus becomes a poly-anionic sheath (50), as described above, with a strong affinity

for cations, and with Ca^{2+} and H^+ more strongly bound than other
monovalent cations (51). They also participate in receptor sites
for neurotransmitter, hormonal and antibody molecules.   For
muscle end-plate, this surface potential is typically about
-50 mV. When the surface potential is modified by increasing
concentration of divalent cations Ca^{2+} or Mg^{2+}, for example, the
effectiveness of tubocurarine as an antagonist for acetyl choline
is reduced (50). Increased divalent cation concentration in the
surrounding fluid decreases the negativity of the surface potential and thereby lowers the concentration of cations at the
membrane-solution interface, suggesting that effects of surface
potential on cationic concentrations at active sites may be
important in drug interactions.

The Singer-Nicolson fluid-mosaic model is also consistent
with two major sequences of events in the transductive coupling
of a wide range of electrochemical stimuli at the membrane surface.   One involves Ca-dependent conformational changes in these
intramembranous particles by which a signal is transmitted to the
interior of the cell (9), as for example, in the activation of
membrane-bound enzymes, such as adenyl cyclase, following binding
of a hormone molecule or an antibody to a membrane surface receptor site.   The second concerns electrochemical interactions
occurring in the length and area of the membrane surface, and
probably involving cross-linking between adjoining molecular
strands, as first suggested by Katchalsky (51) from in vitro
studies of Ca ion binding to polyvinyl chloride.   Clearly, long-
range interactions between charge sites along the membrane surface suggest a mechanisms by which weak oscillating electrochemical gradients may be sensed and "amplified" as steps in a cooperative interaction involving binding and release of Ca ions,
as discussed below.

Evidence for Nonequilibrium Aspects of Field Interactions in Brain Tissue, using $^{45}Ca^{2+}$ Efflux as an Indicator

Efflux of $^{45}Ca^{2+}$ from intact, awake cat cerebral cortex
responds in a highly nonlinear fashion to changing extracellular
Ca^{2+} concentration (53). Increased concentration of Ca^{2+}
resulted in increased efflux of both $^{45}Ca^{2+}$ and ^3H-GABA, but
the effect of a 1 mM increment in Ca^{2+} concentration was only
slightly less than that of a 20 mM increment.   These initial
observations suggested membrane reactions triggering the release
or turnover of calcium.   The observed kinetics are consistent
with displacement of $^{45}Ca^{2+}$ bound to polyanionic sites at the
surface of the membrane (54).

$$Ca^{2+} + {}^{45}Ca - M^{n-} \rightarrow Ca^{45} - Ca\text{-}M^{(n-2)-}$$

$$Ca^{45} - Ca\text{-}M^{(n-2)-} \rightarrow {}^{45}Ca^{2+} + Ca\text{-}M^{n-}$$

where M represents a membrane anionic species. Thus, the efflux of Ca^{2+} from the membrane is proportional to a high power of the concentration of bound Ca^{2+}.

This highly nonlinear pattern of autogenic Ca^{2+} efflux led to a series of studies of EM field interactions with cerebral tissue, in a search for their origins in cooperative mechanisms (55). We proceeded on the premise that if long-range interactions were in-volved at fixed-charge sites on membrane surface macromolecules, major changes in $^{45}Ca^{2+}$ efflux might occur with very weak oscil-lating electric fields around the cells, and that the magnitude of these responses would be comparable with those induced at far higher levels of field intensity. In turn, this led to a search for possible "windows" in the range of field amplitudes inducing a response. A second premise concerning possible long-range interactions was that they might occur in narrow bands of fre-quencies as "windows" in the range from 1 to 100 Hz. This concept arose from possible field interactions with the dominant frequencies of intrinsic EEG rhythms in brain tissue, and from measurements of membrane electrical tissue constants in non-excitable cells, including bone and connective tissue. Based on these criteria, it was hoped to arrive at the levels of cooperativity to be expected in these membrane ion binding mechanisms. Results of these studies have been extensively reviewed elsewhere (29, 30).

Weak, ELF fields at frequencies from 1 to 75 Hz and 5 to 100 V/m in air were tested for their effects on $^{45}Ca^{2+}$ efflux from freshly isolated chick and cat cerebral tissue (23). Tissue gradients were estimated to be in the range of 0.1 μV/cm. Field exposures resulted in a general trend toward a reduction in the release of preincubated $^{45}Ca^{2+}$. Maximum decreases occurred at 6 and 16 Hz and were in the range from 12 to 15 percent. Threshold fields were around 10 and 56 V/m in air for chick and cat tissues, respectively, but sensitivity decreased at 100 V/m. Thus, calcium binding in chick and cat cerebral tissue exhibited frequency and amplitude windows in responses to these extremely weak fields (Figure 2B).

Intrinsic oscillations of the EEG are about six orders of magnitude larger than those just described, typically in the range 10^{-1} to 10^{-2} V/cm in fluid surrounding a neuron. Electri-cal stimulation of awake cat cerebral cortex with 200/sec trains of pulses (1.0 msec duration) at this intensity increased corti-cal efflux of $^{45}Ca^{2+}$ by about 13 percent (26), and simultaneous efflux of the inhibitory neurotransmitter GABA rose by about 12 percent. When freshly isolated chick cerebral tissue was exposed to sinusoidally modulated 147 MHz fields that also pro-duced EEG levels of electric gradient in the tissue, there were striking changes in $^{45}Ca^{2+}$ efflux as the sinusoidal modulation frequency covered the spectrum from 0.5 to 35 Hz (22). No effects were seen from the unmodulated carrier wave, but the $^{45}Ca^{2+}$ efflux followed a smooth "tuning curve," with an increase

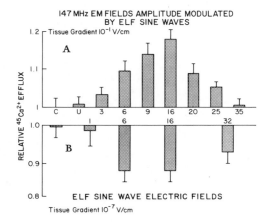

Figure 2. Comparison of (A) $^{45}Ca^{2+}$ from freshly isolated chick cerebral hemi-spheres exposed to a weak radiofrequency field (147 MHz, 0.8 mW/cm^2), ampli-tude-modulated at low frequencies, and (B) $^{45}C^{2+}$ efflux changes from exposure to far weaker electric fields (56 V/m) in the same frequency spectrum from 1 to 32 Hz. The peak magnitude of the efflux change is similar for the two fields, but oppo-site in direction. For the radiofrequency field (A), the unmodulated carrier wave U had no effect when compared with controls C. Field gradients differ by about six orders of magnitude between (A) and (B)(22, 23).

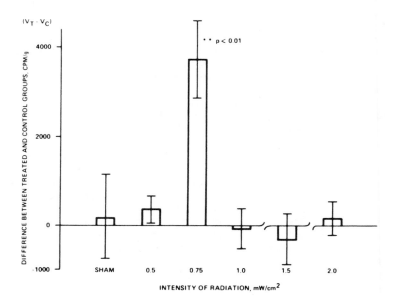

Figure 3. Effects of changing power density of a 147-MHz radiofrequency field, sinusoidally amplitude-modulated at 16 Hz, on $^{45}Ca^{2+}$ efflux from freshly isolated chick cerebral hemispheres. Ordinate shows mean difference (with S.E.) between exposed (V_T) and control (V_C) samples (25).

of about 15 percent in the range from 6 to 20 Hz, and a maximum
effect at 16 Hz (Figure 2A). A similar but sharper efflux curve,
also peaking in the range 9-16 Hz, was found in independent
studies (25). Blackman et al. also reported an amplitude "window"
for this response at incident field energies around 1.0 mW/cm^2,
confirmed independently by Bawin, Sheppard and Adey (56) for
450 MHz fields sinusoidally modulated at 16 Hz (Figure 3).

   The windowed character of these responses in frequency and
amplitude domains unequivocally establishes a series of highly
nonlinear mechanisms in the control of cerebral calcium ion
binding. It also points to long-range interactions requiring
ordered molecular states that persist for appreciable time over
considerable atomic distances (30, 57, 58). It is also clear
that the levels of cooperativity in these interactions must be
high, since for the ELF field effects cited here, the effective
stimuli may appear to be below the level of Boltzmann thermal
noise (kT). Though this is probably not the case (see discussion
on models below), both the biological thresholds cited above and
these chemical thresholds for ELF electric and magnetic fields
are mutually consistent with sensitivities within an order of
magnitude of thermal noise levels (23, 59).

   The search for a physical basis for this cooperativity may
prove difficult. As a prelude to later discussion of possible
models, additional evidence may be cited on modulation of Ca^{2+}
binding and release in cerebral tissue by other ionic species
(17). Increased ^{45}Ca^{2+} efflux from chick cerebral hemispheres
induced by a 450 MHz 0.75 mW/cm^2 field sinusoidally modulated at
16 Hz was insensitive to variations in Ca concentration between
0 and 4.16 mM in the bathing solution. It was enhanced by raised
H$^+$ concentrations (0.108 mM HCl), and inhibited in the absence of
normal levels of HCO$_3^-$ ions. La^{3+} ions added to the NaHCO$_3$-free
medium restored electrical responsiveness, but the 450 MHz field
then reduced ^{45}Ca^{2+} efflux by about 15 percent, compared to the
typical field-induced increase in efflux of about the same size
with normal NaHCO$_3$ levels (2.4 mM). These observations suggest
two conclusions. First, since lanthanum blocks transmembrane
movement of Ca^{2+} in both directions, persisting efflux changes
to field stimulation after La^{3+} perfusion are interpreted as
indicating a site at cell membrane surfaces for EM field interactions with Ca^{2+} binding sites. Second, the influence of H$^+$
concentration suggests that weak, low-frequency extracellular
electric gradients may be transduced in a specific class of
extracellular negative binding sites normally occupied by Ca^{2+}
and susceptible to competitive H$^+$ binding. We may further
hypothesize that, by the windowed character of these interactions, the role of the hydrogen ion may be as a proton in
tunneling interactions (59). These cooperative interactions
in isolated cerebral tissue have suggested two further lines
of research.

Do similar interactions occur in living cortex? Can they be detected in ultrastructural elements of the central nervous system, such as synaptosomes? The $^{45}Ca^{2+}$ efflux was studied in intact awake cat cortex, using a cortical cup technique (18). Tissue fields measured with a miniaturized, implantable electric field probe were of the order of 500 mV/cm with an incident field of 3.0 mW/cm^2, amplitude modulated by a 16 Hz sinewave. Irradiation began 60 min after completion of 90 min incubation of the cortex with $^{45}Ca^{2+}$. Resulting efflux curves were disrupted by waves of increased Ca^{2+} efflux. These waves showed periods of 10 to 30 min. For analysis, the efflux curves were treated by straight-line fits to the logarithmically transformed data, with two epochs for each curve. One curve covered the prefield exposure period, the other from 20 min after field onset to the end of the experiment. Differences associated with the wavelike disruptions between pre-exposure/exposure epochs and control/exposure curves were significant at an 0.96 confidence level, using one-tailed binomial probability statistics. In parallel studies, synaptosomes from male rat cerebral cortex with a typical diameter of 0.5 μm were incubated at 22°C for 10 min in a physiological solution containing $^{45}Ca^{2+}$ (60, 61). They were then applied to Millipore filters and perfused at 2.0 ml/min for 30 min. In experiments in which exposure to 450 MHz fields (as used in experiments with intact cats) began when the synaptosomes were applied to the Millipore filter, and onset of perfusion was delayed until 5-10 min later, continuous exposure to a field of 0.5 mW/cm^2 increased the rate constant of the $^{45}Ca^{2+}$ efflux curve (p < 0.01). Conversely, in experiments at 34°C, where the synaptosomes were continuously perfused from the time of their application to the filter, increased $^{45}Ca^{2+}$ efflux occurred only when field exposure started 10 min after onset of perfusion. Moreover, slow oscillatory perturbations in $^{45}Ca^{2+}$ efflux with periods of 5-10 min followed termination of a 10 min field exposure, resembling those in intact cortex. We may conclude from these studies that responses seen previously in freshly isolated but non-respiring cortex also occur in the intact brain, and that they are a property of tissue elements substantially smaller than a whole cell. Indeed, for a synaptosome with a diameter of 0.5 μm or less, tissue field levels measured in the cat's brain in these studies would not exceed a gradient of 25 μV across its full diameter, far smaller than its membrane potential of the order of 50 mV. From the viewpoint of a cooperative system, this cooperative macromolecular organization at membrane Ca^{2+} binding sites may be presumed functionally effective over dimensions as small as these, since even weaker fields release both $^{45}Ca^{2+}$ and stored transmitter substances, such as GABA, apparently from synaptic stores (26).

Despite this progress in defining some interactions with weak EM fields, particularly in specialized preparations of isolated cells and tissues, we must also take account of recent disclosure of interactions between natural opioid peptides, the enkephalins and endorphins, and the binding of Ca^{2+} to cell membrane surfaces. In the intact brain, they exert powerful modulating influences on states of excitability and associated behavior. Their sites of action are now known to extend to tissues outside the central nervous system, and to include the gastrointestinal tract. In synaptosome fractions, β-endorphin has a regulatory role on Ca^{2+} movement, inhibiting influx and enhancing efflux (62). In thin slices of brain hippocampal tissue, excitatory effects of 200 nM solutions of (D-Ala^2, Met)-enkephalin are strongly modulated by high or low Ca^{2+} concentrations (63). Since amounts of these substances in brain tissue sensitively reflect stressful experiences, we may hypothesize that sensitivity of the intact subject to weak nonionizing EM radiation, as a result of modified Ca^{2+} binding at cell membrane surface sites, may be influenced by concomitant enkephalin levels. These may vary from day to day, and thus become an important determinant of susceptibility to weak fields (64). In a broader context, we may hypothesize that development of realistic safety standards for human exposure, based on needed knowledge of subtle but presumably important neuroendocrine and neurohumoral effects induced by these weak fields, will require close attention to possible variations in thresholds attributable to these natural opioid substances, occasioned by their diurnal and even seasonal variations.

Evidence for Weak Field Effects at Cell Surface Receptor Sites

We have already considered the fluidity of cell membranes, and the long-range mobility of enclosed proteins and lipids in the plane of the membrane. Imposition of weak EM fields offers a tool for study of both receptor mobility and of coupling mechanisms between humoral agents and receptor sites.

Embryonic muscle fibers are initially sensitive to acetyl choline (ACh) over the entire membrane surface, but with the onset of synaptogenesis, ACh receptors are essentially confined to the neurotransmitter function. When a steady electric field of 30 mV is applied across a single spherical embryonic muscle cell of Xenopus, ACh receptors aggregate toward the cathodal pole of the cell within 1 hour. The movement is electrophoretic in nature and results in formation of stable, metabolically independent receptor aggregates (65). In contrast, concanavalin A receptors, which also accumulate toward the cathodal pole, completely resume their general distribution within 10 min of ending of field exposure. At 22°C, the average electrophoretic mobility of the electrophoretically mobile population of the concanavalin A receptors is about $1.9 \times 10^{-3} \mu m/sec/V/cm$, while their average diffusion coefficient is $5.1 \times 10^{-9} cm^2/sec$ (66).

Apart from displacement of receptors by the field, is there evidence of a modification of coupling of signals, usually

associated with binding of humoral and hormonal molecules at
membrane receptor sites, to the chain of intracellular metabolic
sequences? When cultures of a clonal line of osteoblast cells
were exposed to pulsed magnetic fields far weaker than those in
the myosphere experiments (72 Hz pulse train, pulse duration
325 μsec with 5 msec reverse polarity, peak intensity 35 gauss,
induced current density in culture 1.0 μA/cm^2, induced electric
gradient 3 mV/cm), there was a 90–99 percent inhibition of the
adenyl cyclase response to parathyroid hormone (PTH). At the
same time, PTH-specific decreases in collagen synthesis and
alkaline phosphatase release did not occur. Fluoride-activated
adenyl cyclase formation was unchanged, suggesting that the
magnetic field blocked PTH action either by modification of the
PTH receptor on the membrane, or by altered coupling between the
receptor and the enzyme adenyl cyclase inside the membrane (12).
Bone cell cultures from fetal rat calvaria responded to similar
magnetic fields with significantly increased DNA synthesis, but
the response depended on pulse waveform and culture techniques
(14). Cultured chick tibiae showed similar sensitivities in
formation of adenyl cyclase, but differential responses were
noted between shaft and epiphyseal regions in the amount of
collagen formed (13).

Models of Nonequilibrium Phenomena in Bioeffects of Weak EM Fields

    We have considered bioeffects from two quite different levels
of induced electric fields; those occurring with tissue gradients
around 10^{-7} V/cm in extracellular fluid and those at substantially
higher levels from 10^{-3} to 10^{-1} V/cm. In the first class, there
can be no doubt that the coupling process or processes must be
highly cooperative, as discussed below. For bioeffects with
fields in the higher range, it is necessary to evaluate the
possibility that these responses occurred instead by a thermal
energy transfer mechanism.
    This problem has been formulated theoretically by calculating
the minimum electric field strength required to produce the
alteration in Ca^{2+} binding observed in chick cerebral tissue
exposed to 147 and 450 MHz fields (22, 57), if the field interaction occurred by a thermal energy transfer mechanism (67).
This approach involves two stages: (1) a change in the fraction
of Ca^{2+} ion binding sites at the cell surface is related to an
alteration in the temperature and the free energy of binding;
(2) the temperature and free energy changes are related to
absorbed energy from the applied EM field (dependent on the
square of the electric field amplitude). Tenforde concludes
that the value of the absorbed energy predicted theoretically
to achieve the observed release of bound Ca^{2+} from cell membrane
surfaces is at least 100 times greater than the fields actually
present in the exposed brain tissue. Therefore, the altered
Ca^{2+} binding "very likely proceeds by a mechanism other than

thermal energy transfer." Tenforde further points out that
modulation "windows" for these effects suggest a resonant or
cooperative energy transfer mechanism.

However, the path to an acceptable cooperative model is
fraught with difficulty. By comparison with tissue electric
gradients induced by environmental EM fields, the requisite
gradients for some known cooperative macromolecular transitions
are very large. The helix-coil conformational change in
poly(Y-benzyl L-glutamate) can be induced as a cooperative
transition by a gradient of 260 kV/cm (68), based on nearest
neighbor interactions. Long-lasting conformation changes occur
in poly(A).2poly(U) and in ribosomal RNA with pulsed electric
fields of 20 kV/cm and with a decay time of 10 sec (69, 70).
They are viewed as a model for nerve excitability.

It is clear that these phenomena and related models involve
energy levels orders of magnitude greater than those associated
with weak EM fields that elicit such a wide range of proven
bioeffects. We may hypothesize that one or more transductive
steps are necessary before the pericellular electric field
becomes an effective transmembrane signal. Models of these
processes fall into two categories, one considering properties
of polyanionic membrane surface macromolecules, and the other
the behavior of the phospholipid bilayer. They will be summarized (for more extensive review, see 30).

Models of Tissue-Field Interactions at Membrane Surface
Macromolecules. There are no known mechanisms to explain bioeffects at extremely low frequencies (ELF) on the basis of
direct interactions with component dipoles of molecular systems
oscillating at these low frequencies. Grodsky (71) has hypothesized that excitable membranes are energetically equivalent to
sheets of giant dipoles bathed in controlled external fields.
Grodsky's formulation envisaged the outer layer of phospholipid
polar heads as a two-dimensional crystal mosaic of multipolar
charge sites (p-sites), sprinkled with islands of glycoproteins
with cationic binding sites (c-sites). The p-sites are taken to
be occupied by ideal dipoles. Grodsky hypothesized that, with
the addition of an external electric field to the system, when
the frequency of an allowed oscillation mode reaches zero, the
system would become a macroscopic quantum amplification device,
and would exhibit long-range order phase changes that generate
into the zero-frequency mode (Einstein-Bose condensation). The
model has merit in seeking a basis in membrane ultrastructure,
but unfortunately recent reappraisal of the possibilities of an
Einstein-Bose phase transition as the basis for the low frequency
sensitivities indicates that it would not occur with this formulation (I. T. Grodsky and H. Fröhlich, personal communications).
Kaczmarek (72, 73) has considered the possible occurrence of
resonant phenomena in chemical reactions analyzed as linear
systems. For appropriate values of the kinetic constants and

the extent of cooperativity, his model displays multiple steady
states, limit cycle behavior, or both. When the system is in the
limit cycle mode, its dynamics were very sensitive to the frequency of any perturbation. Kaczmarek points out that if calcium
binding in neural membranes can exhibit limit-cycle behavior due
to reaction steps being maintained far from chemical equilibrium,
weak external perturbations could easily disrupt the electrochemical balance. In essence, the status of molecular populations
would then determine low frequency manifestations of field interactions in tissue.

In seeking some form of amplification of initial transductive
steps at an extracellular location, we may presume that it involves systems capable of integrating the weak field over some
distance, and would thus occur in the length and area of the
membrane surface, rather than in a transmembrane axis (74).
This problem has been addressed by Einolf and Carstensen (75)
in a study of the behavior of micron-sized resin particles considered as porous particles with uniformly distributed fixed-
charge sites. Porous charged particles are characterized by a
low frequency dielectric relaxation leading to large static
dielectric constants. This results in polarization of the ionic
atmosphere at the surface of the particle in the presence of an
external electric field. This produces an additional "apparent"
dielectric constant of the particle, exceeding the dielectric
constant by several orders of magnitude at low frequencies. It
is proportional to the diameter of the particle and the square
root of the fixed-charge concentration in the porous material,
with values as high as 10^6 at frequencies below 1 kHz for micron-
sized resin particles. Similar properties may be expected at the
surface of tubular structures with diameters in the micron range,
including dendrites with polyanionic glycoprotein surface layers.

We have considered the Einolf and Carstensen model as a basis
for those bioeffects in which it appears that thermal noise at
normal tissue temperature is substantially larger than the tissue
components of imposed electric fields (23, 30). The Boltzmann
equation may be written in terms that model the cell surface in
the region of the counterion layer as a low-pass filter:

$$e^2 = 4 \text{ kT BR}$$

where the transfer function for the root mean square noise voltage e is a function of the frequency bandwidth B and the specific
resistance of the noise pathway R. With a specific resistance
for brain tissue of the order of 300 $\Omega.cm^{-1}$ and an effective
frequency bandwidth from 0 to 100 Hz, the equivalent noise voltage gradient would be of the order of 10^{-8} V/cm. This is in
close agreement with observed sensitivities in marine vertebrates,
birds and mammals for certain low frequency fields, and these
thresholds are consistent with a thermal "floor" as the limiting
factor.

We have shown that the Einolf and Carstensen model of dielectric dispersion at the surface of small charged spheres also
applied to long, thin cell processes which typify the dendrites
of neurons (76). The degree of polarization induced at the
surface depends on the orientation of the incident field with
respect to the length of the dendrite or axon, radius of the
cylindrical surface, ion mobility, and temperature. We may
speculate that the extraordinary degree of polarization produced
by counterions at the cell surface may bring about a dynamic
distribution of weakly bound ions of reduced momenta. From the
Heisenberg equation relating positional and momentum uncertain-
ties, it is seen that ions of sufficiently low momentum would
exhibit quantum behavior usually not associated with such massive
bodies at biological temperatures. For example, the momentum of
a thermal proton at $300^{\circ}K$ is ordinarily 4.5×10^{24} kg-m/sec. The
resulting positional uncertainty, Δx, is about 10^{-11} m, so small
that classical notions are entirely adequate for dynamic considerations. However, an ion with attenuated momentum $p\varepsilon^{\frac{1}{2}}$ has
a positional uncertainty of $\varepsilon^{\frac{1}{2}}\Delta x$. If we take a value for ε in
the region surrounding the ion of the same order of magnitude as
for the macroscopic ε measured with a cell suspension of 10^4 to
10^6), we see that the ion would have a positional uncertainty of
about 10^{-8} to 10^{-9} m. Tunneling would then be possible from one
potential well to another, because the ionic wave function would
extend through the region of a typical potential barrier and even
over appreciable regions along the surface. If momenta are
sufficiently reduced, smaller ions -- particularly protons --
would have significant probabilities of tunneling from one
potential minimum to another. It is suggested that proton
tunneling may occur between charge sites that interact across
the boundary between coherent and incoherent charge zones on
cell membrane surface glycoproteins (57, 74, 76, 77). Such a
process would be most effective in the axis of the field electric
gradient, along this surface biopolymer sheet. Development of
long-range order among surface macromolecules interacting via
low-momentum ions may induce significant changes over the entire
polarized region.

Models of Tissue-Field Interactions Involving the Cell
Membrane Lipid Bilayer. Although concepts of transductive
coupling of weak electrochemical stimuli by membrane glycoproteins are well supported by available evidence, very little is
known of ways in which events in the glycoprotein layer are
coupled to the underlying lipid bilayer in the ensuing steps of
excitation. Indeed, there remains the possibility that the
external field may interact dierectly with the lipid bilayer,
despite the enormous difference in their respective electric
gradients. Barnes and Hu (78) have estimated shifts in ion
concentration and magnitude of current flow resulting from
membrane rectification of radio and microwave fields, using the

nonlinear Boltzmann equation. In this system, where charged
particle concentrations vary in space, if there is no net current, the field-driven drift current must balance the diffusion
current, so that a potential barrier is formed to maintain the
concentration difference. At equilibrium, even small values of
an alternating field superimposed on this steady potential will
shift equilibrium concentrations. For example, an incident field
of 10 mW/cm^2 produces a gradient of 4.4 V/cm across a membrane
enclosed in an aqueous dielectric medium. This corresponds to an
electric gradient of 9 μV across a 200 Å membrane, with a concentration shift of 1 part in 10^6 and a flow of 400 ions/sec for a
cell with a surface area of 10^{-6} cm^2. The biological significance
of such small shifts is unknown.

     Rather than assuming that changes in ionic permeabilities
through channels in the lipid bilayer in the course of the action
potential account for large transient membrane conductances,
Vaccaro and Green (79) suggest that the sodium permeability
hypothesis be replaced by one attributing the action potential
to nonlinear plasma oscillations and voltage clamp records to
strongly damped oscillatory currents. In this model, the membrane
phase is treated as a semi-electrolyte with connected regions in
which the ionic concentrations are not very different from those
of the adjacent electrolytes. Mobilities of different ionic
species in the membrane are identified with those measured in
the steady state, and are not assumed to have large variations
during excitation. Their solution to the plasma model yields
periods in the millisecond range, consistent with the time course
of the action potential and voltage clamp records. Polyvalent
cations, such as Ca^{2+}, have a more pronounced damping effect on
the electrolyte systems than monovalent cations. Plasma oscillations would allow transfer of ions at a much faster rate than
could be achieved by ordinary conductance, an essential feature
of the action potential. In this initial formulation, the
investigators have not considered the possibility of entrainment
of plasma oscillations by weak imposed fields, although this
would appear a testable aspect of their model.

Summary

     There is good evidence that initial events in coupling of
weak oscillating electrochemical fields to cell membranes occur
on membrane surface polyanions characterized by transient coherent
states of nearest neighbor fixed-charge sites. These coherent
states may exist for considerable distances along the membrane
surface. The first steps in transductive coupling would thus
occur in the length of the membrane. Binding and release of
calcium ions to these membrane surface sites correlates closely
with exposure to certain weak electromagnetic fields. Sensitivity
to these fields in narrow frequency and amplitude "windows" supports a series of models based on highly cooperative interactions

at cell membrane surface glycoproteins. Evidence from calcium-hydrogen ion interactions in the presence of these fields raises the possibility of proton tunneling, perhaps at the margins between coherent and incoherent fixed-charge zones. Recent biophysical models of cell membrane organization are reviewed, with consideration of ionic behavior as a plasma in the lipid bilayer. There is good experimental evidence from a variety of tissues that a form of cell-to-cell communication can occur through weak electrochemical stimuli that are sensed by highly cooperative processes at cell membrane surfaces. In varying degrees, this may be a general property of tissue organization.

Acknowledgments

Studies from our laboratory described here were supported by the Office of Naval Research, the National Institute of Environmental Health Sciences, the Department of Energy, the Bureau of Radiological Health, and the Southern California Edison Company. It is a pleasure to acknowledge their patient help and guidance throughout the difficult initial phases of this research.

Literature Cited

1. Goldman, D. E. Potential, impedance and rectification in membranes. J. gen. Physiol. 1943, 27, 37-60.

2. Hodgkin, A. L.; Huxley, A. F. A quantitative description of membrane current and its application to conduction and excitation in nerve. J. Physiol., London 1952, 117, 500-544.

3. Eccles, J. C. "The Neurophysiological Basis of Mind: The Principles of Neurophysiology"; University Press: Oxford, 1953; 314 pp.

4. Reisin, I. L.; Gulati, J. Cooperative critical thermal transition of potassium accumulation in smooth muscle. Science 1972, 176, 1137-1139.

5. Ling, G. N. All-or-none adsorption by living cells and model protein-water systems: discussion of the problem of "permease-induction" and determination of secondary and tertiary structure of proteins. Fed. Proc. 1966, 25, 958-978.

6. Gulati, J.; Reisin, I. L. Cooperative thermal effects on the accumulation of potassium and sodium in frog muscle. Science 1972, 176, 1140-1143.

7. Keynes, R. D. Evidence for structural changes during nerve activity and their relation to the conduction mechanism. In: "The Neurosciences"; F. O. Schmitt, Ed.; Rockefeller University Press: New York, 1970; pp. 707-714.

8. Bass, L.; Moore, W. J. A model of nervous excitation based
on the Wien dissociation effect. In: "Structural Chemistry and
Molecular Biology"; A. Rich; C. M. Davidson, Eds.; Freeman:
San Francisco, 1968; pp. 356-368.

9. Edelman, G. M. Surface modulation in cell recognition and
cell growth. Science 1976, 192, 218-226.

10. Edelman. G. M.; Yahara, I.; Wang, J. L. Receptor mobility
and receptor-cytoplasmic interactions in lymphocytes. Proc.
Nat. Acad. Sci. USA 1973, 70, 1442-1446.

11. Yahara, I.; Edelman, G. M. Restriction of the mobility of
lymphocyte immunoglobulin receptors by concanavalin A. Proc.
Nat. Acad. Sci. USA 1972, 69, 608-612.

12. Luben, R. A.; Chen, M.; Rosen, D.; Pilla, A. A.; Adey,
W. R. Effects of therapeutic electromagnetically induced current
on hormone responsiveness of bone cells in vitro. American
Electrochemical Society, 157th Meeting, St. Louis, Missouri, May
1980. J. Electrochem. Soc. 1980, 127, 129c (abstract).

13. Fitten-Jackson, S. Chick tibia-osteogenesis-calcification.
Personal communication.

14. Norton, L.A.; Shteyer, A.; Rodan, G. A. Electromagnetic
field effects on DNA synthesis in bone cells. American
Electrochemical Society, 157th Meeting, St. Louis, Missouri,
May 1980. J. Electrochem. Soc. 1980, 127, 129 (abstract).

15. Kurtz, R. J. Modulation of white blood cell activity
in vitro. Personal communication.

16. Sisken, B. F.; Lafferty, J. F.; Pilla, A. A. The effects of
inductively coupled current on sensory and sympathetic ganglia
in vitro. Comparison with Nerve Growth Factor (NGF). American
Electrochemical Society, 157th Meeting, St. Louis, Missouri,
May 1980. J. Electrochem. Soc. 1980, 127, 130c (abstract).

17. Bawin, S. M.; Adey; Sabbot, I. M. Ionic factors in release
of $^{45}Ca^{2+}$ from chick cerebral tissue by electromagnetic fields.
Proc. Nat. Acad. Sci. USA 1978, 75, 6314-6318.

18. Bawin, S. M.; Adey, W. R.; Lawrence, A. F.; Bassen, H. I.
Weak amplitude-modulated radiofrequency fields modify $^{45}Ca^{2+}$
release from cat cerebral cortex, in vivo. Bioelectromagnetics
Society, Second Annual Meeting, San Antonio, Texas, September
1980. Bioelectromagnetics 1980, 1(2), 211 (abstract).

19. Schwan, H. P. Some tissue determinants of interactions with electric fields. Neurosci. Res. Program Bull. 1977, 15, 88-98.

20. Elul, R. Dipoles of spontaneous activity in the cerebral cortex. Exptl. Neurol. 1962, 6, 285-299.

21. Elul, R. The genesis of the EEG. Internat. Rev. Neurobiol. 1972, 15, 227-272.

22. Bawin, S. M.; Kaczmarek, L. K.; Adey, W. R. Effects of modulated VHF fields on the central nervous system. Ann. New York Acad. Sci. 1975, 247, 74-81.

23. Bawin, S. M.; Adey, W. R. Sensitivity of calcium binding in cerebral tissue to weak environmental electric fields oscillating at low frequency. Proc. Nat. Acad. Sci. USA 1976, 73, 1999-2003.

24. Bawin, S. M.; Lin-Liu, S.; Adey, W. R. Influence of weak electromagnetically induced pulsating current on Ca binding in isolated cerebral tissue. American Electrochemical Society, 157th Meeting, St. Louis, Missouri, May 1980. J. Electrochem. Soc. 1980, 127, 129c (abstract).

25. Blackman, C. S.; Elder, J. A.; Weil, C. M.; Eichinger, D.C.; and House, D. E. Induction of calcium-ion efflux from brain tissue by radio frequency radiation: effects of modulation frequency and field strength. In: "International Union of Radio Science, Symposium on Bioeffects of Electromagnetic Waves, Washington, D. C., 1977." Radio Science 1979, 14, 93-98.

26. Kaczmarek, L. K.; Adey, W. R. Weak electric gradients change ionic and transmitter fluxes in cortex. Brain Res. 1974, 66, 537-540.

27. Bawin, S. M.; Gavalas-Medici, R.; Adey, W. R. Effects of modulated very high frequency fields on specific brain rhythms in cats. Brain Res. 1973, 58, 365-384.

28. Takashima, S.; Onoral, B.; Schwan, H. P. Effects of modulated RF energy on the EEG of mammalian brains. Rad. and Environm. Biophys. 1979, 16, 15-27.

29. Adey, W. R. Frequency and power windowing in tissue interactions with weak electromagnetic fields. Proc. Inst. Electrical Electronics Eng. 1980, 68, 119-125.

30. Adey, W. R. Tissue interactions with nonionizing electromagnetic fields. Physiol. Rev. 1980, in press.

294   BIOLOGICAL EFFECTS OF NONIONIZING RADIATION

31. Kalmijn, A. J. The detection of electric fields from
inanimate and animate sources other than electric organs.
In: "Handbook of Sensory Physiology III/3. Electroreceptors
and Other Specialized Receptors in Lower Vertebrates"; A.
Fessard, Ed.; Springer-Verlag: New York, 1974; pp. 147-200.

32. Parker, G. H.; vanHeusen, A. P. The responses of the
catfish, Amiurus nebulosus, to metallic and non-metallic
rods. Am. J. Physiol. 1917, 44, 405-420.

33. Keeton, W. T. The orientational and navigational basis
of homing in birds. In: "Recent Advances in the Study of
Behavior"; Academic Press: New York, 1974.

34. Southern, W. E. Orientation of gull chicks exposed to
Project Sanguine's electromagnetic field. Science 1975, 189,
143-145.

35. Wever, R. Einfluss schwacher electro-magnetischer Felder
auf die circadiane Periodik des Menschen. Naturwissenschaften
1968, 55, 29-33.

36. Wever, R. Effects of low-level, low-frequency fields on
human circadian rhythms. Neurosci. Res. Program Bull. 1977, 15,
39-45.

37. Gavalas, R. J.; Walter, D. O.; Hamer, J.; Adey, W. R. Effect
of low-level, low-frequency electric fields on EEG and behavior in
Macaca nemestrina. Brain Res. 1970, 18, 491-501.

38. Gavalas-Medici, R.; Day-Magdaleno, S. R. Extremely low
frequency, weak electric fields affect schedule-controlled
behavior of monkeys. Nature 1976, 261, 256-258.

39. Sagan, P. M.; Adey, W. R.; Sabbot, I. M.; Bystrom, B. G.
Effects of 60 Hz environmental electric fields on the central
nervous system of laboratory rats. Bioelectromagnetics, in press.

40. Kalmijn, A. J. Electromagnetic guidance systems in fishes.
In: "Biomagnetics Effects Workshop"; T. Tenforde, Ed.; Lawrence
Berkeley Laboratory: Berkeley, Publication LBL-7452, 1978;
pp. 8-10.

41. Blakemore, R. P. Magnetotactic bacteria. Science 1975,
190, 377-379.

42. Goldman, A. I.; O'Brien, P. J. Bees have magnetic remanence.
Science 1978, 201, 1026-1027.

43.   Presdi, D.; Pettigrew, J.D. Ferromagnetic coupling to muscle receptors as a basis for geomagnetic field sensitivity in animals. Nature 1980, 285, 99-101.

44.   Sagan, P. M.; Medici, R. G. Behavior of chicks exposed to low-power 450 MHz fields sinusoidally modulated at EEG frequencies. Radio Science 1979, 14, 239-254.

45.   Dumanskiy, J. D.; Shandala, M.G. The biologic action and hygienic significance of electromagnetic fields of superhigh and ultrahigh frequencies in densely populated areas. In: "Biologic Effects and Health Hazards of Microwave Radiation"; P. Czerski, Ed.; Polish Medical Publishers: Warsaw, 1974; pp. 289-293.

46.   Thomas, J. R.; Burch, L. S.; Yeandle, S. S. Microwave radiation and chlordiazepoxide: synergistic effects on fixed interval behavior. Science 1979, 203, 1357-1358.

47.   Schmitt, F. O.; Samson, F. E., Eds. Brain cell micro-environment. Neurosci. Res. Program Bull. 1969, 7, 277-417.

48.   Singer, S. J.; Nicolson, G. L. The fluid mosaic model of the structure of cell membranes. Science 1972, 175, 720-731.

49.   McConnell, H. M. Coupling between lateral and perpendicular motion in biological membranes. In: "Functional Linkage in Biomolecular Systems"; F. O. Schmitt, D. M. Crothers, D. M. Schneider, Eds.; Raven Press: New York, 1975; pp. 123-131.

50.   Elul, R. Fixed charge in the cell membrane. J. Physiol. London 1967, 189, 351-365.

51.   Katchalsky, A. Polyelectrolytes and their biological interactions. In: "Connective Tissue. Intercellular Macro-molecules"; New York Heart Association, Eds.; Little, Brown: Boston, 1964; pp. 9-41.

52.   Van der Kloot, W. G.; Cohen, I. Membrane surface potential changes may alter drug interactions: an example, acetyl choline and curare. Science 1979, 203, 1351-1352.

53.   Kaczmarek, L. K.; Adey, W. R. The efflux of $^{45}Ca^{2+}$ and ^{3}H-gamma-aminobutyric acid from cat cerebral cortex. Brain Res. 1973, 63, 331-342.

54.   Hafemann, D. R.; Costin, A.; Tarby, T. J. Electrophysiological effects of enzymes introduced into the lateral geniculate body of the cat. Exptl. Neurol. 1970, 27, 238-247.

55. Haken, H. Cooperative phenomena in systems far from thermal equilibrium and in nonphysical systems. Rev. Modern Physics 1975, 47, 67-120.

56. Bawin, S. M.; Sheppard, A. R.; Adey, W. R. Possible mechanisms of weak electromagnetic field coupling in brain tissue. Bioelectrochem. Bioenergetics 1978, 5, 67-76.

57. Adey, W. R. Long-range electromagnetic field interactions at brain cell surfaces. In: "Magnetic Field Effect on Biological Systems"; T. Tenforde, Ed.; Plenum Press: New York, 1979; pp. 57-78.

58. Schwarz, G. Cooperative binding to linear biopolymers. II. Fundamental static and dynamic properties. Eur. J. Biochem. 1970, 12, 442-453.

59. Kalmijn, A. Biophysics of geomagnetic field detection. In press, 1980.

60. Adey, W. R.; Bawin, S. M.; Lin-Liu, S. Increased calcium efflux from cerebral tissue exposed to weak modulated microwave fields. Physiological Society, London, July 1980. Proceedings, 23P.

61. Lin-Liu, S.; Adey, W. R. Effect of ELF-modulated 450 MHz field on calcium efflux from rat synaptosomes. Bioelectromagnetics Society, Second Annual Meeting, San Antonio, September 1980. Bioelectromagnetics 1980, 1(2), 211 (abstract).

62. Lin-Liu, S.; Bawin, S. M.; Adey, W. R. Role of β-endorphin on calcium effluxes in synaptosomes. Society for Neuroscience, Annual Meeting, Cincinnati, Ohio, November 1980. Proceedings, p. 766 (Abstract No. 260.5).

63. Bawin, S. M.; Adey, W. R.; Lin-Liu, S.; Mahoney, M. D. Calcium sensitivity of enkephalin response in the hippocampal slice. Society for Neuroscience, Annual Meeting, Cincinnati, Ohio, November 1980. Proceedings, p. 765 (Abstract No. 260.4).

64. Iversen, L. L.; Nicoll, R. A.; Vale, W. W., Eds. Neurobiology of peptides. Neurosci. Res. Program Bull. 1978, 16, 211-376.

65. Orida, N.; Poo, M.-M. Electrophoretic movement and localisation of acetylcholine receptors in the embryonic muscle cell membrane. Nature 1978, 275, 31-35.

66. Poo, M.-M.; Robinson, K. R. Electrophoresis of concanavalin A receptors along embryonic muscle membrane. Nature 1977, 265, 602-605.

67. Tenforde, T. S. Thermal aspects of electromagnetic field interactions with bound calcium ions at the nerve cell surface. J. theor. Biol. 1980, 83, 517-521.

68. Schwarz, G.; Seelig, J. Kinetic properties and electric field effect of the helix-coil transition of poly(gamma-benzyl l-glutamate) determined from dielectric relaxation measurements. Biopolymers 1968, 6, 1263-1277.

69. Neumann, E.; Katchalsky, A. Long-lived conformation changes induced by electric impulses in biopolymers. Proc. Nat. Acad. Sci. USA 1972, 69, 993-997.

70. Neumann, E.; Nachmansohn, D.; Katchalsky, A. An attempt at an integral interpretation of nerve excitability. Proc. Nat. Acad. Sci. USA 1973, 70, 727-731.

71. Grodsky, I. T. Neuronal membrane: a physical synthesis. Math. Biosci. 1976, 28, 191-219.

72. Kaczmarek, L. K. Frequency sensitive biochemical reactions. Biophys. Chem. 1976, 4, 249-252.

73. Kaczmarek, L. K. Cation binding models for the interaction of membranes with EM fields. Neurosci. Res. Program Bull. 1977, 15, 54-60.

74. Adey, W. R. Models of membranes of cerebral cells as substrates for information storage. BioSystems 1977, 8, 163-178.

75. Einolf, C. W.; Carstensen, E. L. Low-frequency dielectric dispersion in suspensions of ion-exchange resins. J. Phys. Chem. 1971, 75, 1091-1099.

76. Sheppard, A. R.; Adey, W. R. The role of cell surface polarization in biological effects of extremely low frequency fields. U. S. Department of Energy Symposium Series 50, "Biological Effects of Extremely Low Frequency Electromagnetic Fields"; DOE: Washington, D. C., 1979; pp. 147-158.

77. Adey, W. R.; Bawin, S. M. Brain cell surfaces in cooperative binding and release of calcium by low-level electromagentic fields; a review. Radio Science 1980, in press.

78. Barnes, F. S.; Hu, C.-L. J. Model for some nonthermal effects of radio and microwave fields on biological membranes. Inst. Electrical Electronics Engineers, Trans. Microwave Theory and Techniques 1977, 25, 742-746.

79. Vaccaro, S. R.; Green, H. S. Ionic processes in excitable membranes. J. theor. Biol. 1979, 81, 771-802.

RECEIVED October 31, 1980.

Calcium Ion Efflux Induction in Brain Tissue by Radiofrequency Radiation

C. F. BLACKMAN, W. T. JOINES, and J. A. ELDER

Experimental Biology Division, Health Effects Research Laboratory,
U.S. Environmental Protection Agency, Research Triangle Park, NC 27711

One of the most interesting and controversial papers on
the biological effects of nonionizing radiation was published
by Bawin, Kaczmarek and Adey in 1975 (1). They found a 147
MHz carrier wave could elicit an enhanced efflux of calcium
ions from chick brain tissue only when amplitude modulated at
certain sub-ELF frequencies. In addition to being one of the
few U. S. reports at that time which described a biological
response to an exposure at a power density below 10 mW/cm^2,
the results demonstrated a modulation frequency-specific
response with a maximum effect at 16 Hz. This response was
particularly significant because the effective modulating
frequencies were within the range of frequencies found in the
electroencephalogram (EEG) of the intact animal.

An important feature of the research was the relatively
simple biological procedure: halves of chick brains were
labeled with a radioisotope ($^{45}Ca^{++}$), exposed to RF fields for
a short time, and the amount of $^{45}Ca^{++}$ released into the
medium during irradiation was measured. In 1979, we reported
our success in replicating the essential characteristics of
the frequency response curve (2). However, success was achieved
only after exploring a range of power densities at 147 MHz
carrier frequency, 16 Hz amplitude modulation. This result
demonstrated the existence of a power density window at 0.83
mW/cm^2 in that no enhanced calcium efflux was found at either
higher or lower power densities. Subsequent to this work, we
examined the effect of 9 Hz modulation on the power density
response and found that the location of the window was unchanged
(3).

More recently, the power density response of the calcium-
ion efflux at 50 MHz, modulated at 16 Hz, was examined (4).
In comparison to the above results, two power-density windows
were found, both of which occurred at higher exposure fields
than the single effective power density at 147 MHz. With a
carrier frequency of 450 MHz, Sheppard et al. (5) located a
power density window that occurred within the general power

density range shown to be effective in producing calcium-ion
efflux at the 147 MHz carrier frequency.

These results led us to analyze the relationship between
carrier-wave frequency and power density. We developed a
mathematical model (6) which takes into account the changes in
complex permittivity of brain tissue with frequency. This
model predicted that a given electric-field intensity within a
brain-tissue sample occurred at different exposure levels for
50-, 147-, and 450-MHz radiation. Using the calculated electric-
field intensities in the sample as the independent variable,
the model demonstrated that the RF-induced calcium-ion efflux
results at one carrier frequency corresponded to those at the
other frequencies for both positive and negative findings. In
this paper, we present two additional experiments using 147-MHz
radiation which further test both negative and positive predictions of this model.

In addition to highlighting the basic results of the
mathematical analysis outlined above, this paper presents the
results of some important ancillary findings. Oxygen consumption of the sample was measured as an indication of the physiological state of the brain tissue. Requirements for certain
components in the exposure medium are emphasized. Finally, we
discuss mechanisms that may be responsible for the RF-induced
calcium-ion efflux from brain tissue.

Experimental Procedures

The experimental procedures have been described in detail
(3,4), but are briefly described here for completeness. Chick
forebrains were removed, separated at the midline, and incubated
at 37°C in a physiological buffer containing radioactive
calcium ions ($^{45}Ca^{++}$). Any radioactivity not tightly associated
with the tissue was then removed by rinsing and the samples
(one forebrain half per tube) were placed in fresh buffer (1.0
ml) without the radioactive tracer. Following a 20 minute
treatment in a stripline exposure system, an aliquot of the
bathing solution was removed from each tube and assayed for
the amount of radioactive calcium that was released from the
tissue. Forebrain halves from the same chicken served as a
treatment/control pair to simplify the subsequent statistical
analysis. Two treatment conditions were compared in order to
reduce the influence of data variability: exposure of tissue
samples to radiation was alternated within a one hour period
with identically prepared samples which were exposed to zero
power density radiation (sham exposure). This experimental
design substantially increased the sensitivity of the test.
For example, the results of our previous study (2) were repeated
with a much higher level of statistical significance (3), i.e.
p<.001 compared to p<.05.

A detailed description of the exposure system is presented elsewhere (3). Either 50-MHz or 147-MHz radiation, sinusoidually amplitude modulated (>95%) at 16 Hz, was used to treat the samples. During treatment, the samples were maintained in a 37°C environment. In new experimental results presented here, chick forebrains were exposed at 0.37 and 0.49 mW/cm^2 to 147-MHz radiation, modulated at 16 Hz.

In an ancillary experiment, the influence of the buffering agent was tested on the ability of modulated 147-MHz radiation to enhance calcium-ion efflux. The standard medium used for these experiments was composed of 155 mM NaCl, 5.6 mM KCl, 2.16 mM CaCl$_2$, 11.1 mM glucose, and 2.4 mM NaHCO$_3$, at a pH of 7.6 to 7.8. Two other media were used, which were identical to the standard medium except for the replacement of NaHCO$_3$ with either 10 mM Tris (pH 7.4) or 10 mM HEPES (pH 7.4). The labeling, washing and exposure of the tissues were all done in medium with the same buffering agent. Exposures were conducted using 147 MHz, sinusoidally, amplitude modulated at 16 Hz, at a power density of 0.83 mW/cm^2.

The respiratory activity of the brain tissue was determined by measuring the rate of oxygen uptake with a Clark oxygen electrode (7). The sample of tissue (a brain half) was treated exactly as if used in a calcium efflux experiment except no radioactivity or RF power was used. Following this procedure which required about 55 minutes, the tissue was placed in the oxygen electrode cell containing 1.6 ml of the standard medium (pH 7.8) at 37°C and the rate of oxygen uptake was recorded.

Theoretical and Experimental Results

Outline of Mathematical Analysis. We have described the basis for the mathematical model in detail elsewhere (6). The brain tissue plus buffer was assumed to approximate a spherical object in order to simplify the mathematical development. This assumption is reasonable because the tissue rests in the hemispheric portion of the test tube (Figure 1).

Several mathematical relationships have been developed using the vector electric field intensity induced inside a sphere as a function of the incident electric field intensity (8,9). The square of the average internal electric field intensity, $|\bar{E}|^2_{av}$, was derived and related to the time-average power density incident upon the sample within the stripline. A relationship was then developed that defines the power densities at various carrier frequencies which would give the same average internal electric field intensity in the sample. These developments were necessary because the relative complex permittivity of the tissue and the wavelength of radiation change with carrier frequency. Finally, using the complex permittivity values reported by Foster et al. (10), relationships were derived for incident power densities at 50, 147,

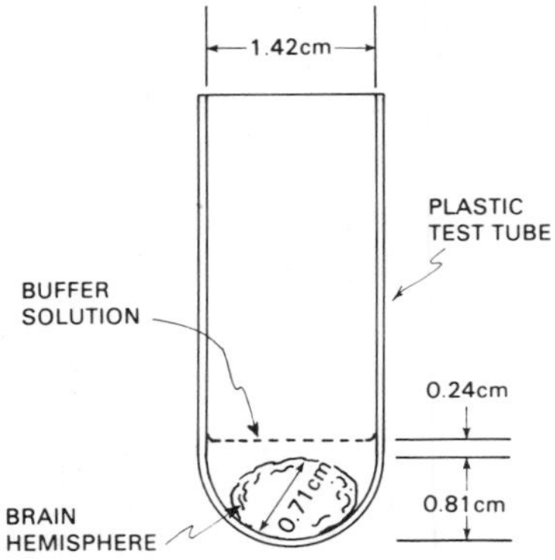

Figure 1. Schematic of the brain tissue in buffer at the bottom of the test tube used in our experiments. The mean height from the top of the tissue to the surface of the solution is 0.24 cm, and the meniscus of the solution is essentially flat across the entire diameter.

Table I. Values of P_i used in previously reported experiments on calcium-ion efflux from chick-brain samples at carrier-wave frequencies of 50, 147, and 450 MHz. The P_i values in each horizontal row are related by Equations (3) and (4) to yield the same average electric field intensity within the sample, as shown in the last column. Values of P_i yielding statistically significant results are bracketed by solid bars, cross-hatched bars bracket insignificant results, and untested values of P_i are not bracketed.

50 MHz	147 MHz	450 MHz	$|E|_{av}$, V/m
0.37	0.08	0.03	0.79
0.49	0.11	0.04	0.91
0.72	0.16	0.05	1.10
1.44	0.32	0.11	1.56
1.67	0.37	0.12	1.68
2.17	0.49	0.16	1.92
2.45	0.55	0.18	2.04
3.64	0.83	0.28	2.50
4.32	0.97	0.32	2.71
4.95	1.11	0.37	2.90
6.15	1.38	0.46	3.23
7.40	1.66	0.55	3.54
13.4	3.00	1.00	4.77
26.8	6.00	2.00	6.75
66.9	15.0	5.00	10.7

and 450 MHz to give the same internal electric field intensity. To augment the theoretical development and for later reference, some of the mathematical relationships are concisely stated in the following sub-section.

<u>Equivalent Incident Power Densities at Different Frequencies.</u>
The average electric field intensity squared that is induced within a spherical sample of radius (a) much less than the wavelength (λ) of the radiofrequency field in air is

$$|\bar{E}|^2_{av} = \left|\frac{3}{2+\varepsilon^*_r}\right|^2 E^2_o + 0.1 \left(\frac{2\pi a}{\lambda}\right)^2 E^2_o \tag{1}$$

where

$$\varepsilon^*_r = \frac{\varepsilon}{\varepsilon_o} - j\frac{\sigma}{\omega\varepsilon_o}$$

is the relative complex permittivity, σ is sample conductivity, ω is the radian frequency, and $e^{j\omega t}$ time dependence is assumed for all fields. The first term in Equation (1) is due to the uniform incident electric field (E_o), and the second term is due to the uniform incident magnetic field ($H_o = E_o/\eta_o$) in the stripline, where $\eta_o = 377$ ohms, the intrinsic impedance of free space. The time-averaged power density (P_i) incident upon the sample within the stripline is

$$P_i = \frac{1}{2} E^2_o/\eta_o \tag{2}$$

To make $|E|_{av}$ within the sample the same at different carrier frequencies, we calculate from Equations (1) and (2):

$$P_{i50} = 4.46\ P_{i147} \tag{3}$$

and

$$P_i 147 = 3.00\ P_{i450} \tag{4}$$

where P_{if} denotes the incident power density at carrier frequency f.

Specific values of P_i used in previously reported experiments on calcium-ion efflux from chick-brain samples are listed in Table I under the carrier wave frequency used in the experiment (3,4,11). In addition, values of P_i which result in the same $|E|_{av}$ in the sample have been calculated for the other carrier frequencies using Equations (3) and (4). For example, 3.64 mW/cm^2 at 50 MHz, 0.83 mW/cm^2 at 147 MHz, and

0.28 mW/cm^2 at 450 MHz all produce the same $|E|_{av}$, 2.50 V/m, within a spherical brain tissue sample according to our model. For the incident power densities in each horizontal row, $|E|_{av}$ is calculated and shown as the last column of Table I. As indicated in Table I, positive test results have been obtained for 3.64 mW/cm^2 at 50 MHz and 0.83 mW/cm^2 at 147 MHz, while 0.28 mW/cm^2 at 450 MHz has not been tested.

If the internal electric field intensity is indeed a common factor for equality of results at each carrier frequency, then each three P_i values in a horizontal row would be bracketed by the same symbols. Since the unbracketed P_i values have not been tested in calcium-ion efflux experiments, we predict that they will yield the same results as a tested value in the same horizontal row.

Based on the positive and negative findings at 1.67 and 2.17 mW/cm^2, respectively, at 50 MHz, further studies were performed at power densities corresponding to the same $|E|_{av}$ at 147 MHz. The predictions that exposure at 0.37 mW/cm^2 would produce a positive finding and exposure at 0.49 mW/cm^2 would produce a negative finding were confirmed by these experimental results (Table II).

Table II. Mean relative quantity of calcium ions released by brain tissue pairs as a function of exposure to 147-MHz radiation, amplitude modulated at 16 Hz.

Power density mW/cm^2	Sham			Exposed			P
	n	Mean	S.E.	n	Mean	S.E.	
0.37	32	1.079	.035	32	1.221	.057	.037
0.49	32	1.150	.044	32	1.115	.041	.568

Figure 2 displays the percent difference in mean efflux between the exposed and sham groups at different power densities of 50- and 147-MHz radiation, as well as lines connecting those power densities which would produce the same value of internal electric field intensity in the samples. These results support the mathematical model and demonstrate its usefulness in defining effective power densities over a range of carrier frequencies.

The relationship between effective power densities at different carrier frequencies can be viewed in a different manner by plotting carrier frequency versus incident power density (Figure 3). Lines connecting P_i values which produce the same internal electric field intensity at 50, 147, and 450 MHz are as shown. This figure serves to illustrate the smaller range of P_i values as carrier-wave frequency is increased from

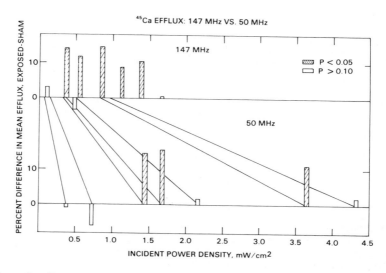

Figure 2. *Percent difference in mean efflux between the exposed and sham groups vs. power density at 50 and 147 MHz. The lines connect power densities at 50 and 147 MHz, which are calculated to produce the same value of internal electric field intensity in the samples.*

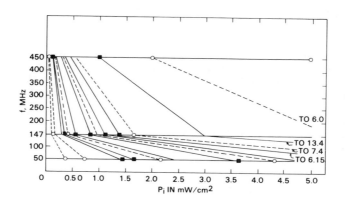

Figure 3. *Results indicated in Table I at 50, 147, and 450 MHz plotted vs. P_i values (values of P_i yielding significant results (■) and insignificant results (○)). Solid and dashed lines connect P_i values that produce the same internal electric field intensity at 50, 147, and 450 MHz.*

50 to 450 MHz. The implication is that better resolution
between tested values of P_i should be obtained at the lower
frequencies.

Table I and Figure 3 highlight another intriguing feature
of the results obtained to date. The experimental results at
50 and 147 MHz have demonstrated two effective power density
ranges separated and bracketed by regions of no effect. The
mathematical model, applied to this data, predicts an additional
effective power density range at each carrier frequency.
Moreover, if the experimental results of Adey (11) are evaluated
in this manner, a fourth effective power density window is
predicted for each of the carrier frequencies. Confirmation
of the predictions of the mathematical model resulting from
these data is necessary in order to ensure that these results
reflect a true response of the biological tissue.

Absorbed Power and Effect of Temperature. The square of
the average internal field intensity, $|\bar{E}|^2_{av}$, can be used to
compute an estimated thermal load to the sample at the various
carrier frequencies. Using $|\bar{E}|^2_{av}$, the average power per unit
volume absorbed within an isolated spherical sample is

$$P_a = \frac{1}{2} \sigma |\bar{E}|^2_{av} \tag{5}$$

where P_a is in W/cm^3 for σ in mhos/cm and $|\bar{E}|^2_{av}$ in V/cm. The
initial slope of temperature rise within the tissue is related
to P_a by

$$P_a = K \rho c \, \Delta T/t \tag{6}$$

where K is 4.186 joules/cal, ρ is the tissue density in g/cm^3,
c is the specific heat of the tissue in cal/g°C, ΔT is the
temperature change in °C, and t is the time in seconds. From
Equations (5) and (6), we have

$$\Delta T/t = \frac{\sigma |\bar{E}|^2_{av}}{2K\rho c} \tag{7}$$

or

$$\Delta T/t = \frac{\sigma |\bar{E}|^2_{av}}{7.74} \tag{8}$$

taking the density and specific heat of brain tissue as 1.05
g/cm^3 and 0.88 cal/g°C (12). The use of these conservative
values gives rise to an overestimate of ΔT. As an example
using Equation (8), 3.64 mW/cm² at 50 MHz yields a $\Delta T/t$ of
3.93×10^{-7} °C/sec, and 1.00 mW/cm² at 450 MHz yields a $\Delta T/t$
of 2.20×10^{-6} °C/sec. Neglecting the loss of thermal energy,

the corresponding temperature rises for a 20-min exposure are 0.0005°C and 0.0026°C, respectively.

For these typical exposure conditions, the rate of energy absorption is too low to produce gross or generalized heating of the sample, or for that matter, to be measured by any readily available method. In the experiments at 147 MHz, the absorption of radiofrequency energy by the sample was so small that no difference could be detected in the amount of power incident upon the sample and the power transmitted through the exposure system. These results indicate that the effect was not due to generalized heating caused by absorption of RF energy.

In other experiments, the effect of temperature has been determined by measuring Ca^{++} efflux from chick brain tissue incubated at 32°C and 41°C (3). When compared to 37°C, the efflux was 9% lower at 32°C and 15% higher at 41°C. The temperature difference in control and irradiated samples could be experimentally controlled to less than 1°C, therefore temperature variations in the samples do not account for the 15-24% change in Ca^{++} efflux caused by exposure to 16 Hz modulated carrier waves.

Most biological effects of radiofrequency radiation are attributed to a response to the thermalized absorbed energy. However, two very important experimental results make it difficult to interpret enhanced calcium ion efflux in terms of thermal mechanisms: (a) for a given effective incident power and carrier frequency, the effect is dependent on the frequency of the modulation (1,2); and (b) there are positive-effect ranges of internal electric field intensity which are separated by no-effect regions (4). These results strongly suggest a frequency-specific phenomenon and provide evidence against gross thermal mechanisms.

Proposed Mechanism Responsible for Calcium Efflux.
Calcium-ion efflux from brain tissue does not appear to be a function of carrier frequency, since equivalent results are obtained at carrier frequencies of 50, 147, and 450 MHz provided the internal electric field intensity is the same in each brain. However, an important question remains: why should there be alternate ranges, or windows, of internal electric field intensity which cause efflux enhancement? An hypothesis that is consistent with and helps explain this finding is: The internal electric field $|E|_{av}$ in Equation (1) has a linear as well as a nonlinear dependence on the external electric field (E_o) for the specific values of E that yield enhanced efflux.

With regard to this hypothesis, only the first term in Equation (1) is a function of tissue properties, since

$$\varepsilon_r^* = \frac{\varepsilon}{\varepsilon_o} - j \frac{\sigma}{\omega \varepsilon_o}.$$

Hence, ε_r^* may have a small nonlinear dependence upon E_o. Biological membranes are known to have a nonlinear response to a static or low-frequency electric field (13,14,15), and many researchers have suggested a nonlinear response for biological materials due to RF fields (16-20). Neglecting the second term of Equation (1), the simplest linear plus nonlinear dependence of $|E|_{av}$ on E_o may be expressed as

$$|E|_{av} = k_1 E_o + k_2 E_o^2 = k_1 (1 + \frac{k_2}{k_1} E_o) E_o \qquad (9)$$

where $k_1 = 3/(2 + \varepsilon_r^*)$ and k_2 is a parameter to be determined as a function of k_1 and E_o.

The external field (E_o) is a modulated carrier wave represented by

$$E_o = E_{oc} (1 + m \cos \omega_m t) \cos \omega_c t \qquad (10)$$

where E_{oc} is the amplitude of the unmodulated carrier, m is the modulation index, $\omega_m/2\pi = f_m$ is the modulation frequency (typically 16 Hz), and $\omega_c/2\pi = f_c$ is the carrier frequency (typically 50, 147, or 450 MHz). Substituting Equation (10) into Equation (9), and using trigonometric identities, yields

$$|E|_{av} = k_1 E_{oc} \cos \omega_c t + k_2 E_{oc}^2 m \cos \omega_m t + \frac{k_2 E_{oc}^2}{4} (2 + m^2) +$$

$$\frac{k_1 E_{oc}}{2} m \cos (\omega_c + \omega_m) t + \frac{k_1 E_{oc}}{2} m \cos (\omega_c - \omega_m) t +$$

$$\frac{k_2 E_{oc}^2}{2} \cos 2\omega_c t + \frac{k_2 E_{oc}^2}{4} m^2 \cos 2\omega_m t +$$

$$\frac{k_2 E_{oc}^2}{2} m \cos (2\omega_c + \omega_m) t + \frac{k_2 E_{oc}^2}{2} m \cos (2\omega_c - \omega_m) t +$$

$$\frac{k_2 E_{oc}^2 m^2}{4} \cos 2\omega_c t + \frac{k_2 E_{oc}^2 m^2}{8} \cos (2\omega_c + 2\omega_m) t +$$

$$\frac{k_2 E_{oc}^2 m^2}{8} \cos (2\omega_c - 2\omega_m) t \qquad (11)$$

The first term in Equation (11) is the unmodulated carrier wave, of amplitude $k_1 E_{oc}$, and the second term is a signal at the modulation frequency, of amplitude $k_2 E_{oc}^2 m$, generated by the nonlinear dependence of E on E_o.

The field intensities, or wave amplitudes, that have produced changes in calcium-ion efflux at typical carrier frequencies and at typical modulation frequencies may be used to estimate the amount of nonlinearity that would be required to conform with observed results. Adey (11) has reported that a relatively small internal electric field intensity, on the order of 10^{-7} V/cm, at 16 Hz is sufficient to alter the binding of calcium ions in brain tissue. The internal field intensity of the carrier waves shown in Table 1 are on the order of 10^{-2} V/cm. From these observations, the ratio of the amplitudes of the first two terms in Equation (11) is

$$\frac{k_2 E_{oc}^2 m}{k_1 E_{oc}} = \frac{10^{-7}}{10^{-2}} = 10^{-5} \qquad (12)$$

and assuming a modulation index of m = 1,

$$\frac{k_2}{k_1} E_{oc} = 10^{-5} \qquad (13)$$

By substituting 10^{-5} for $k_2 E_o / k_1$ in Equation (9), it is apparent that the suggested amount of nonlinearity is very small and would not be detectable by conventional measurements of ε_r^* versus $|E|_{av}$.

To account for the alternate ranges of effective incident power densities, the internal field $|E|_{av}$ need only have a small nonlinear dependence upon the external field (E_o) at specific values of internal electric field (E) that yield enhanced efflux. At all other values of E, the dependence of $|E|_{av}$ on E_o may be entirely linear. A plot of $|E|_{av}$ versus E_o from Equation (1), at the carrier frequencies 50, 147, and 450 MHz, is shown in Figure 4. Obviously, a deviation from linearity of the amount estimated earlier (1 part in 10,000) would not be noticed on the straight lines of Figure 4. However, the $|E|_{av}$ values where the relationship is assumed to be slightly nonlinear are indicated by the solid horizontal lines. These solid lines indicate the $|E|_{av}$ values from Table 1 which correspond to P_i (or E_o) values that produced efflux enhancement. The dashed horizontal lines in Figure 4 indicate $|E|_{av}$ values corresponding to P_i (or E_o) values that were not effective. At these points, the dependence of $|E|_{av}$ on E_o may be entirely linear. At present, we have no firm hypothesis to describe the postulated multiple regions of nonlinear dependence of the internal field, E, on the external field, E_o.

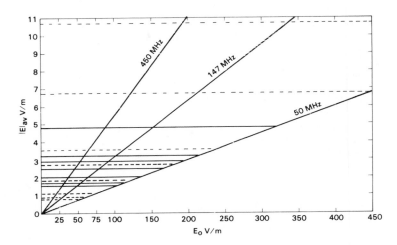

Figure 4.   Average internal electric field intensity ($|\mathrm{E}|_{av}$) as a function of the external electric field intensity (E_o) for 50-, 147-, and 450-MHz carrier frequencies.

Solid horizontal lines indicate values of $|\mathrm{E}|_{av}$ that correspond to E_o (or P_i) values that produce efflux enhancement. The dashed horizontal lines indicate similar values where no significant enhancement of efflux has been observed.

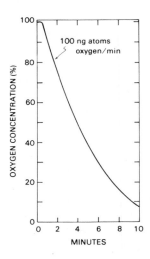

Figure 5.   Respiratory activity of chick brain tissue.

A sample (brain half) was treated exactly as if used in a calcium efflux experiment except no radioactivity or RF power was used. Following this procedure, which required about 55 min, the tissue was placed in an oxygen electrode cell containing 1.6 mL of the medium (pH 7.8) at 37° C, and the rate of oxygen consumption was measured (7, 23).

An additional hypothesis that is consistent with and helps explain the role played by the 16 Hz amplitude modulation is as follows: the nonlinear medium demodulates the carrier releasing a 16-Hz signal within the brain tissue, and it is the 16-Hz signal that causes changes in the calcium binding. This change in calcium binding may occur by Maxwell-Wagner relaxation (21) at the polarized interface between the Ca^{++} ions and the brain tissue. This hypothesis is not developed here. Alternative hypotheses have been offered (cf. Adey, this volume) to explain the fundamental role played by the sub-ELF (1,2,22). Obviously, more theoretical and experimental work must be performed before a clear choice can be made regarding the most likely hypothesis.

Ancillary Experiments

Effect of Buffer Solution. An essential component of the medium in potentiating enhanced calcium-ion efflux due to RF radiation appears to be bicarbonate. We have substituted both Tris and HEPES buffers for bicarbonate and have failed to observe enhanced calcium efflux at 0.83 mW/cm² (147 MHz). The same result has been reported by Bawin (personal communication) when bicarbonate was replaced by imidazole or MOPS buffers. Although the significance of this finding is not yet apparent, these results should be of interest to other investigators who attempt to replicate or extend the studies on RF-induced calcium-ion efflux from brain tissue. One should also note that the initial report by Bawin et al. (1) incorrectly listed the bicarbonate concentration at $\overline{24\ mM}$ instead of 2.4 mM (22).

Respiratory Activity of Brain. Questions concerning the metabolic state of the isolated brain tissue are frequently posed. Figure 5 shows the respiratory activity of a brain half which had undergone the same treatment as a sample used in calcium efflux experiments. The initial linear portion of the curve represents a respiratory rate of about 100 ng atoms oxygen/min. The rate decreased with time and more than 90% of the oxygen in the medium was depleted in less than 10 min. When the oxygen-depleted solution was repeatedly replaced with fresh medium, very similar curves were obtained. For example, the initial respiratory rates in the second and third replacement volumes were 6% and 15% less than the first trial, respectively. The tissue was therefore capable of respiratory activity throughout the 55 to 60 minute experimental period. Freshly excised brain samples exhibited similar responses at slightly higher respiratory rates. One should recall that Bawin et al. (1) added cyanide to the samples and found that the respiratory poison (inhibitor) did not affect enhanced calcium efflux.

Summary and Conclusion

Keeping the average electric field intensity the same
within a spherical model of chick-brain in buffer solution at
different incident carrier wave frequencies requires that
incident power density be changed with frequency to compensate
for the change in complex permittivity and wavelength with
frequency. The resulting Equations (3) and (4) relate corresponding values of P_i at carrier frequencies of 50, 147, and
450 MHz.

Very few results are available to test this mathematical
model. Circumstances have lead to two tests comparing a
negative and a positive finding at 147 MHz with results at 450
MHz. One test was performed at 50 MHz (3.64 mW/cm^2) to test a
prediction of this model based on the result of 147 MHz (0.83
mW/cm^2). All these tests have provided results that agree
with the model. In this paper, we describe the results of two
tests at 147 MHz which agree with the predictions, one positive
and one negative, made from the 50 MHz data. Thus, all the
results to date support the predictions of the theoretical
analysis. Further support for the theory is the fact that no
result is contradicted by a corresponding experiment at a
different carrier frequency. A more complete test of the
theory will be obtained when additional experiments are conducted
at the untested values of P_i.

The experimental results suggest that radiofrequency
radiation may be useful as an investigative tool to learn more
about the electrical properties of the central nervous system.

The specific carrier-wave amplitudes (field intensities)
which have been found to be effective in producing Ca^{++} ion
efflux are discussed in terms of tissue properties and relevant
mechanisms. The brain tissue is hypothesized to be electrically
nonlinear at specific field intensities; this nonlinearity
demodulates the carrier and releases a 16 Hz signal within the
tissue. The 16 Hz signal is selectively coupled to the Ca^{++}
ions by some mechanism, perhaps a dipolar-type (Maxwell-Wagner)
relaxation, which enhances the efflux of Ca^{++} ions. The
hypothesis that brain tissue exhibits a slight nonlinearity
for certain values of applied RF electric field intensity is
not testable by conventional measurements of ε_r^* because changes
in this factor on the order of 1 part in 10,000 are not detectable. However, the Ca^{++} ion efflux experiment itself may
prove to be the most sensitive and discriminating indicator to
date of nonlinear electrical behavior in biological tissue.
The specific values of electric field intensity where the
tissue may be electrically nonlinear (e.g., 2.5 V/m) should be
tested in other experiments where a tissue nonlinearity could
release a low frequency or a DC signal (the third term in
Equation 11) which could in turn interact with on-going biological activities.

Literature Cited

1. Bawin, S. M.; Kaczmarek, L. K.; Adey, W. R. Effects of modulated VHF fields on the central nervous system. Ann. N.Y. Acad. Sci., 1975, 247, 74-81.
2. Blackman, C. F.; Elder, J. A.; Weil, C. M.; Benane, S. G.; Eichinger, D. C.; House, D. E. Induction of calcium-ion efflux from brain tissue by radio-frequency radiation: Effects of modulation frequency and field strength. Radio Science, 1979, 14(6S), 93-98.
3. Blackman, C. F.; Benane, S. G.; Elder, J. A.; House, D. E.; Lampe, J. A.; Faulk, J. M. Induction of calcium-ion efflux from brain tissue by radio frequency radiation: Effect of sample number and modulation frequency on the power-density window. Bioelectromagnetics, 1980, 1, 35-48.
4. Blackman, C. F.; Benane, S. G.; Joines, W. T.; Hollis, M. A.; House, D. E. Calcium-ion efflux from brain tissue: Power density vs. internal field intensity dependencies at 50-MHz RF radiation. Bioelectromagnetics, 1980, 1(3).
5. Sheppard, A. R.; Bawin, S. M.; Adey, W. R. Models of long-range order in cerebral macromolecules: Effects of sub-ELF and of modulated VHF and UHF fields. Radio Science, 1979, 14(6S), 141-145.
6. Joines, W. T.; Blackman, C. F. Power density, field intensity, and carrier frequency determinants of RF-induced calcium-ion efflux from brain tissue. Bioelectromagnetics, 1980, 1(3).
7. Lessler, M. A.; Brierley, G. P. Oxygen electrode measurements in biochemical analysis. Methods Biochem. Anal., 1969, 17, 1-29.
8. Lin, J. C.; Guy, A. W.; Johnson, C. C. Power deposition in a spherical model of a man exposed to 1-20 MHz electromagnetic fields. IEEE Trans. Microwave Theory Tech., 1973, 21, 791-797.
9. Spiegel, R. J. ELF coupling to spherical models of man and animals. IEEE Trans. Biomed. Eng., 1976, 23 387-391.
10. Foster, K. R.; Schepps, J. L; Stoy, R. D.; Schwan, H. P. Dielectric properties of brain tissue between 0.01 and 10 GHz. Phys. Med. Biol., 1979, 24, 1177-1187.
11. Adey, W. R. Frequency and power windowing in tissue interactions with weak electromagnetic fields. Proc. IEEE, 1980, 68(1), 119-125.
12. Cooper, T. E.; Trezek, G. J. A probe technique for determining the thermal conductivity of tissue. J. Heat. Transfer, 1972, 94, 133-140.
13. Goldman, D. E. Potential impedance and rectification in membranes. J. Gen. Physiol., 1943, 27, 37-60.

14. Hamel, B. B.; Zimmerman, I. A dipole model for negative
     steady-state resistance in excitable membranes. Biophys.
     J., 1970, 10, 1029-1056.
15. Arndt, R. A.; Bond, J. D.; Roper, L. D. A fit to nerve
     membrane rectification curves with a double-dipole-layer
     membrane model. Bull. Math. Biophys., 1972, 34, 151-172.
16. Spiegel, R. J.; Joines, W. T. A semiclassical theory for
     nerve excitation by a low intensity electromagnetic
     field. Bull. Math. Biophys., 1973, 35, 591–605.
17. Wachtel, H.; Seaman, R. L.; Joines, W. T. Effects of
     low-intensity microwaves on isolated neurons. Ann. N. Y.
     Acad. Sci., 1975, 247, 46-52.
18. Joines, W. T. Reception of microwaves by the brain.
     Med. Res. Eng., 1976, 12, 8-12.
19. Barnes, F. S.; Hu, C. L. Model for some non-thermal
     effects of radio and microwave fields on biological
     membranes. IEEE Trans. Microwave Theory Tech., 1977,
     MTT-25, 742-746.
20. Berkowitz, G. C.; Barnes, F. S. The effects of nonlinear
     membrane capacity on the interaction of microwave and
     radio frequencies with biological materials. IEEE Trans.
     Microwave Theory Tech., 1979, MTT-27, 204-207.
21. Pethig, R. "Dielectric and Electronic Properties of
     Biological Materials"; John Wiley & Sons, New York, 1979;
     p. 153.
22. Bawin, S. M.; Adey, W. R.; Sabbot, I. M. Ionic factors
     in release of $^{45}Ca^{2+}$ from chicken cerebral tissue by
     electromagnetic fields. Proc. Nat. Acad. Sci. (US),
     1978, 75, 6314-6318.
23. Elder, J. A.; Ali, J. S. The effect of microwaves (2450
     MHz) on isolated rat liver mitochondria. Ann. N.Y. Acad.
     Sci., 1975, 247, 251-262.

RECEIVED December 1, 1980.

A PROTOTYPE SENSORY-SYSTEM EFFECT

The Microwave Hearing Effect

JAMES C. LIN[1]

Department of Electrical and Computer Engineering, Wayne State University, Detroit, MI 48202

Human subjects exposed to pulse-modulated microwave energy can perceive a sound which seems to occur from within or near the subject's head. The sensation has been described as a click, buzz or chirp depending on the modulation characteristics of the impinging radiation. The effect was first described by Frey in 1961 ([1]). Although Frey published a series of papers over the next few years ([2],[3],[4]), his findings attracted little attention and were almost totally neglected during the decade that followed. In 1973 Guy et al. ([5],[6]) confirmed Frey's observations and many other papers that followed also supported his findings ([7], [8],[9]).

This microwave acoustic or auditory phenomenon which may be briefly defined as hearing of microwave pulses is now attracting the interest of those studying biological effects of radio and microwave radiation. Not only is the phenomenon impressive in itself but it has important ramifications for understanding neurological and behavioral activities of microwave radiation. The study of microwave acoustic effects also leads us to realize that an increment of temperature of only about 10^{-6} °C can elicit physiologically significant responses from human beings. Furthermore, since the mechanism of microwave acoustic effect is probably better understood than those of any other biological effects of microwaves, it has a special theoretical interest. It is not unreasonable to assume that the more completely we understand the microwave acoustic phenomenon, the more likely we will be able to assess the biological effects of microwave radiation and to devise rational biomedical applications of the microwave acoustic effect.

The microwave acoustic effect may be defined as the auditory perception of microwave radiation which is a form of electromagnetic energy which occupies the part of spectrum between ordinary radio waves and infrared and optical waves. This definition may

[1]Current address: Bioengineering Program, University of Illinois at Chicago Circle, Chicago, Illinois 60680.

seem surprising, and one might even question whether such sensation could exist. Let me therefore begin by citing some well
documented observations.

Human Perception

Human subjects, whose heads were irradiated with rectangular
pulse modulated microwave energy, with peak incident power density on the order of 300 mW/cm^2, perceived an audible sound.
The frequencies of these microwaves ranged from 200 to 3000 MHz,
while the pulsewidths varied from 1 to 150 μs ([1],[6],[9],[10],[11]).
The sensation appeared as a barely audible click, buzz or chirp
depending on such factors as pulsewidth and repetition frequency
of the incident radiation, and usually was perceived as originating from within or near the head. When earplugs were used to
attenuate ambient noise, the subject would indicate an apparent
increase in the level of microwave-induced sound. The sensation
occurred instantaneously and was independent of the subject's
orientation in the microwave field.

Subjects with air-conduction hearing loss, but with good
bone conduction, could hear the microwave-induced sound at
about the same incident power density as normal subjects could.
In contrast, subjects with clinically normal hearing but poor
bone conduction for frequencies above 5 kHz, would usually have
difficulty perceiving pulse-modulated microwave energy. It appears reasonable to argue, on the basis of these findings and
other observations given in more detail in the afore-mentioned
papers, that the perception of microwave pulses depends on the
presence of an intact neural hearing apparatus, especially for
high-frequency sound. But, how does the perception occur?

Auditory Pathways

In order to understand this phenomenon, let us consider
briefly the anatomical pathways by which sonic energy is perceived. The auditory system can be conveniently divided into two
components: the peripheral portion consisting of the external,
middle and inner ears (Figure 1); and the central portion, comprising of the auditory nerve and pathways to various central
neural structures (Figure 2).

When a sound pressure wave impinges on the ear, it is amplified by the external auditory meatus and causes the tympanic membrane to vibrate in a characteristic manner. This vibration is
transformed by the auditory ossicles of the middle ear into movements of the stapedial footplate. These movements create pressure waves in the fluids of the inner ear which displace the
basilar membrane of the cochlear duct and cause the hair cells
located on the top of the basilar membrane to generate electrical
potentials. This potential elicits impulses in the auditory
nerve. After the auditory nerve, the nerve impulses are transmitted through the cochlear nuclei, the trapezoid body, the

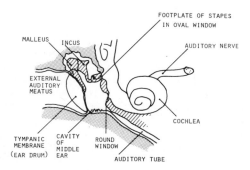

Figure 1.   Simplified representation of the human external, middle, and inner ears
(13)

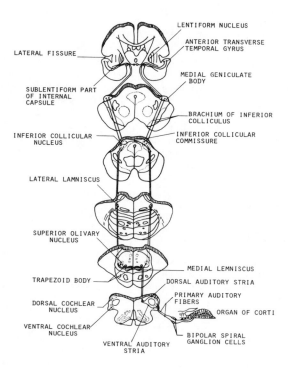

Figure 2.   Schematic of the auditory pathways (13)

superior olivary complex, the inferior colliculus, the medial geniculate body and finally the auditory cortex. The primary auditory cortex receives the nerve impulses and interprets them as different sounds. The impulses are also conveyed to the surrounding auditory associative areas for recognition.

In addition to the usual course through the external auditory meatus and the middle ear ossicles described thus far, hearing may also be mediated by way of the bones of the skull. The latter has been designated as bone conduction to distinguish it from the air conduction route reserved for the former. Under ordinary conditions, sound pressures in the air cause almost no vibration in the skull bones, therefore bone conduction is less significant than air conduction in hearing. Holding vibrating devices such as a tuning fork against the skull can cause vibrations of sufficient amplitude in the skull to elicit bone-conducted sound. Intense airborne sound can also impart sufficient energy to the skull to initiate bone conduction hearing. In this case vibration of the skull is transmitted directly to the fluid of the inner ear and causes the basilar membrane to move. After it reaches the organ of Corti, the transmission of sound to the auditory cortex is the same as that for air conduction.

There are three widely accepted routes by which bone-conducted sound stimulates the cochlea. These are the compressional, inertial and osseotympanic theories of bone conduction (12). Compressional bone conduction implies that the cochlear shell is compressed slightly in response of the pressure variation caused by a sound. Inertial bone conduction alludes to a relative motion between the ossicular chain and the temporal bone for low frequency vibrations. The osseotympanic theory denotes a mechanism by which relative movement of the skull, with respect to the mandible, sets up pressure variation in the air present in the auditory meatus. Since perception of microwave pulses are correlated with the capacity to hear high-frequency sound, it rules out inertial or osseotympanic bone conduction as potential mechanisms for microwave acoustic effect.

Site of Interaction

A vast amount of electrophysiological evidence has accumulated over the past several years demonstrating that auditory responses to microwave pulses are similar to those evoked by conventional acoustic pulses (6,7, 11,13,14,15). Furthermore, they show that microwave acoustic effect is mediated by an electromechanical interaction which is initiated outside or at the cochlea. An alternative hypothesis involves direct stimulation of the cochlear nerve or neurons at higher levels along the auditory pathway. This latter mechanism is probably not at work as I shall presently demonstrate.

If the external meatus of guinea pigs was blocked by cotton balls soaked in mineral oil, the amplitude of microwave-evoked brainstem potentials (the electrophysiological response of brain-

stem auditory nuclei recorded from an electrode placed on the
scalp at the vertex) would remain unaltered. Similarly, filling
the middle ear cavity with mineral oil which impeded ossicular
movement, had no effect on microwave-evoked responses. Furthermore, disablement of both tympanic membrane and middle ear ossicles only led to a reduced brainstem potential (16). This
indicated that the middle ear was not the route primarily used by
microwave-induced sound and that the decrease in brainstem potential probably stemmed from a small relative motion between the
stapes and the cochlear oval window. In contrast, destruction of
the cochlea by perforating the round window would completely
abolish the response (7,16). These results suggest that the site
of initial interaction of pulse-modulated microwave energy with
the auditory system is either outside or at the cochlea.

This interpretation finds support in systematic studies of
responses from brainstem nuclei following successive coagulative
lesion production in the auditory loci (17). The effect of
brainstem lesions on electrical potentials recorded from the
superior olivary (SO) nucleus in response to microwave pulse
stimulation is shown in Figure 3. Lesions in proximal nuclei
(inferior colliculus, IC and lateral lemniscus, LL) had negligible influence on the response recorded from superior olivary
nucleus. The response, however, disappeared after a lesion was
made in its nucleus, thus, confirming the peripheral nature of
the primary site of transduction.

Perceptive Mechanism

A peripheral interaction should involve displacement of
tissues and initiation of pressure waves in the head that are
transferred into the inner ear, where they are converted into
electrical potentials and then transmitted into the central
nervous system. I will briefly describe two classes of transduction mechanisms that have been suggested whereby mechanical
displacement of tissues in the head might be induced by pulse-
modulated microwave radiation (13). A number of coupling mechanisms between the incident microwave energy and the cochlea have
been suggested in the last few years. Included in this category
are movements involving basilar membrane structures (18) and
thermoelastic expansions involving the cochlear apparatus (19).
These hypotheses seem to make perception of microwave pulses
highly dependant on the subject's orientation, which is contrary
to psychophysical observations referred to earlier. Furthermore,
they ignored experimental facts that showed microwave energy does
not need to be deposited in the cochlea to initiate the microwave
auditory effect (20,21). Thus as a narrow-beam, direct-contact
microwave applicator was moved around the head of a cat, the
evoked brainstem responses would show remarkable preservation of
amplitude and time characteristics (Fig. 4).

Another class of mechanisms pertains to movements in gross
anatomical entities of the head such as scalp, muscle, skull and

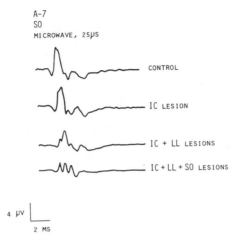

Figure 3.   Effects of brainstem lesions on the microwave pulse-evoked auditory responses from the vertex of a cat (17)

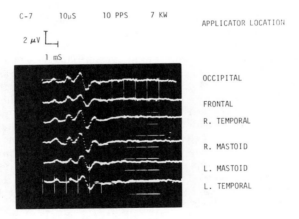

Figure 4.   Brainstem auditory responses from the vertex of a cat as a small, narrow-beam, direct-contact applicator is moved around the head

brain. For example, radiation pressure exerted by impinging
microwave pulses on the scalp has been suggested as a potential
transduction mechanism (22). Data now available tend to discount
this mechanism (6,13,24,26). According to the radiation pressure
hypothesis, higher microwave frequencies would be more effective
in producing auditory effects. Experimental evidence revealed
however, that human beings and laboratory animals either failed
to respond to 10 GHz microwaves or the incident power density
must be increased to inordinately high values for a barely per-
ceptible response, while they had little difficulty in responding
to 2.45 GHz radiation (2,6).

At frequencies which the auditory effect can easily be
detected, microwave energy can penetrate deeply into tissues of
the head. The absorbed energy produces a volumic strictive force
which sets up a pressure wave that propagates throughout the
cranial tissue media (6). This electrostrictive force mechanism
is probably not very important, because, the calculated acoustic
pressure in the head is about 100 to 1000 times smaller than
another volumetric transduction mechanism, namely thermoelastic
expansion (6,13,23,24,26). This thermoelastic expansion mechanism suggests that when microwave radiation impinges on the
head, a portion of the absorbed energy is converted into heat
which generates a miniscule but rapid rise of temperature in the
tissues. This rise of temperature (10^6 °C) occurring in a very
short time (10 μs) produces rapid thermoelastic expansion of the
brain or other tissues in the head which then launches a wave of
pressure that is detected by the hair cells in the cochlea (6,
13,23,27).

It appears reasonable to argue that the auditory perception
of pulsed microwave is due to thermoelastic expansion. This view
receives strong support from several avenues of evidence which I
will presently summarize.

Experimental and Theoretical Corroboration

A mathematical analysis of pressure waves created by thermoelastic expansion of brain matter showed that the sound pressure
required for human subjects to barely perceive microwave pulses
is about the same as the known minimum audible sound pressure for
bone conduction (13,27). The frequency of sound provides another
line of evidence. It was shown that the fundamental frequency of
sound is given by

$$f_s = 3.14 \ v/(2\pi a) \text{ for stress-free surface, or}$$

$$f_c = 4.49 \ v/(2\pi a) \text{ for constrained surface.}$$

Thus, microwave-induced sound is a function of sound propagation
speed (v), and the radius (a) or circumference ($2\pi a$) of the head.
Figure 5 illustrates measured cochlear microphonic frequency in
cats and guinea pigs (8,15) and calculated fundamental sound

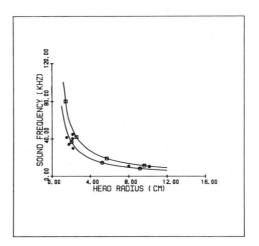

*Figure 5. Microwave-induced sound fre-
quency as a function of head radii or circumference ((□) constrained surface;
(○) stress-free)*

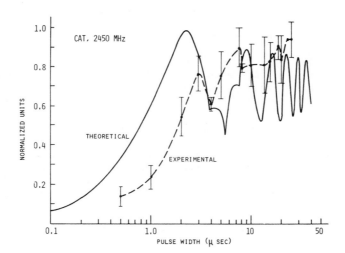

Proceedings of the Institute of Electrical and Electronics Engineers

*Figure 6.   Variation of microwave-induced sound pressure and brainstem potential
amplitudes as a function of pulse width (21)*

frequency (27). It also includes the well documented requirement
for human perception of pulsed microwaves: the ability to hear
sonic energy above 8 kHz (9,11). Clearly, there is agreement
between observed and calculated sound frequency. Furthermore,
the theory predicts the frequency of sound perceived by a subject
exposed to microwave pulses to be the same regardless of the
frequency of impinging microwaves and is independent of the
pattern of absorbed energy. This is supported by the report that
the same cochlear microphonics were produced by 918- and 2450-MHz
radiation (15).

     There is another avenue of support for the theory that
predicted a sound pressure that initially increased with pulsewidth but soon reached a peak and then gradually oscillated to a
lower value with further increase in pulsewidth (27). The theory
would be strengthened if this could be demonstrated in laboratory
animals and human subjects. Several recent publications presented supportive evidence from cat (20,21,28) and guinea pigs (29)
as well as human beings (11). Figure 6 shows the calculated
sound pressure amplitude and the variation of microwave-induced
auditory brainstem response in cats with the width of impinging
microwave pulses while keeping constant the peak power and repetition rate. Similar relationships between calculated sound
pressure or relative loudness in guinea pigs and pulsewidth is
given in Figure 7. The characteristics of these curves are remarkably similar. The sound pressure, loudness or brainstem
response increased and then decreased as suggested by the theory.
Furthermore, this nonmonotonic dependence of the response on
pulsewidth was also seen in some single auditory neurons of the
cat (30). Measurements in human subjects are presented in
Figure 8 along with calculated sound pressure. The nonlinear dependence on pulsewidth is as evident as the similarity between
these curves. The slight difference between the pulsewidths at
which sound pressure or loudness reached a maximum probably stemmed from a difference in actual and assumed head radii or circum-
ferences. In general, sound pressure peaks at wider pulsewidths
for larger head radii (13,27). Thus there exists a vast amount
of evidence that supports the thermoelastic mechanism of microwave-induced acoustic effect.

Resolution of a Dilemma

     It should be mentioned that a recent publication (11) showed
that the pitch (frequency) of sound induced by microwave pulses
of widths less than 50 μs persisted as the subject's head was
lowered into saline water, while the loudness diminished roughly
in proportion to the depth of immersion. Upon complete immersion, auditory sensation disappeared. For pulse widths longer
than 50 μs, even partial immersion resulted in loss of perception. This was interpreted as being at odds with the thermoelastic theory. There is, however, an explanation that does
seem to fit the data.

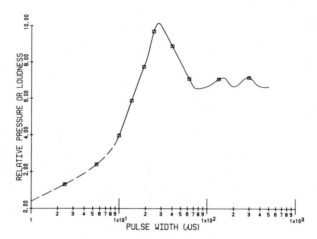

Figure 7. Relative sound pressure induced by microwave pulses in the heads of guinea pigs as a function of pulse width (computed from data in Ref. 29)

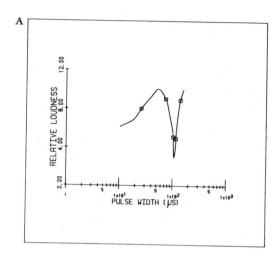

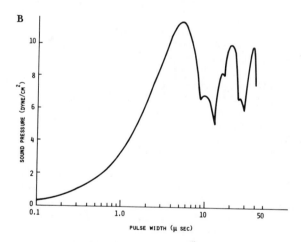

Figure 8.   Comparison of measured loudness and calculated sound pressure as functions of microwave pulse width for human subjects. (A) Relative loudness at 800 MHz (11); (B) calculated sound pressure for a 7-cm-radius head sphere at 918 MHz (13).

The theory suggests that the frequency of sound (pitch) evoked by microwave pulses is the same regardless of absorbed energy distribution and that the amplitude of sound (loudness) increases in proportion to the rate of energy absorption. Moreover, the amplitude of sound or loudness rises, peaks and then falls as the pulse width increases from a low to a high value. Thus, as the subject's head was lower into water, the absorbed energy and its distribution would change (decrease), but the acoustic property would remain unaltered (since skull and water differ by a large margin, immersion would not alter the acoustic characteristic by an appreciable amount). Therefore, the perceptual quality of microwave-induced sound persisted while the loudness diminished in proportion to the depth of immersion. The reason for the disappearance of auditory sensation upon complete immersion is that the impinging microwave energy was greatly attenuated by water before reaching the head. The small fraction that does reach the head most likely was below the threshold of perception. The observation that even partial immersion resulted in loss of perception for pulsewidths greater than 50 μs could be resolved by recalling that 50 μs was reported as being the optimal pulsewidth for auditory perception by their subjects. Hence, microwave pulses of widths greater than 50 μs would not be as effective in eliciting an acoustic sensation and could easily be disrupted by lowering the head partially into water. Clearly, these findings would strengthen rather than weaken the thermoelastic theory of microwave acoustic effect.

There are two alternate routes that might be taken by the microwave-induced thermoelastic pressure wave to reach the cochlea: the well-known bone conduction route and a yet unspecified but perhaps a direct route from brain matter to the cochlea. While current information precludes elaboration of the latter, compressional bone-conduction appears to be the most likely candidate for the former, since the frequency of microwave-induced sound is very high and is inversely proportional to the radius or circumference of the head (15,26,27).

Discussion

The results presented demonstrate that auditory systems of animals and humans respond to pulsed microwaves. However, there is little likelihood of the microwave acoustic effect arising from direct interaction of microwave pulses with the cochlear nerve or neurons at higher structures along the auditory pathway. The pulsed microwave energy, instead, initiates a thermoelastic wave of pressure in the head that travels to the cochlea and activates the hair cells in the inner ear. This theory covers many experimental observations, but it may be incomplete and thus require further extension to account for certain additional experimental findings. Tyazhelov, et al. (11) found in their beat frequency experiment that matching of microwave pulses (10 μs, 8000 pps) to a phase-shifted 8 kHz sinusoidal sound input resulted in loss of auditory perception, as the theory would suggest. However, cancellation also occurred when a 5000 pps train of pulses was properly phased with a 10 kHz sound signal. Seemingly, some modification is necessary to account for this finding. It may turn out that the discrepancy was related to harmonic generation by the audio equipment.

One strength of the theory is that it stimulates new questions and permits a more precise statement of new problems. The thermoelastic mechanism is apparently adequate to characterize the acoustic effect occurring in heads of humans and animals exposed to pulsed microwaves. The precise location in the head (scalp, skull or brain) microwave pulses are transformed into the acoustic wave of pressure however is at present not specifiable. Several speculations can be advanced, but there is little direct physiological data that would identify the possible gross tissue structures involved. Clearly, this is an area still requiring study.

Acknowledgment

I thank Vivian Chen for help with some of the figures, and the National Science Foundation for its support of my research in this area.

Literature Cited

1. Frey, A.H., Aerosp. Med., (1961), 32: 1140-1142.
2. Frey, A.H., J. Appl. Physiol., (1962), 17: 689-692.
3. Frey, A.H., Psychol. Bull., (1965), 63: 322-337.
4. Frey, A.H., J. Appl. Physiol., (1967), 23: 984-988.
5. Guy, A.W., Taylor, E.M., Ashleman, B. and Lin, J.C., IEEE Int. Microwave Symp. Digest, (1973), 321-323.
6. Guy, A.W., Chou, C.K., Lin, J.C. and Christensen, D., Annu. NY Acad. Sci., (1975), 247: 194-218.
7. Taylor, E.M. and Ashleman, B.T., Brain Res., (1974), 74: 201-208.
8. Chou, C.K., Galambos, R. Guy, A.W. and Lovely, R.H., J. Microwave Power, (1975), 10: 361-367.
9. Cain, C.A. and Rissmann, W.J., IEEE Trans. Biomed. Eng., (1978), 25: 288-293.
10. Frey, A.H. and Messenger, R., Jr., Science, (1973), 181: 356-358.
11. Tyazhelov, V.V., Tigranian, R.E., Khizhniak, E.O. and Akoev, I.G., Radio Science, (1979), 14(6/S): 259-263.
12. Tonndorf, J., Acta. Oto-Laryn. Supplement, (1966), 213: 1-132.
13. Lin, J.C., "Microwave Auditory Effects and Applications", Thomas, Springfield, Ill., 1978, 19, 33, 165.
14. Lin, J.C., Meltzer, R.J. and Redding, F.K., Proc. San Diego Biomed. Symp., (1978), 17: 461-465.

15. Chou, C.K., Guy, A.W. and Galambos, R., *Radio Science*, (1977), 12(6/S): 221-228.
16. Chou, C.K. and Galambos, R., *J. Microwave Power*, (1979), 14: 321-326.
17. Lin, J.C., Meltzer, R.J. and Redding, F.K., *J. Microwave Power*, (1979), 14: 291-296.
18. Sharp, J.C., Grove, H.M. and Gandhi, O.P., *IEEE Trans. Microwave Theory Tech.*, (1974), 22: 583-584.
19. Frey, A.H. and Coren, E., *Science*, (1979), 206: 232-234.
20. Lin, J.C., Meltzer, R.J. and Redding, F.K., *URSI Open Symp. Biol. Effects Electrom. Waves*, (1978, Finland); *Radio Science*, to appear.
21. Lin, J.C., *Proc. IEEE*, (1980), 68: 67-73.
22. Sommer, H.C. and Von Gierke, H.E., *Aerosp. Med.*, (1964), 35: 834-839.
23. Foster, K.R. and Finch, E.D., *Science*, (1974), 185: 256-258.
24. Borth, D.E. and Cain, C.A., *IEEE Trans. Microwave Theory Tech.*, (1977), 25: 944-954.
25. Lebovitz, R.M., *Annu. NY Acad. Sci.*, (1975), 247: 182-193.
26. Lin, J.C., *J. Microwave Power*, (1976), 11: 295-298.
27. Lin, J.C., *IEEE Trans. Microwave Theory Tech.*, (1977), 25: 605-613 and 938-943.
28. Lin, J.C., "Studies on Microwave-Induced Auditory Effect", Sci. Rpt. RES-1, Dept. of Elect. Engg., Wayne State University, Detroit, MI, 1979.
29. Chou, C.K. and Guy, A.W., *Radio Science*, (1979), 14(6/S): 193-197.
30. Lebovitz, R.M. and Seaman, R.J., *Brain Res.*, (1977), 126: 370-375.

RECEIVED December 1, 1980.

INDEX

A

Absorption
  coefficient
    of lysozyme, far-infrared 87, 88f
    of myoglobin, far-infrared 87, 88f
    of a paste of yeast cells vs.
      temperature 90f, 91
  cross section for water in the
    microwave frequency range 103
  of dipole oscillators in aqueous
    solution 85, 86f
  and emission of a photon, spectro-
    scopic transition associated with 30
  and emission of radiation in
    ordinary molecular fluids
    (equilibrium systems) 1–17
  of radiation, Einstein coefficient of 102
Acetyl choline (ACh) receptors 285
Acoustic effect, microwave 317–329
  thermoelastic mechanism of 321–325
Adenyl cyclase 286
Air conduction hearing 319–320
Algae, single-cellular 84
  chlorella pyrenoidosa, temperature
    dependence of the millimeter-
    wave absorption of 89
Alternating current electric field(s)
  on the Hodgkin–Huxley model of
    squid axon membrane,
    effects of 147–158
  membrane sensitivity to 149
  movement of ions in 124
Ampullae Lorenzini 122
Antibody molecules, receptors for 275
Attenuation function 29–33
  for ($\alpha_{TOT}(\omega)$), for water at milli-
    meter- and far-infrared wave-
    lengths, total 7f
  bulk ($\alpha_{TOT}(\omega)$) 19
  effects of the Bose-condensation on 29–33
  for molecular fluids 3
  for structural and free water in the
    microwave and far-infrared 9
  for water 6f
Attenuation of water to EM fields in
  the millimeter-wave and
  far-infrared 5–8
Auditory
  pathways, anatomical 318–320
  perception of microwave pulses 321–323

Auditory (*continued*)
  responses to microwave pulses 320
  frequency response of membrane
    components in nerve 133–144
  squid, giant
    membranes, effects of alternating
    current electric fields on the
    Hodgkin–Huxley model
    of 147–158
  relations between ionic con-
    ductance and membrane
    potential in 156
  at various frequencies, membrane
    capacity and conductivity of 138f
  at various membrane potentials,
    membrane capacitance
    of 140f, 142f

B

Bacteria, movement of magnetotactic 125
Belousov–Zhabotinskii mixture 199
Benoit, theory 72
Bicarbonate 311
Bifurcation(s) 165
  imperfect 183–184, 185f, 208
  plot for *Fucus* 176f
  secondary 179
  theory 171–174
    for a spherical cell 174
    TDGL-type theory compared to 176f
Biochemical
  origin, cellular oscillator of 254
  oscillations, autonomous 250
  reaction systems to oscillating
    stimuli, response of 243–254
Bioeffects of weak EM fields, models
  of nonequilibrium phenomena
  in 286–290
Bioelectric
  organization of nervous tissue 277–278
  patterning in cell aggregates 184–199
  patterning in the integral
    operator formalism 197–198
  sensitivities of organisms to envi-
    ronmental EM fields 278–279
Bioelectricity, developmental 163–210
Bioelectricity, self-organizing 164–165
Bioelectrics, growth in developmental 209

Biological
    membrane, electrical properties of 18–20
    membranes, capacitance of 120
    response function(s) 19, 27–29
    at millimeter wavelengths, fre-
        quency-dependence of 36
    solutions, viscosities of 266
    systems
        coherent modes in 219–240
        coherent processes in 213–217
        dissipative structures in 18–20
        free and structural water in 8–12
        interactions of an EM-field with 239
        in the far-infrared region 1–37
        in the microwave region 1–37
        nonthermal action of electric
            fields on 126
        thresholds 123t
    tissue, dielectric properties of 109–129
    tissues in vitro 16–17
Biology components and their
    relaxation mechanisms 114t
Biomolecules in aqueous solution 85
Biomolecules, nonlinear polarization
    oscillations in 229
Biomorphogenesis, effects of electric
    fields in 163
Biophysical mechanisms of EM-field
    interaction 109–129
Biophysics 220
Biopolymer(s)
    β relaxation of 74
    rotational diffusion and quasi-lattice
        vibrations 14–16
    solutions, dispersion regions in 76f
    solutions, frequency-dependent
        behavior of 65
Biopolymeric systems, effect of the
    membrane electrostatic field on
    the vibrational states of 34
Biopolymeric systems, quasi-lattice
    vibrations of 8
Birefringence, optical 71
Birefringence, transient 64
Blood, α- and β-dispersions in 114
Boltzmann equation 288
Bone conduction
    compressional 320
    hearing 320
    inertial 320
    osseotympanic 320
Bose-condensation 20
    on the attenuation function, effects
        of 29–33
    Einstein– 287
    -like excitation 224
Brain
    current densities in 124
    electrochemical oscillations in 272

Brain (*continued*)
    respiratory activity of 311–312
    tissue 272
        absorbed power and effect of
            temperature on 306–307
        evidence for nonequilibrium
            aspects of EM field inter-
            actions in 280–285
        with frequency, mathematical
            model for changes in com-
            plex permittivity of 300
        mechanism for calcium efflux
            from 307–311
        by radiofrequency radiation,
            calcium ion efflux induc-
            tion in 299–312
        respiratory activity of 301
        thermoelastic expansion mecha-
            nism of 323
Brainstem lesions on the microwave
    pulse-evoked auditory responses,
    effects of 322f
Brillouin scattering 84

C

Calcium 280
    to cell membrane, binding of 285
    efflux from brain tissue, mecha-
        nism for 307–311
    ion binding, cerebral 283
    ion efflux induction in brain tissue
        by radiofrequency radiation 299–312
    -mediated membrane feedback
        models, quasi-steady state ..167–171
    from the membrane, efflux of 280–285
Calf thymus DNA, aqueous solutions
    of 67
Capacitance, membrane 134
    of artificial membranes 135–137
    of lecithin–hexadecane 135
    of nerve membrane 137–143
    of squid giant axon at various
        membrane potentials 140f, 142f
Capacitance, voltage dependence of
    lipid bilayer 147
Carrier-wave frequency and power
    density, relationship between 300
Cell(s)
    aggregates, bioelectric pattern-
        ing in 184–199
    -to-cell communication by electro-
        chemical perturbations 272
    -to-cell transport phenome-
        nology 186–187
    in external gradients 181–184
    low-frequency dynamics of biologi-
        cal polymers and 83–91
    mass, spherical 193

Cell(s) (continued)
  membrane(s)
    binding of Ca^{2+} to 285
    lipid bilayer, models of tissue–
      EM field interactions
      involving 289–290
    models of transductive coupling
      of weak EM fields 279–280
    in the polarization processes of
      biological media in the
      radiofrequency range,
      role of 117
    states, nonlinear transitions in 273–276
  nerve 276
    effects of extracellular tissue EM
      fields in excitation of 276
  spontaneous generation of electro-
    chemical patterns in single 164
  surface receptor sites, evidence for
    weak EM field effects at ...285–286
  transport, nonlinear integral oper-
    ator model of effective 190–192
Cellular
  growth rate, effect of low-level EM
    fields at millimeter wave-
    lengths on 35
  membranes, a perturbation model
    for EM-field interaction with
    excitable 147–158
  oscillator of biochemical origin 254
  self-organization
    electrophysiological 165–181
    mechanisms 178–181
    nonlinear aspects of 171–174
  systems, frequency dependence of
    the growth rate function for 37
  systems, Raman spectroscopic
    measurements on in vivo 35
Cerebral calcium ion binding 283
Cerebral cortex, intrinsic oscillating
  EM field in 277
Channel opening, mechanism of 134
Chemical
  effect, thermal 267
  wave systems, phenomena in 199
  waves and steady electric fields,
    interaction of 201
Chlorella pyrenoidosa (monocellular
  algae), temperature dependence
  of the millimeter-wave absorp-
  tion of 89
Chromatin, DNA in 105
Circular arc function, Cole–Cole 66
Cochlea 320
Coherent
  electric oscillations 221, 239
  electric polarization waves 214–217
  modes in biological systems 219–240

Coherent (continued)
  oscillations in membranes 224–229
  processes in biological systems 213–217
Cole–Cole
  circular arc function 66
  dispersion equation 48, 58
  distribution function of relaxation
    times 111
Collision broadening, general theory
  of 1–3
Complex permittivity
  of brain tissue with frequency,
    mathematical model for
    changes in 300
  of globular proteins 69
  $\kappa^*(\omega)$ of a molecule 2
  for a relaxation process 6f
  of water 46, 49t, 52f
Concanavalin A receptors 285
Condensation, Bose- 20
Conductance 79
  effect, nonlinear 256
Conduction, bone
  compressional 320
  hearing 320
  inertial 320
  osseotympanic 320
Conduction hearing, air 319–320
Conductivity 209
  dielectric ($\sigma(\omega)$) 4
  of erythrocytes, internal 115
  for a relaxation process 6f
Cortex, intrinsic oscillating EM fields
  in cerebral 277
Counterion
  displacements in relaxation of
    globular proteins, role of 69
  polarization models 67
  polarizations of DNA and polypep-
    tides, relaxation of 68
Current
  densities in the brain 124
  loops in the egg of the seaweed
    Fucus, self-organized ionic 172f
  –voltage sampling technique, thin-
    film 256–261
Cystine, low-frequency Raman spec-
  trum of 15

D

Debye
  dispersion 53, 58
  equation 3, 50
  –Perrin theory 69
  relaxation function 66
  theory for polar liquids and
    solutions 65
  -type equation 109

n-Decane 135, 137
Depolarization effects, kinetic 64
Dielectric
  behavior of tissues 109, 110*f*
  conductivity ($\sigma(\omega)$) 4
  constant 109
    of muscle tissue, frequency of
      dependence of 110*f*
    relaxation regions of 109
  dispersion at the surface of charged
    spheres 287–289
  increments and relaxation fre-
    quencies for myoglobin
    solution 58*t*
  polarization at radiofrequencies,
    mechanism for 117
  properties
    of biological tissue 109–129
    of electrolytes 115
    of water in the microwave and
      far-infrared regions 46–55
    of water in myoglobin solution ..57–61
  response of molecular fluids 3
  theory 17
Dielectrics in the biological context,
  aqueous 13–14
Dielectrophoresis 125
Diffusion equation, forced rotational .. 71
Diffusion and quasi-lattice vibrations,
  biopolymers, rotational 14–16
Dipole(s)
  effects 111
  moments, fluctuating 69
  oscillators in aqueous solution,
    absorption of 85, 86*f*
  permanent and fluctuating 65–71
  torques 72
Dispersion(s)
  α- 111, 113
  β- 75, 111
    in blood, α- and 114
  γ- 74, 111, 113
    of water 114
  δ- 75,116
  Cole–Cole 58
    equation 48
  Debye 58
    regions 53
  effects
    characteristic frequencies
      observed with biological
      material for
      α- 113*t*
      β- 113*t*
      γ- 113*t*
    high-voltage 265
    of a polyelectrolyte under high
      sinusoidal electric fields,
      low-frequency 255–269

Dispersion(s) (*continued*)
  in muscle tissue, α- and β- 114
  regions in biopolymer solutions 76*f*
DNA
  aqueous solutions of calf thymus 67
  calculated microwave absorption
    by double-helical 101–106
  chain, lowest frequency vibrational
    bands of a helical 101–102, 104*f*
  in chromatin 105
  fibers and films, longitudinal acous-
    tic mode in oriented 95
  long-range forces in 95–99
  low-frequency relaxation in 69
  normal mode frequencies of poly-
    (dG)–poly(dC) double
    helix 102, 104*f*
  and polypeptides, relaxation of
    counterion polarizations of 68
  solutions, polarization of aqueous .. 65

E

Ear, anatomy of 318–320
Ear, human 319*f*
EEG (electroencephalogram) 272, 277
Eggs, developing 208
Einstein–Bose condensation 287
Einstein coefficient of absorption of
  radiation 102
Electric
  field(s)
    on biologic systems, nonthermal
      action of 126
    effects (of)
      in biomorphogenesis 163
      imposed 198
      on wave propagation 203
    on the Hodgkin–Huxley model of
      squid axon membranes,
      effects of alternating
      current 147–158
    interaction of chemical waves and
      steady 201
    membrane intrinsic 239
  signal propagation under
    imposed 199–207
  sinusoidal
    electrical properties of poly-
      electrolyte solutions
      under 255–269
    low-frequency dispersion
      effects of polyelectrolyte
      under high 255–269
    nonlinear impedance of a
      polyelectrolyte under
      high 255–269
  moment density (Maxwell
    polarization) 63
  oscillations, coherent 221, 239

Electrical
   field effects on membranes 121*t*
   fields, membrane interactions
      with 120–124
   properties 109–120
      of the biological membrane 18
   of polyelectrolyte solutions under
      sinusoidal electric fields ..255–269
   relaxation mechanism 111*t*
   response of polymers in solution 63–80
   and viscous properties of tissue
      water 115
Electrified periodic precipitation 203
Electro-banding phenomenon 205
Electrochemical
   oscillations in brain 272
   patterns in single cells, spontaneous
      generation of 164
   perturbations, cell-to-cell commu-
      nication by 272
Electrochemistry, concentration
      effect in 266
Electrode polarization 67
Electroencephalogram (EEG) 272
Electrolyte(s)
   dielectric properties of 115
   impedance of thin-film 256
   solution, polarization 75
Electrolytic solvents, effects of ion
      concentrations in 75
Electromagnetic (EM)
   fields
      behavioral responses to 278–279
      bioelectric sensitivities of orga-
         nisms to environmental ..278–279
      in cerebral cortex, intrinsic
         oscillating 277
      with the dissipative subsystem
         in the Fröhlich vibrational
         model, interaction of an
         external 26*f*
      in excitation of nerve cells, effects
         of extracellular tissue 276
      interaction(s)
         with biological systems 239
         in the far-infrared region 1–37
         in the microwave region 1–37
         biophysical mechanisms of ..109–129
         in brain tissue, evidence for
            nonequilibrium aspects
            of 280–285
         with excitable cellular mem-
            branes, a perturbation
            model for 147–158
         involving the cell membrane
            lipid bilayer, models
            of tissue– 289–290
         external
            with the dissipative sub-
               system 22*f*

Electromagnetic (EM) (*continued*)
   fields (*continued*)
      interactions (*continued*)
         external (*continued*)
            with the equilibrium system   22*f*
            among the free and
               structural water and 12*f*
            at membrane surface macro-
               molecules, models of
               tissue– 287–289
         intrinsic membrane 13
         ionic nonequilibrium phenomena
            in tissue interactions
            with 271–291
         in the millimeter-wave and far-
            infrared, attenuation of
            water to 5–8
         at millimeter wavelengths on
            cellular growth rate, effect
            of low level 35
         Raman-active transitions as a
            function of perturbation by
            millimeter-wave 36
      weak
         cell membrane models of trans-
            ductive coupling of 279–280
         effects at cell surface receptor
            sites, evidence for 285–286
         models of nonequilibrium
            phenomena in bioeffects
            of 286–290
         tissue sensitivities and mem-
            brane models of trans-
            ductive coupling to 276–280
   interactions, resonant 128
   theory 3
Electrophysiological patterns gen-
      erated by the outer
      membrane 192–197
Electrophysiological self-organization,
      cellular 165–181
Electrostatic field on the vibrational
      states of biopolymeric systems,
      effect of the membrane 34
Emission of radiation in ordinary
      molecular fluids, absorption and
      (equilibrium systems) 1–17
Endorphins 285
Enkephalins 285
Enzyme–substrate reactions 128, 227
Equilibrium system, external EM field
      interaction with 22*f*
Equilibrium systems (absorption and
      emission of radiation in ordinary
      molecular fluids) 1–17
Erythrocytes, internal conductivity
      of 115
Excitation, Bose condensation-like 224
Excitation model, local 235, 239

F

Far-infrared
  attenuation function for structural
    and free water in microwave
    and 9
  attenuation of water to EM fields in
    the millimeter-wave and 5–8
  region, EM-field interaction with
    biological system in 1–37
  regions, dielectric properties of
    water in the microwave and 46–55
  wavelengths, total attenuation func-
    tion ($\alpha_{TOT}(\omega)$) for water at
    millimeter- and 7f
Ferromagnetic bodies, intracellular 278
Field(s)
  -generated force effects 124–126
  on the Hodgkin–Huxley model of
    squid axon membranes, effects
    of alternating current
    electric 147–158
  on a nerve membrane system, effect
    of oscillating 147
Fluid(s)
  attenuation function for molecular   3
  dielectric response function of
    molecular 3
  mosaic model 279
  Singer–Nicolson 280
Force effects, field-generated 124–126
Fourier-transform spectrometer 87
Frequency dependence of the dielec-
    tric constant of muscle tissue 110f
Frequency-dependent behavior of
    biopolymer solutions 65
Fröhlich vibrational model 20–27
  interaction of an external EM field
    with the dissipative subsystem
    in 26f
  spectroscopic properties of 31
  vibrational states and photon-
    induced transitions in 22f
Fucus
  bifurcation plot for 176f
  development 166
  seaweed 164

G

Ginzburg–Landau, time-dependent
    (TDGL) equations 175–178
Glycoproteins 279
  membrane surface 275
Gradient theory, small 187–189

H

Hearing
  air conduction 319–320
  bond conduction 320
  effect, microwave 317–329

Heat damage, ohmic 255
Hexadecane 135, 137
  membrane, capacitance of lecithin– 135
Hodgkin–Huxley
  equation(s) 133, 151t
  model 271
    of squid axon membranes, effects
      of alternating current elec-
      tric fields on 147–158
  theory of nerve propagation 164
Human ear 319f
Hydrogen-bonded bridge-heads, vibra-
    tional excitation of 10
Hydrogen-bonded interactions among
    water molecules 8
Hyperpolarizability 181–182, 208
Hysteresis behavior, oscillating
    phenomena and 220

I

Impedance
  membrane 134
  of a polyelectrolyte under high
    sinusoidal electric fields,
    nonlinear 255–269
  resonance of polymer 265
  of thin-film electrolyte 256
Insulator 266
Ion(s)
  in an alternating current field,
    movement of 124
  channels in lipid bilayer membrane,
    voltage-sensitive 147
  concentrations in electrolytic
    solvents, effects of 75
  effects, kinetic 77
  gating 157
Ionic
  channel(s) 133, 141–143
    voltage sensor for 148
  conductance and membrane poten-
    tial in the squid giant axon,
    relation between 156
  current loops in the egg of the sea-
    weed *Fucus,* self-organized 172f
  nonequilibrium phenomena in tissue
    interactions with EM fields 271–291
  solutions, permittivity decreases of   77
IUator models, comparison of velocity
    response of Oregonator and 204f

K

Kerr effect 70f, 263
  relaxation 71–74
  transient or dynamic 64
Kinetic depolarization effects 64
Kinetic ion effects 77
Kramers–Kronig relations 113

L

β-Lactoglobulin, relaxation of 66
Langevin equation 116
Laplace equation 64, 169
Laser–Raman effect 217
Lecithin bilayers, membrane capaci-
    tance and conductance of 136f
Lecithin–hexadecane membrane,
    capacitance of 135
Liesegang configuration 205
Liesegang experiment, schematic of .. 206f
Limit cycle(s) oscillation(s) 221–222, 245
    nonlinear 221
Linear response theory 63, 73
Liouville equation 72
Lipid(s)
    bilayer capacitance, voltage
        dependence of 137
    bilayer models of tissue–EM field
        interactions involving the cell
        membrane 289–290
    membrane 134
    bilayer 135
        voltage-sensitive ion channels in 147
Liquid crystals, space-charge-limited-
    current (SCLC) effect in 266–267
Liquids, space charge effect of elec-
    trical properties of 266
Lubricants 266
Luminescence 84
Lymphocyte membrane 275
Lysozyme 87
    far-infrared absorption coefficient
        of 87, 88f
    low-frequency Raman spectra of .. 15

M

Magnetotactic bacteria, movement of 125
Maxwell
    polarization (electric moment
        density) 63
    –Wagner relaxation 311
    –Wagner effect 111
    –Gibbs theory for molecular
        weights 68
Membrane(s) 117–120
    binding of Ca^{2+} to cell 285
    capacitance 134
        of artificial membranes 135–137
        and conductance of lecithin
            bilayers 136f
        of lecithin–hexadecane 135
        of nerve membrane 137–143
        of squid giant axon at various
            membrane potentials 140f, 142f
    capacity and conductivity of squid
        giant axon at various
        frequencies 138f

Membrane(s) (*continued*)
    coherent oscillations in 224–229
    components in nerve axon, fre-
        quency response of 133–144
    effects of alternating current electric
        fields on the Hodgkin–Huxley
        model of squid axon 147–158
    efflux of Ca^{2+} from 280–285
    electrical properties of biological ..18–20
    electrophysiological patterns gen-
        erated by the outer 192–197
    extended high-polarization model
        of 229, 235
    feedback models, quasi-steady state
        Ca^{2+} mediated 167–171
    field(s)
        electrostatic, on the vibrational
            states of biopolymeric
            systems, effect of 34
        EM, intrinsic 13
        interactions with electrical 120–124
        intrinsic electric 239
        sensitivity to an alternating
            current 149
    flux law feedback 179
    impedance 134
    lipid(s) 134
        bilayer 135
        models of tissue–EM field
            interactions involving
            the cell 289–290
        voltage-sensitive ion channels
            in 147
    lymphocyte 275
    models of transductive coupling
        of weak EM fields, cell 279–280
    models of transductive coupling to
        weak EM fields, tissue sensi-
        tivities and 276–280
    neuronal 276
    a perturbation model for EM-field
        interaction with excitable
        cellular 147–158
    potential 133
        microwave-induced 122
        perturbations 158
    in the squid giant axon, relation
        between ionic conductance
        and 156
    proteins 134
    receptor sites 285
    states, nonlinear transitions
        in cell 273–276
    surface glycoproteins 275
    surface macromolecules, models of
        tissue–EM field interactions
        at 287–289
    system, effect of oscillating fields
        on a nerve 147

Metabolites through oscillating reactions, flux of labeled 247–253
Microwave
absorption by double-helical DNA, calculated 101–106
acoustic effect 317–329
fields, transmembrane potentials induced by 120
hearing effect 317–329
-induced
acoustic effect, thermoelastic mechanism of 321–325
membrane potential 122
sound 323
pulses
amplitude of sound (loudness) evoked by 328
auditory perception of 321–323
auditory responses to 320
frequency of sound (pitch) evoked by 328
region, EM field interaction with biological systems in 1–37
sensitivities 122
spectroscopy 87
water in
and far-infrared, attenuation function for structural and free 9
and far-infrared regions, dielectric properties of 46–55
frequency range, absorption cross section for 103
Millimeter
and far-infrared wavelengths, total attenuation function ($\alpha_{TOT}(\omega)$) for water at 7f
-wave
absorption of monocellular algae (Chlorella pyrenoidosa), temperature dependence of 89
absorption of yeast (Saccharomyces cerevisiae), temperature dependence of 89
EM fields, Raman-active transitions as a function of perturbation by 36
and far-infrared, attenuation of water to EM fields in 5–8
spectroscopy, sub-millimeter and 85–87
techniques, quasi-optical 87–91
wavelengths on cellular growth rate, effect of low-level EM fields at 35
wavelengths, frequency-dependence of biological response functions at 36
Molecular
biology, membrane 279
fluids, attenuation function for 3

Molecular (continued)
fluids, dielectric response function of 3
vibration, modes of 101
Muscle
potassium in smooth 273
tissue, α- and β-dispersions in 114
tissue, frequency dependence of the dielectric constant of 110f
Myoglobin 87
far-infrared absorption coefficient of 87, 88f
relative permittivity of an aqueous solution of 59f
solution
dielectric increments and relaxation frequencies for 58t
dielectric properties of water in ..57–61
water of hydration in 61
sperm whale 58

N

NaPSS, i-v curves for 258f–259f
Nerve
axon, frequency response of membrane components in 133–144
cells 276
effects of extracellular tissue EM fields in excitation of 276
excitation 133
membrane, membrane capacitance of 137–143
membrane system, effect of oscillating fields on 147
propagation, Hodgkin–Huxley theory of 164
Nervous tissue, bioelectric organization of 277–278
Neuronal membrane 276
Newtonian fluid, non- 265–266
Nucleic acids 66
dielectric properties of 116–117
Nucleosomes 105

O

Ohmic heat damage 255
Opioid peptides 285
Oregonator and IUator models, comparison of velocity response of .. 204f
Oscillating
phenomena and hysteresis behavior 220
reactions, flux of labeled metabolites through 247–253
stimuli, perturbation of nonlinear reaction schemes by 243–247
stimuli, response of biochemical reaction systems to 243–254

Oscillation(s)
  autonomous biochemical 250
  in brain, electrochemical 272
  coherent electric 221, 239
  limit cycle(s) 221–222, 245
    nonlinear 221
  in membranes, coherent 224–229
  nonlinear internal 239
  nonlinear plasma 290
Oscillator of biochemical origin,
    cellular 254
Oscillator, generalized Van der Pol 222–224
Ostwald–Prager theory 205

P

Pacemakers 124
Parathyroid hormone (PTH) receptor 286
PBLG (poly-γ-benzyl-L-glutamate) .. 116
Peptides, opioid 285
Permittivity
  of an aqueous solution of myo-
      globin, relative 59f
  complex
    of brain tissue with frequency,
        mathematical model for
        changes in 300
    of globular proteins 69
    $\kappa^*(\omega)$ of a molecule 2
    for a relaxation process 6f
    of water 46, 49t, 52f
  data fitted to various models, water 51t
  decreases of ionic solutions 77
  static 67
Phase fluctuation optical heterodyne
    spectroscopy 15
Photon, spectroscopic transition asso-
    ciated with absorption and
    emission of 30
Photons, Planck-type distribution of .. 17
Planck-type distribution of photons 17
Plasma oscillations, nonlinear 290
Polarization(s)
  of aqueous DNA solutions 65
  of DNA and polypeptides, relaxa-
      tion of counterion 68
  electrode 67
  electrolyte solution 75
  high-frequency 74–77
  Maxwell (electric moment density) 63
  models, counterion 67
  oscillations in biomolecules,
      nonlinear 229
  polyion 67
  processes of biological media in
      radiofrequency range, role of
      cell membranes in 117
  at radiofrequencies, mechanism
      for dielectric 117
  waves, coherent electric 214–217

Poly-γ-benzyl-L-glutamate (PBLG) .. 116
Polyaminoacids 87
Poly(dA) · poly(dT) 97
Poly(dG) · poly(dC) 96, 101
  absorption cross section per base
      pair vs. frequency for the lon-
      gitudinal, torsional, and bend-
      ing acoustic modes for chains
      of 104f
  double helix DNA, normal mode
      frequency of 102, 104f
Polyelectrolyte(s) 66
  under high sinusoidal electric fields,
      low-frequency dispersion
      effects of 255–269
  under high sinusoidal electric fields,
      nonlinear impedance of 255–269
  solutions under sinusoidal electric
      fields, electrical properties
      of 255–269
Polyion polarization 67
Polymer(s)
  and cells, low-frequency dynamics
      of biological 83–91
  impedance, resonance of 265
  in solution, electrical response of 63–80
Polypeptides 66
  relaxation of counterion polariza-
      tions of DNA and 68
Ponderomotive forces 124
Potassium channels 133, 141–143
Potassium in smooth muscle 273
Potential perturbations, membrane 158
Power density(ies)
  at different frequencies 303–306
  relationship between carrier-wave
      frequency and 300
  window 299
Prolate spheroid 195
Prolate spheroidal coordinates to
    describe an elongated cell mass .. 194f
Protein(s)
  dielectric properties of 116–117
  gate 141
  globular 65, 87
    complex permittivity of 69
    role of counterion displacements
        in relaxation of 69
  membrane 134
  tissue 111
Proton tunneling 289

Q

Quasi-
  lattice vibrations of biopolymeric
      systems 8
  lattice vibrations, biopolymers, rota-
      tional diffusion and 14–16

Quasi- (continued)
  optical millimeter-wave techniques 87–91
  steady state Ca^{2+} mediated mem-
    brane feedback models 167–171

R

Radiation
  calcium ion efflux induction in
    brain tissue by radio-
    frequency 299–312
  Einstein coefficient of absorption of   102
  in ordinary molecular fluids,
    absorption and emission of
    (equilibrium systems) 1–17
  pressure hypothesis 323
Radiofrequency(ies)
  mechanism for dielectric polariza-
    tion at 117
  radiation, calcium ion efflux induc-
    tion in brain tissue by 299–312
  range, role of cell membranes in the
    polarization processes of bio-
    logical media in 117
Radiometer 263
Raman
  -active transitions as a function of
    perturbation by millimeter-
    wave EM fields 36
  effect, laser- 217
  scattering, high-frequency 84
  scattering, low-frequency 83–84
  spectroscopic measurements on in
    vivo cellular systems 35
  spectroscopy 83
Receptor(s)
  acetyl choline (ACh) 285
  for antibody molecules 275
  concanavalin A 285
  parathyroid hormone (PTH) 286
  sites, membrane 285
Relaxation
  of biopolymers, β 74
  of counterion polarizations of DNA
    and polypeptides 68
  in DNA, low-frequency 69
  frequencies for myoglobin solution,
    dielectric increments and 58t
  frequency, bulk water 61
  function, Debye 66
  γ 74
  of globular proteins, role of
    counterion displacements in .. 69
  Kerr effect 71–74
  Maxwell–Wagner 311
  mechanism, electrical 111t
  mechanisms, biology components
    and their 114t
  phenomena 46

Relaxation (continued)
  process(es) 4
  complex permittivity for 6f
  conductivity for 6f
  time domain measurements of 77–80
  regions of the dielectric constant   109
  times, Cole–Cole distribution
    function of 111
Resonant electromagnetic interactions   128
Resonance of polymer impedance   265
Resonances, nonlinear   239
Respiratory activity of brain 311–312
  tissue   301
Response theory   72
  linear   73
Rotational diffusion equation, forces ..   71

S

Saccharomyces cerevisiae, growth rate
    of cells of   28
Saccharomyces cerevisiae (yeast),
    temperature dependence of the
    millimeter-wave absorption of ..   89
Scattering, low-frequency Raman 83–84
SCLC (space-charge-limited-current)
    effect in liquid crystals 266–267
Seaweed Fucus   164
Semiconductor   266
Separatrix   245
Singer–Nicolson fluid-mosaic model ..   280
Sinusoidal electric fields, low-fre-
    quency dispersion effects of a
    polyelectrolyte under high 255–269
Sinusoidal electric fields, nonlinear
    impedance of a polyelectrolyte
    under high 255–269
Sodium channels 133, 141–143
Sound
  frequency of   323
  (loudness) evoked by microwave
    pulses, amplitude of   328
  microwave-induced   323
  (pitch) evoked by microwave pulses,
    frequency of   328
Squid giant axon
  membranes, effects of alternating
    current electric fields on the
    Hodgkins–Huxley model of 147–158
  relation between ionic conductance
    and membrane potential in   156
  at various frequencies, membrane
    capacity and conductivity of ..   138f
  at various membrane potentials,
    membrane capacitance of 140f, 142f
Space charge effect of electrical prop-
    erties of liquids   266
Space-charge-limited-current (SCLC)
    effect in liquid crystals 266–267

Sperm whale myoglobin 58
Spheroid, prolate 195
Spheroidal coordinates to describe an
    elongated cell mass, prolate 194*f*
Spectrometer, Fourier-transform 87
Spectroscopic theory 17
Spectroscopic transition associated
    with the absorption and emission
    of a photon 30
Spectroscopy
    microwave 87
    phase fluctuation optical heterodyne 15
    Raman 83
    sub-millimeter and millimeter wave 85–87
Steady-state (nonequilibrium) systems,
    chemically-pumped 17–33
Substrate reactions, enzyme 128
Synaptosomes 284

T

TDGL (*see* Time-dependent Ginz-
    burg–Landau equations)
Tetrodotoxin (TTX) 134
Thermal chemical effect 267
Thermocouple 263
Thermoelastic expansion mechanism
    of the brain 323
Thermoelastic mechanism of micro-
    wave-induced acoustic effect ..321–325
Time-dependent Ginzburg–Landau
    (TDGL) 175–178
    equations 175–178
    -type theory compared to
        bifurcation theory 176*f*
    domain measurements of relaxation
        processes 77–80
    domain reflection measurements,
        schematic of apparatus for 76*f*
Tissue(s)
    bioelectric organization of
        nervous 277–278
    brain 272
        absorbed power and effect of
            temperature on 306–307
        evidence for nonequilibrium
            aspects of EM field inter-
            actions in 280–285
        with frequency, mathematical
            model for changes in com-
            plex permittivity of 300
        mechanism for calcium efflux
            from 307–311
        by radiofrequency radiation,
            calcium ion efflux induc-
            tion in 299–312
        respiratory activity of 301
    dielectric properties of biological 109–129
    α- and β-dispersions in muscle 114

Tissue(s) (*continued*)
    –EM field interactions
        in excitation of nerve cells, effect
            of extracellular 276
        involving the cell membrane lipid
            bilayer, models of 289–290
        ionic nonequilibrium phenomena
            in 271–291
        at membrane surface macro-
            molecules, models of 287–289
    in vitro, biological 16–17
    proteins 111
    sensitivities and membrane models
        of transductive coupling to
        weak EM fields 276–280
    water, dielectric properties of 115
    water, electrical and viscous
        properties of 115
Torques, dipole 72
Transmembrane potentials induced
    by microwave fields 120
Transmission line theory 78
Transverse displacement bending
    modes 102
TTX (tetrodotoxin) 134
Turing models, classic 179
Turing pattern formation
    phenomenon 164

V

Van der Pol oscillator,
    generalized 222–224
Van Vleck–Weisskopf Karplus–
    Schwinger line-shape function 17
Vibration, biopolymers, rotational
    diffusion and quasi-lattice 14–16
Vibration modes of molecular 101
Vibrational
    bands of a helical DNA chain,
        lowest frequency 101–102, 104*f*
    excitation of hydrogen-bonded
        bridge-heads 10
    model, Fröhlich 20–27
        interaction of an external EM
            field with the dissipative
            subsystem in 26*f*
        vibrational states and photon-
            induced transitions in 22*f*
    states of biopolymeric systems,
        effect of the membrane electro-
        static field on 34
Viscous properties of tissue water,
    electrical and 115
Voltage sensing 157
Voltage sensor for an ionic
    channel 148

W

Water 113
  attenuation function for 6f
  at millimeter- and far-infrared
    wavelengths, total ($\alpha_{TOT}(\omega)$) 7f
  complex permittivity of 46, 49t, 52f
  dielectric properties of 115
  in the microwave and far-infrared
    regions 46–55
  γ-dispersion of 114
  to EM fields in the millimeter-wave
    and far-infrared, attenuation of 5–8
  free and structural
    in biological systems 8–12
  and an external EM field, inter-
    actions among 12f
  in the microwave and far-infrared
    attenuation function for   9
  of hydration in myoglobin solution   61
  in the microwave frequency range,
    absorption cross section for .. 103
  molecules, hydrogen-bonded inter-
    actions among 8

Water (continued)
  in myoglobin solutions, dielectric
    properties of 57–61
  permittivity data fitted to various
    models 51t
  relaxation frequency, bulk 61
Wave(s)
  -field interaction in Belousov–
    Zhabotinskii, theory of 201–203
  propagation 202
    electric field effects on 203
  and steady electric fields, inter-
    action of chemical 201
  systems, phenomena in chemical 199
Wayne–Kerr admittance bridge 135
Wien effects 255

Y

Yeast cells vs. temperature, absorption
  coefficient of a paste of 90f, 91
Yeast (Saccharomyces cerevisiae),
  temperature dependence of the
  millimeter-wave absorption of   89